D0745299

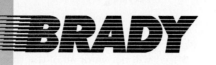

VEHICLE RESCUE

Second Edition

Harvey D. Grant

James B. Gargan

PRENTICE HALL, Upper Saddle River, New Jersey 07458

Library of Congress Cataloging-in-Publication Data

Grant, Harvey D. (date)
    Vehicle rescue / Harvey D. Grant, James B. Gargan.
    —2nd ed.
      p.   cm.
    Includes index.
    ISBN 0-8359-8374-9
    1. Traffic accidents.   2. First aid in illness and injury.
3. Crash injuries.   4. Transport of sick and wounded.
I. Gargan, James B., 1932-   . II. Title.
    RD96.6.G7   1997
    617.1'028—dc20   96-1797
                                          CIP

Acquisition Editor: *Susan Katz*
Production Editor: *Karen Fortgang, bookworks*
Copy Editor: *Nancy Savio–Marcello*
Designer: *Amy Rosen*
Cover Designer: *Laura Ierardi*
Manufacturing Buyer: *Ilene Sanford*
Editorial Assistant: *Carol Sobel*
Marketing Manager: *Judy Streger*

© 1997 by Prentice-Hall, Inc.
A Simon & Schuster Company
Upper Saddle River, New Jersey 07458

Printed in the United States of America

10 9 8 7 6 5 4 3 2 1

ISBN 0-8359-8374-9

Prentice-Hall International (UK) Limited, *London*
Prentice-Hall of Australia Pty. Limited, *Sydney*
Prentice-Hall Canada Inc., *Toronto*
Prentice-Hall Hispanoamericana, S.A., *Mexico*
Prentice-Hall of India Private Limited, *New Delhi*
Prentice-Hall of Japan, Inc., *Tokyo*
Simon & Schuster Asia Pte. Ltd., *Singapore*
Editora Prentice-Hall do Brasil, Ltda., *Rio de Janeiro*

NOTICE

The procedures described in this book have been theo-
rized, developed, refined, taught, and used over a period
of years. They work, but make no mistake about it, they
will not work all of the time.

If every accident were the same, rescue personnel
would be able to use just a few tools with predictable results. However, many variables influence the outcome of a
vehicle rescue effort, including the nature and extent of the
damage to the vehicle, the nature and degree of entrapment
of occupants, the types of hazards produced by the accident, the availability and usability of supplies and equipment, the positions of injured patients within the vehicle,
the nature and extent of injuries, the weather, and so on.

Accordingly, rescue personnel must be able to use
many tools in various ways to achieve certain objectives.
A fundamental knowledge of tools and techniques can be
gained from reading a book such as this, but proficiency
in vehicle rescue operations results from learning to com-
bine tools and techniques under the tutelage of a qualified
instructor and then periodically practicing the skills
under the supervision of a competent rescue officer.

GENDER USAGE

Past attitudes have allowed our language to develop with
the pronouns "he" and "his" being used in general to sig-
nify persons of either gender. Since some readers object to
the constant use of masculine pronouns, many writers
have elected to use plural pronouns such as "they" and
"them" and other non-sexist terms.

Authorities in both professional journals and popular
publications have stated that the "quick-fix" approach
should be discouraged. They maintain that the repeated
use of "he or she" and "him and her" is not proper in a long
manuscript, and that the use of "(s)he" is incorrect in all
cases. They recommend different sentence structures
when appropriate and the traditional use of "he" and "his"
when necessary. Hence, in this text you will find "he" often
used when referring to the actions taken by a rescuer.

In doing so, neither the authors nor the publisher
imply that women should not serve on rescue squads, or
that they act in any less professional manner than men
when participating in rescue efforts.

A WORD ABOUT SUPPLIES AND EQUIPMENT

This book lists about half of the more than 500 items that
can be used for rescuer and victim protection, and dozens
of hazard management, gaining access, emergency care,
disentanglement, patient packaging, removal, and transfer activities that may be necessary during a vehicle rescue operation.

The fact that a manufacturer's name and model number is included with the lists and descriptions of supply
items and tools in Phase One, or that a certain tool or appliance is illustrated, does not suggest that the item is the
only one that can be used for a particular vehicle rescue
operation. These are supply items, tools and appliances
with which the authors are familiar and which are known
to be dependable. Equivalent items available from other
manufacturers should be equally dependable.

To their credit, the manufacturers of hydraulic- and
pneumatic-powered rescue tools have taken great pains to
develop products that will give years of dependable service.

I would like to dedicate this book to my old friend and partner

Harvey D. Grant.

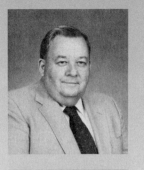

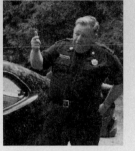

Harvey was dispatched to Rescue Heaven on January 24, 1993, having established himself as the father of vehicle rescue and EMS by the time his contract ran out on planet Earth.

For those who never had the opportunity to hear him speak or direct a training session, the loss is magnified.

There have surely been a few "pileups" at the "Pearly Gates!" I hope Harvey saves at least one for me to work on.

—JIM GARGAN

CONTENTS

PHASE FIVE Managing Incident Scene
Hazards   83

PHASE SIX Gaining Access to Trapped
Persons   123

PHASE SEVEN Caring for Life-Threatening Conditions   171

PHASE EIGHT Disentangling Trapped Patients   183

PHASE ELEVEN Transferring Injured Patients
to Ambulances 269

PHASE TWELVE Terminating the Rescue
Operation 281

FOREWORD

As you read this, thousands of rescuers are working to extricate hundreds of people trapped by the tangled wreckage of motor vehicle accidents. A safe, systematic approach to rescue operations is essential to provide a positive outcome for both the rescuers and their patients. From preparing for the alarm to terminating the incident, each step must be carefully planned and each rescuer must be properly trained to perform the duties necessary to efficiently complete each task.

The first edition of this book was published in 1975. Since then it has been the foundation for nearly every vehicle rescue training class conducted around the world. Harvey Grant and his close friend, Jim Gargan, spent decades researching and improving their techniques with one goal in mind: to improve the chance of survival for the very next person involved in a serious automobile accident. Harvey and Jim's pioneering approach to presenting the information has made it possible for their students to save thousands of people from needless pain, crippling injuries, and death. Their style of presenting the information meets the most important of all criteria: It is easy to remember when you need it . . . when you are facing the rescue in the street.

The rescue community lost its most valuable mentor when Harvey Grant died an untimely death in 1993. He had nearly completed this long-awaited edition of *Vehicle Rescue*. Fortunately his close friend, business partner, and coauthor, Jim Gargan, picked up the work and continued. Jim now brings us his nearly half-century experience in the emergency services and shares his unparalleled expertise in vehicle rescue by completing this book.

My personal philosophy is that you should never rely on any single source of information for vehicle rescue. However, the one source that cannot be overlooked is *Vehicle Rescue*. It has served as the foundation for all that have followed, and with this latest edition, will serve as the foundation for years to come. Use it as a safety guide, a reference source, a training outline, and an example of how any well-disciplined vehicle rescue effort should be conducted.

Work safely;
Lt. Steve Kidd
Orange County (FL) Fire/Rescue Division
Squad-1

Coauthor:
The Carbusters Video Rescue Series

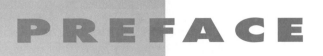

PREFACE

Vehicle accidents are a big business, if one can consider calling pain, disability, death, and related economic loss a big business.

The following statistics are derived from the *1994 Traffic Safety Facts,* published by the National Highway Traffic Safety Administration, U.S. Department of Transportation:

Overview

- In 1994, 40,676 people lost their lives in motor vehicle crashes, an increase of 1.3 percent from 1993.
- The fatality rate per 100 million vehicle miles of travel in 1994 was 1.7. The fatality rate per 100,000 population was 15.62 in 1994, 0.3 percent higher than 1993 (15.57).
- An average of 111 persons died each day in motor vehicle crashes in 1994— one every 13 minutes.
- Motor vehicle crashes are the leading cause of death for every age from 6 through 28 years old.
- Vehicle occupants comprised almost 84 percent of fatalities in 1994; the remaining 16 percent were pedestrians, pedalcyclists, and other nonoccupants.

Occupant Protection

- In 1994, 47 states and the District of Columbia has safety belt use laws in effect. Use rates vary widely from state to state, reflecting factors such as differences in public attitudes, enforcement practices, legal provisions, and public information and education programs.
- From 1982 through 1994, it is estimated that safety belts saved 65,290 lives (9,175 in 1994).
- In 1994, it is estimated that 308 children under age 5 were saved as a result of child restraint use. An estimated 2,655 lives were saved by child restraints from 1982 through 1994.
- In 1994, 47 percent of occupants of passenger cars and 54 percent of occupants of light trucks involved in fatal crashes were unrestrained.
- In fatal crashes, 73 percent of passenger car occupants who were totally ejected were killed. Safety belts are very effective in preventing total ejections; only 1 percent of the occupants reported to be using restraints were totally ejected, compared with 20 percent of the unrestrained occupants.

Motorcycles

- The 2,304 motorcyclist fatalities accounted for 6 percent of total fatalities in 1994.
- The motorcycle fatality rate per 100 million vehicle miles traveled is about 20 times that of passenger cars.
- Motorcycle operator error was identified as a contributing factor in 76 percent of fatal crashes involving motorcycles in 1994. Excessive speed was the contributing factor most often noted.
- Forty-three percent of fatally injured operators and 48 percent of fatally injured passengers were not wearing helmets at the time of the crash.
- Approximately one out of every five motorcycle operators involved in a fatal crash in 1994 was driving with an invalid license at the time of the collision.
- Motorcycle operators involved in fatal crashes in 1994 had a higher blood alcohol concentration (BAC) level (28.9 percent higher) than any other type of motor vehicle driver.
- NHTSA estimates that 518 lives were saved by the use of motorcycle helmets in 1994.

Medium and Heavy Trucks

- Eleven percent (5,544) of all motor vehicle traffic fatalities reported in 1994 involved heavy trucks (gross vehicle weight rating greater than 26,000 pounds) and 1.5 percent (608) of the fatalities involved medium trucks (gross vehicle weight rating of 10,000 to 26,000 pounds).
- Seventy-eight percent of fatalities involving a medium or heavy truck were occupants of another vehicle. Thirteen percent were occupants of the medium or heavy truck.
- Medium and heavy trucks accounted for 8 percent of all vehicles involved in fatal crashes in 1994.

- Three-quarters of the medium and heavy trucks in fatal crashes in 1994 collided with another motor vehicle in transport.
- Only 1.4 percent of the drivers of medium and heavy trucks involved in fatal crashes in 1994 were intoxicated. (Compared with 19.4 percent for passenger cars, 22.9 percent for light trucks, and 28.9 percent for motorcycles.)

Cars, Light Trucks, and Vans

- There were 30,780 occupant fatalities in passenger vehicles in 1994. This is approximately 90 percent of total occupant fatalities (passenger cars 64 percent; light trucks 26 percent).
- Single-vehicle crashes accounted for 41 percent of all fatal crashes, multi-vehicle crashes 42 percent, and the remaining 17 percent were nonoccupant crashes.
- Frontal impacts accounted for 62 percent of passenger vehicle occupant fatalities where the impact of the vehicle is known.
- Ejection accounted for 27 percent of occupant fatalities in passenger vehicles. Occupants of light trucks experienced almost twice the ejection rate of passenger cars.
- Utility vehicles experienced the highest rollover involvement rate of any vehicle type in fatal crashes (37 percent) compared to 25 percent for pickups, 18 percent for vans, and 15 percent for passenger cars.
- Sixty-six percent of passenger vehicle occupant fatalities were unrestrained.
- Drivers of light trucks have a higher intoxication rate (22.9 percent) than that of passenger car drivers (19.4 percent).

In view of these staggering figures, it would be interesting to know how many times fire departments, rescue squads, and EMS units were called upon to respond to the locations of vehicle accidents. Sadly, there are no such statistics; however, if emergency service units responded only to accidents that resulted in injuries and death, they would have answered well over 6 million calls for help. Vehicle rescue is a big business also.

The more than 6 million police-reported accidents that occurred in 1994 ranged in severity from "fender benders" to multiple-vehicle, multiple-casualty, multiple-fatality incidents, and the activities of responding rescuers were similarly varied. In some cases, arriving emergency service personnel discovered that their services were not needed; in other cases, they discovered situations that would take the combined personnel of many organizations hours to control. At times, the rescuers were well trained to cope with the emergencies at hand; at other times, they were woefully ill-prepared.

Countless articles and books have been written on techniques of extrication and disentanglement. This text is not one of them. In our view, vehicle rescue constitutes not just a few activities but a complete system of operations. Extrication is but one activity within this system, and disentanglement is but one aspect of that activity. This text treats the system of vehicle rescue in terms of its component parts, each one of which builds on those that precede it and leads into those that follow. The system of vehicle rescue operations as we see it includes twelve phases of activity:

- Preparing for Rescue Operations
- Responding to the Location of the Accident
- Assessing the Situation
- Reaching Off-Road Rescue Sites
- Managing Incident Scene Hazards
- Gaining Access to Trapped Patients
- Caring for Life-Threatening Conditions
- Disentangling Trapped Patients
- Packaging Injured Patients for Removal and Transfer
- Removing Injured Patients from Vehicles
- Transferring Injured Patients to Ambulances
- Terminating the Rescue Operation

If emergency service personnel are to perform competently at an accident scene, they must understand the theories and techniques associated with each phase of this system of operations. Firefighters may be well trained in fire prevention and suppression, but less experienced in gaining access, emergency care, and disentanglement procedures. Emergency medical personnel may be quite knowledgeable on the subject of patient care, but they may have had little training in hazard management and rescue operations. Squad members, although well versed in rescue procedures, may not be experienced in providing support to EMS personnel.

We have prepared this book to make readers aware of the many activities for which fire, rescue, and ambulance personnel may be responsible at the locations of vehicle accidents. We do not suggest that it provides the ultimate answer to the needs of the emergency services. Just as one cannot precisely predict the injuries and damages that an incident will produce, neither can one predict which specific rescue activities will be required.

The performance of vehicle rescue procedures requires a wide-ranging knowledge of skills, some of which are simple and some complex. Thus this book includes in-depth descriptions of the wide variety of operations that can be accomplished with the tools and appliances carried on rescue vehicles regardless of their size. The days when rescuers could shrug off failures to perform efficiently at the scene with the excuse "I cannot do because I do not have" are gone.

It is our hope that this book will guide fire, rescue, ambulance, and police personnel in the training and performance of vehicle rescue activities. If it does no more than stimulate thinking about the varied requirements for service at the location of vehicle accidents, it will have served a worthy purpose.

Harvey D. Grant
James B. Gargan

ACKNOWLEDGEMENTS

As I contemplate the task of acknowledgement, ever hopeful of not forgetting someone, I must first refer to the Acknowledgement pages of Vehicle Rescue I. All of those people contributed to the final outcome of Vehicle Rescue II, along with those mentioned here.

Whether it be the scheduling of classes, a different use of a tool, procuring tools, or perhaps helping me find wrecked vehicles to play with, all of these and more are contributions to the success of this book. And there are so many to thank! We started in 1988 and I reluctantly wrapped it up on the prodding of my publisher in 1995.

Harvey would have liked you all to know how much we appreciate your support. From the early days at Southwest Virginia EMS with Vassie Vaught, Jamie Smyth, and Steve White, to Richmond with EMS Director Terry Wright, Captain Dan Barry, and Sergeant Terri Jo McDowell of West End Rescue Squad and Jim Fitch of Forest View Rescue Squad and more recently Chesterfield County Fire/ Rescue, over to West Virginia EMS Director, Terry Shore, now heading up the National EMT Registry in Columbus, OH.

Georgia's EMS Directors, Bob Carpenter, Terry McBride, David Moore, Dennis Lockridge, and Keith Wages; the old Rescue Training Associates gang, Robert H. Murray, Jr., now Chief of Meadowwood (NH) Fire Department; Arthur W. Reid, Jr., of Allentown, PA; Peter Friend and Peter Hayes of Wolfeboro, NH; Dwight Lodge, now General Manager of National Accounts for Laerdal; Charles B. Gillespie, M.D., of Albany, GA; Mike Moore and John Perry of the Claymont (DE) Fire Department; and Dick Marshall of Hudson, NH; and on to the present Rescue Training Consultants involved in Vehicle Rescue: Joe Vattilana, Frank Puoci, Jr., Tony Talamonti, Richard Rawls, Rocky Walker, John Whited, Harry Metcalfe, and Bob Gargan; with associates, Sam Sealy of Chatham, NJ; Jessie Smith, Apopka, FL; Jim Eidenberg, Downingtown, PA; Lt. John Czajkowsky, Orange County (FL) Fire/Rescue; Howard Dawley, Loudoun County, VA; Dwight Clark, Forsyth, GA; Karl Marzolf, Rockville, MD; and Lt. Tom Carr of Montgomery County (MD) Fire/ Rescue.

Others who provided assistance along the way are Jim Masters, Bethesda Chevy

Chase (MD) Rescue Squad; Chief Bob Goeltz, Hermitage (PA) Fire Department; Ron Lehman, of the "Old Paratech Days"; Ellen Manson, Washington, VA, a founder of CISD; Al Perry, former Chief, GM Proving Grounds, Midland, MI; Franco Gomero, Jamie Obermeyer, and Pete Jerabek of General Motors; my nephew and dear friend, John Ostien; and Roy Alson, M.D., F.A.C.E.P., Bowman Gray School of Medicine, Winston-Salem, NC.

Our Canadian connection includes Donna Hastings McGeady, EMT-P, and Bruce Patterson, EMT-P, both of Grant MacEwan Community College, Edmonton; Bernie Van Tighem and Bob Fisher of the Alberta Fire Training School; Ray and Bruce Cole formally with Airshore International of British Columbia, the developers of my Jimmi-Jak Rescue System; and Steve Cudmore, the new owner of Airshore, who brings new ideas for the Jimmi-Jak System.

I appreciated the help of Chief Robert Walker, Cocoa Beach (FL) Fire Department; Chief Robin Shetzler, Odessa (DE) Fire Company; P.J. Richardson of Reeves Manufacturing; Tom Wehr, Wehr Engineering; Chuck Sheaffer, Fire and Rescue Products; Ellen Dorsett, of Southport, NC; the Southport (NC) Fire/Rescue Department; and John Clegg of Lakes Entrance, Australia.

For reviewing the book, I am indebted to: Lou Jordan, Emergency Training Associates, Union Bridge, MD; Lieutenant Clyde Coble, Fairfax County (VA) Fire/Rescue; Lieutenant Steve Kidd, Orange County (FL) Fire/Rescue; Walter Idol, EMT-P, Chief Flight Paramedic for UT Lifestar, Knoxville, TN; Charles "Brother" Smith, Jr., of Saltville, VA; and Bob Elling, EMT-P, from Colonie, NY.

Pictures are by Les Lougheed, Chief Flight Mechanic, UT Lifestar, Knoxville, TN, and posed by members of the Knoxville (TN) Volunteer Rescue Squad.

A special thank you to Katherine West, BSN, MSED, CIC, Infection Control Consultant, who did a superb job on "Cleaning Contaminated Tools and Equipment."

And finally, to the ladies who put up with us and helped put it all together, my wife, Barbara; my secretary, Deanna "Dee" Belay; Editorial Production Manager, Karen S. Fortgang; Carol Sobel, Assistant Publisher; and the boss lady, Susan Katz, V.P./Publisher.

Jim Gargan

ABOUT THE AUTHORS

Harvey D. Grant

A life-long resident of Claymont, Delaware, Harvey D. Grant was involved with emergency services for over 42 years. He served as President of Rescue Training Associates, Ltd., for 12 years and was a former Chief of Claymont (DE) Fire Company.

Harvey Grant was the first Senior Instructor for the Delaware State Fire School, where he was responsible for developing and conducting training courses in emergency medical services, rescue and instruction.

Mr. Grant was Chairman of the American Society for Testing Materials Task Group Committee, charged with developing standards for rescue equipment for ambulances. He was a former President of the New Castle County (DE) Vol. Firemen's Association, a former Director of the Delaware Volunteer Firemen's Association and Secretary of the National Fire Protection Association Committee, which developed the first standards for fire service instructors.

Harvey Grant was a member of the International Association of Fire Chiefs, serving on its Transportation Emergency Rescue Committee. He was also a member of the Eastern Association of Fire Chiefs.

Mr. Grant spoke at many national seminars and training programs and wrote numerous articles for emergency service publications.

Harvey D. Grant was the author of the first edition of *Vehicle Rescue* and coauthor of the second edition of *Vehicle Rescue, Emergency Care, The Handbook of Procedures for EMS Personnel,* and the *Action Guide for Emergency Service Personnel.*

James B. Gargan

A resident of Kure Beach, North Carolina, where he serves as President of Rescue Training Consultants.

1996 marks Mr. Gargan's 48th anniversary in the emergency services. He served as Chief of the Prospect Park (PA) Fire Department and was active for many years as an instructor for the Pennsylvania State Fire School. He was Director of the Delaware County (PA) Fire School, teaching fire and rescue skills throughout eastern Pennsylvania.

Mr. Gargan is a member of the International Association of Fire Chiefs, the Eastern Association of Fire Chiefs, and the Delaware County (PA) Firemen's Association. Mr. Gargan also serves on the Advisory Council to the Urban Search and Rescue Task Force of the Congressional Fire Services Caucus in Washington, D.C.

Jim Gargan served as Technical Director for the First Due Rescue Company Series on Trench Collapse, Advanced Trench Collapse Operations, and Building Collapse-Heavy Construction by American Safety Video Publishers, a subsidiary of Mosby Lifeline.

Mr. Gargan has appeared on many national seminars and training programs, and has written numerous articles for emergency service magazines.

James B. Gargan is the author of *Trench Rescue, First Due Trench Rescue* and *BTLS Access.* He is the coauthor of the second edition of *Vehicle Rescue* and the *Action Guide for Emergency Service Personnel.*

Mr. Gargan is the inventor of the Jimmi-Jak pneumatic/mechanical stabilization system, and he also has his own company, J & B Equipment Company, Inc., of New Castle, Delaware.

PHASE ONE

Preparing
for
Rescue Operations

THE RESCUE SQUAD: A SYSTEM OF PEOPLE AND MACHINES

How does a rescue squad function as a system? What, in fact, is a system? According to one reference source, a system comprises interrelated elements that form a collective whole. This definition is obscure unless you understand the words used, so let's pin down the meaning of "system" in terms of things to which we can easily relate.

We ourselves are part of many systems. The ones in which we are included depend on where we live, how we live, what we do, what we earn, and many other factors. In our daily lives, we become involved in many varied systems. Communications systems allow us to talk to each other across vast distances. Transportation systems provide the means to travel from one place to another. We are all in the data banks of many computer systems. The goods that we buy and use come from manufacturing and distribution systems. If we break the law, or if someone breaks laws meant to protect us, we come into contact with judicial systems.

Our school-age children are part of educational systems. If we become sick or injured, we pass through a community EMS system.

These systems have one thing in common: They are made up of people and machines that function together to achieve a desired result. Similarly, a rescue squad is a system. Whether it is an independent unit, part of a large municipal fire department, part of a small rural department, or part of an EMS organization, a rescue squad is a collection of people, equipment, and machines dedicated to saving lives and property.

If you are a provider of pre-hospital care, such as an EMT or a paramedic, as well as a rescuer, you are familiar with another system of people, equipment, and machines that has been put together to save lives: your community's EMS system.

An EMS system can be compared to a chain of physical and human resources. Just as the emergency department of a hospital is an extension of the hospital itself, so an ambulance is a mobile extension of the emergency department. Likewise, ambulance personnel extend services provided by the emergency department physician. In all cases the quality of care available to the sick and injured depends on the integrity of the chain that connects the physical plant facilities with the human resources.

Under many circumstances, the rescue squad system becomes part of the EMS system. The rescue squad forms an important link in an extensive emergency care chain. In some communities, the rescue squad is responsible only for extricating people from wrecked vehicles. In other communities, the rescue squad also has the responsibility for delivering injured persons to medical facilities. Survival often depends on how well this combination of people and machines that is known as a rescue squad functions.

Needless to say, a rescue squad will not be effective at the time of an emergency unless it is ready to respond quickly and perform competently.

THE RESCUE VEHICLE

Rescue squad vehicles range in size and construction from pickup trucks with cross-body tool boxes to extra-heavy-duty, tandem wheel, custom-built units that have a large walk-in body mounted on a custom fire apparatus chassis. Combinations of body styles, chassis sizes, and compartment configurations are limited only by the designer's imagination and the buyer's budget. While there is certainly a place for imagination and innovation in the design of a rescue vehicle, they must be subordinate to other guiding influences. Some of the penalties for substituting imagination for good judgment and logic are:

- An unnecessarily large vehicle
- Poor use of storage space
- Unnecessary expense
- The need to make costly modifications soon after purchase
- Early obsolescence

Types of Rescue Vehicles

Rescue vehicles have for some time been categorized as heavy-duty, medium-duty, or light-duty units. While those designations were supposed to be made on the basis of the tasks that might be accomplished with the tools and appliances carried on the unit, they were more often than not descriptive of the size of the truck. Even though they carry a great deal of equipment for salvage, ventilation, and fire ground support, many heavy-duty rescue vehicles have only a few items intended for or suitable for rescue. On the other hand, small trucks are being equipped with complete inventories of hydraulic rescue tools, air bags, and other equipment designed for heavy rescue operations. Perhaps it would be better to give rescue units designations more suited to the class of service rather than size.

A **Limited Service Rescue Vehicle,** as the name suggests, might be a small vehicle that is stocked with supplies and equipment for just one rescue specialty—vehicle rescue, for example. Such a unit might be operated by a fire department that has an aerial apparatus equipped for structural rescue operations or by an independent EMS organization (Figure 1.01).

A **General Service Rescue Vehicle** might be a medium-sized truck that has supplies and equipment for rescue operations

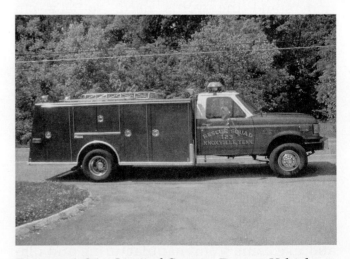

FIGURE 1.01   Limited Service Rescue Vehicle, Knoxville (TN)

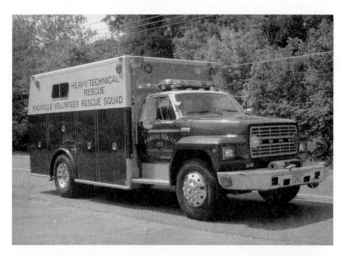

FIGURE 1.02   General Service Rescue Vehicle, Knoxville (TN)

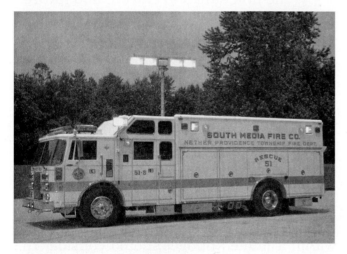

FIGURE 1.03   All Service Rescue Vehicle, South Media (PA)

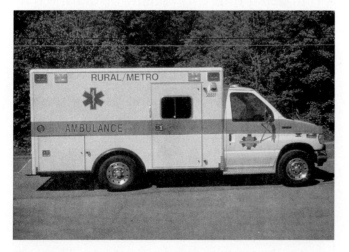

FIGURE 1.04   Box Ambulance, Knoxville (TN)

most likely to be undertaken in the response area, at the locations of vehicle accidents, building fires, machinery entrapments, and the like (Figure 1.02).

An **All Service Rescue Vehicle** might be one that has just about everything needed for just about every type of emergency, including a wide variety of powered tools, lifting devices, and fire ground support equipment. In most cases the unit can be self-sustaining at emergency locations (Figure 1.03).

Trucks specially equipped for rescue operations are not the only rescue vehicles. Ambulances may also be equipped to serve as rescue vehicles. In response areas where an ambulance is likely to arrive at the locations of motor vehicle accidents at the same time or shortly after a rescue unit, the rescue equipment inventory can be minimal. When an ambulance crew is responsible for all phases of a vehicle rescue operation, as in a very remote area, the unit should have supplies and equipment for hazard management, vehicle stabilization, gaining access, and disentanglement (Figure 1.04).

Selecting the Most Appropriate Rescue Vehicle

When planning for a new squad vehicle, rescue officers would do well to consider the primary purpose for which the vehicle is intended, the kind of terrain over which it must travel, the availability of rescue personnel, the funds available for the vehicle, and the community's future needs.

Primary Use of the Vehicle. Larger rescue vehicles generally serve three purposes. First, they carry the hazard management equipment, support equipment, tools for gaining access and disentanglement, and patient transfer devices that will probably be needed at the locations of motor vehicle accidents. Second, they carry tools and appliances that will probably be needed at the location of a building collapse, cave-in, underground emergency, water-related accident, and incidents other than motor vehicle accidents. Third, they carry supplies and equipment for supporting suppression activities at fire locations.

If the rescue vehicle will respond to all kinds of emergencies, it must be large enough to accommodate the wide variety of supplies and equipment that might be needed. If the vehicle will be used only for a particular purpose, as for vehicle rescue operations, chassis and body sizes can be held to a minimum.

Topography. Land features, water features, seasonal weather conditions, and the character of roads within the rescue squad's response area should all play an important part in the ultimate selection of a rescue vehicle. Consideration should be given to the need for a four-wheel drive vehicle.

In predominantly hilly country where two-lane winding roads are common, smaller and lighter rescue units are usually preferred. Although a high-performance engine enables a heavy truck to climb steep grades easily, the weight of the larger rig and its higher center of gravity may make it difficult and even dangerous to drive on narrow, winding roads.

In rural areas that have many two-lane bridges, the weight of a heavy truck may be a serious problem. Some older bridges were not designed for trucks that weigh 10 to 15 tons or more. More than one fire department has been embarrassed when one of its vehicles plunged through the deck of an old bridge. Likewise, many departments have been embarrassed to find that a new unit is too high to pass under low bridges in a response area.

Personnel Availability. When an emergency service unit transports its personnel, it should consider a rescue vehicle with crew-carrying capabilities. Vehicle weight and height are two other important considerations. Large cab-forward units have space for crew members on each side of the engine compartment and in the body of the vehicle.

Many rescue squads do not have personnel transportation needs. When this is the case, rescue officers often elect either to use

the space that would normally be allotted to crew members for equipment storage or to reduce the overall size of the unit.

Cost. Large rescue vehicles can easily fall within the $200,000 to $300,000 range, while a super-large, fully equipped rescue vehicle can cost as much as half a million dollars. Such an expenditure cannot be considered lightly, and a commitment to purchase should be made only after the following questions can be answered affirmatively.

- Do we need such a large unit?
- Do we need all the equipment that the unit will be able to carry?
- Is the unit suited to current and future needs of the response area?
- Can we afford the unit?

Money, like adequate personnel, is a luxury that few emergency service units have. If funds do not permit the purchase of a custom squad vehicle, care exercised in the selection of a vehicle and its equipment can produce a rig that will be completely functional if not quite as beautiful as the squad members would like.

Rescue officers who are responsible for fitting the purchase of a new squad vehicle within a limited budget should consider the various construction and utility truck bodies offered by a number of truck manufacturers. A completed unit can usually be delivered at a cost of under $30,000 and will give years of reliable service. Moreover, one of these units can usually be placed in service much sooner than a custom-constructed vehicle.

Future Community Needs. The purchase of a rescue squad vehicle is a long-term investment that requires consideration of the vehicle's adaptability to changing needs. A fire department might elect to purchase a small vehicle, only to find in just a few years that it is too small. Consider what happens when a superhighway is built through a community that previously had a need for only a small, minimally equipped rescue vehicle. The new highway inspires builders to erect industrial facilities near interchanges, and all of a sudden there are trucks and construction vehicles operating on areas that once were open fields.

Manufacturing facilities, new homes, and shopping centers spring up around interchanges and traffic flow becomes a problem. With the increase in traffic there is an increase in traffic accidents and consequently the need for a larger rescue unit.

Planning for a new rescue truck, as for any emergency vehicle, must include consideration of the potential for new roads, new industries, new housing, and all other growth factors that might impose new requirements on the local emergency services.

Fire and rescue officials in areas that have a considerable amount of land available for development should seek the advice of the city or county planner when deliberating about the purchase of a new vehicle. Land-use plans are prepared for many years and are generally dependable.

A rescue vehicle, even a big expensive one, is of little value to injured people trapped in wrecked vehicles unless it has supplies and equipment suited for vehicle rescue operations.

SUPPLIES AND EQUIPMENT FOR VEHICLE RESCUE OPERATIONS

Because of the nature of rescue activities, squad vehicles must carry various supplies and equipment, some highly specialized and others quite ordinary. Whatever is carried, rescue equipment *must* be maintained in peak operating condition at all times, and each crew member *must* be fully trained in the operation of each item. These two points are emphasized for an important reason: When a life hangs in the balance during a rescue operation, there is no room for halfway measures. Survival often depends on how well a tool or appliance functions and, most assuredly, on a rescuer's ability to use the equipment most efficiently.

It is virtually impossible to list here all the supplies and equipment available for ve-

hicle rescue operations, and it is difficult to state which items should be carried on any particular squad vehicle. Certain basic tools should be carried on every squad truck, along with essential life-support equipment, but the need for highly specialized equipment is often dictated by circumstances.

- Rescue squads operating in heavily traveled truck transportation corridors where serious accidents are common should certainly have hydraulic rescue tools, air bags, large-capacity lifting and supporting devices, and other equipment suited for "heavy" rescue operations.
- Fire departments that operate rescue vehicles in addition to rescue-equipped engines or aerial units are not likely to buy supplies and equipment already carried on those units.
- Rescue units that operate in predominantly rural areas that have no major transportation arteries might not carry more than minimal extrication equipment.

Following are supplies and equipment identified as useful for vehicle rescue operations. Again, the selection of items should be based on such factors as need, available storage space, and cost.

Supplies and Equipment for Personal Protection

Consider some of the many things that make accident locations dangerous work places for rescue personnel.

- Shards and fragments of broken glass, jagged metal and plastic edges, and sharp-pointed objects are mechanisms of injury that can abrade, puncture, incise, lacerate, avulse, and even amputate a rescuer's unprotected body parts.
- Particles of glass, plastic, metal, hydraulic fluid, bloodborne pathogens, and paint can enter a rescuer's

unprotected eyes during a rescue operation.

- An unstable vehicle or machine can topple onto a rescuer and crush the life from him.
- Smoke, noxious fumes, toxic gases, and dusts can poison a rescuer's unprotected respiratory system.
- Contact with an energized power conductor can result in lethal electrocution.
- Flames, radiant heat, exhaust pipes, catalytic converters, and other hot objects can burn a rescuer's unprotected skin surfaces, as can a variety of dangerous chemicals.
- Powerful rescue tools can generate twisting forces sufficient to break bones.
- Even contact with hand tools can result in injury when body parts are unprotected.

The elements can contribute to a hazardous environment. Rain and snow make tools and work surfaces slippery, and ice makes road surfaces treacherous. Heat and cold can adversely affect a rescuer's performance.

Mechanisms of injury and the elements are not the only threats to personal safety at accident locations, however. A number of human factors can increase the potential for injury, including

- A poor attitude toward personal safety
- Little or no training in rescue procedures, or poor training
- A lack of skill in tool use
- Physical problems that prevent a rescuer from performing strenuous activities

Unsafe acts also result in injuries at accident locations, as when rescuers

- Have "tunnel vision," or do not size up the overall picture
- Fail to manage or control hazards
- Fail to select the correct tools for gaining access and disentanglement operations
- Use unsafe tools and techniques
- Use tools improperly
- Work at an unsafe speed
- Fail to recognize mechanisms of injury and unsafe surroundings
- Lift heavy objects improperly
- Deactivate safety devices designed to prevent injury

However, the unsafe act that contributes most to accident scene injuries is *the failure of emergency service personnel to wear personal protective gear during rescue operations!* While there's not a great deal you can do to reduce the number of existing injury-producing mechanisms at accident locations, and while there's certainly nothing you can do to control the elements, there are at least three things you can do to reduce the potential for injury: (1) Learn the value of personal protective gear, (2) acquire some if none is provided, and (3) use it!

Scalp and Skull Protection

To be effective, a rescuer's headgear should protect the wearer from water, impact from a blunt object, penetration by a sharp-pointed object, laceration by a sharp-edged object, heat, cold, and contact by dangerous materials (chemicals, hot oil, tar, etc.). Trendy baseball caps, uniform hats, wool watch caps, and similar headgear often seen on rescue personnel do little other than to protect the wearer from sunlight and cold.

An **Approved Firefighter's** or **Rescuer's Helmet** affords the greatest head protection during vehicle rescue operations. However, the rear brim of many fire helmets often gets in the way during rescue operations in close quarters. Some manufacturers are now offering helmets more suited to the needs of rescue personnel. The "Commando" helmet, manufactured by Cairns and Brother, Inc., is an example of a "rescue" helmet. It has a tough shell that resists impact, penetration, and cutting, a foam and web suspension, and a secure chin strap, but not the objectionable rear brim projection (Figure 1.05).

As an alternative to a firefighter's helmet, a **Hard Hat** is favored by many rescuers because of its light weight and compact design. If you prefer to wear a hard hat, select a construction model with a full suspension and a secure chin strap—a helmet that meets the standards set by the American National Standards Institute (ANSI) and the Occupational Safety and Health Administration (OSHA).

Whatever your choice of helmet, select a bright-colored model and affix reflective stripes and lettering so it is highly visible at all times (Figure 1.06).

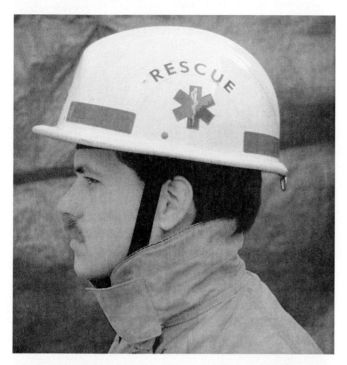

FIGURE 1.05   Cairns "Commando" Helmet

Face and Neck Protection

While a helmet protects the head and a turned-up coat collar affords a degree of protection for the neck, a rescuer's face is often left unguarded.

A **Nomex® Hood** of the type used by firefighters affords excellent protection not only from radiant heat but also from cold during rescue operations. A hood can be worn in two ways: with just the eyes exposed when maximum protection is desired, or with the lower margin of the eye slot tucked under the chin, as when it is necessary to wear the hood under the face piece of a breathing apparatus.

A one-size-fits-all protective hood can be easily carried in the pocket of a turnout coat (Figure 1.07).

Eye Protection

A hinged plastic shield does not provide adequate eye protection during aggressive vehicle rescue efforts. Depending on the type of shield used, flying particles of debris can strike the wearer's face from underneath the shield and from the side.

Safety Goggles afford both wraparound protection and a full field of vision. A soft vinyl frame closely conforms to the contours of the wearer's face. There are many types of safety goggles. Select a pair that protects you not only from impact and flying particles but also from chemical splashes, dusts, and other contaminants. Be sure that the goggles have indirect venting to keep the lens fog-free (Figure 1.08).

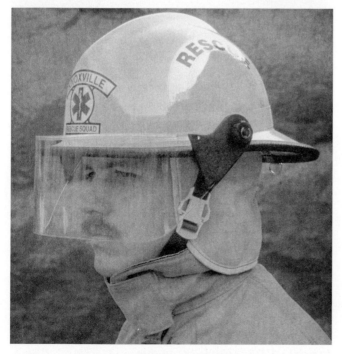

FIGURE 1.06   Fire/Rescue Helmet

If you decide to wear goggles for eye protection, resist the temptation to store them on your helmet. The headband will lose its elasticity when continually stretched.

Safety Glasses also afford good protection against impact and flying objects. If you prefer to wear this form of eye protection, select a pair of safety glasses with large lenses and side shields (Figure 1.09). Safety glasses are available in several colors; amber or yellow lenses are especially good for rescue operations. They make objects appear remarkably sharp on dull days or in low-light situations.

Ear Protection

While a helmet will protect your scalp and skull, and safety goggles or glasses will protect your eyes, your ears will remain vulnerable unless you wear a hood or earflaps during rescue operations.

An **Earmuff-Style Industrial Hearing Protector** will protect your ears in two ways. It will reduce the level of high-frequency noises common to rescue operations, but not speech and other low-frequency sounds. Moreover, the rigid shells will protect your ears from contact with tools and debris, and flying objects that can become lodged in your ear canals. Gel-filled cushions or foam pads assure comfort (Figure 1.10).

Select a hearing protector that has a metal headband rather than a plastic one. Plastic headbands sometimes lose their "spring" after long periods of storage, and thus fail to keep the shells pressed firmly against the sides of the wearer's head.

Upper-Body Protection

It's amazing that a rescuer will take steps to protect his scalp, skull, eyes, ears, and hands during a rescue operation and leave his upper body unprotected except for ordinary clothing. A T-shirt, uniform shirt, or lightweight jacket does little to protect the wearer from jagged metal and plastic parts and sharp-pointed pieces of debris.

A **Firefighter's** or **Rescuer's Turnout Coat** affords several layers of protection. The

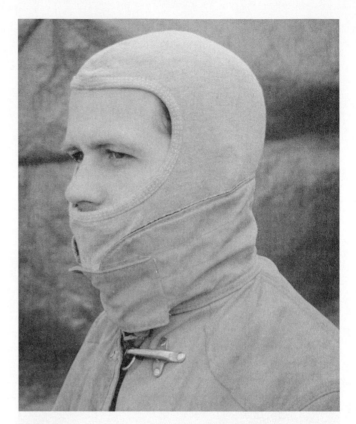

FIGURE 1.07 Protective Nomex Hood

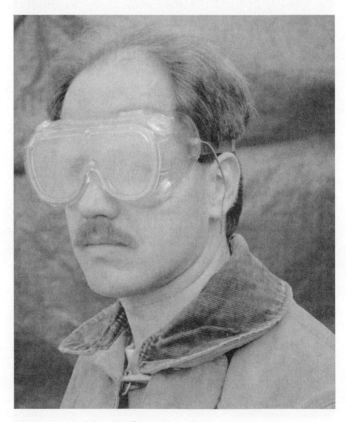

FIGURE 1.08 Safety Goggles

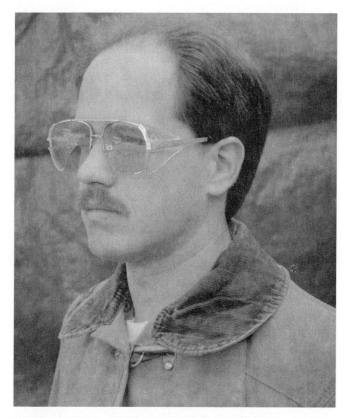

FIGURE 1.09 Safety Glasses

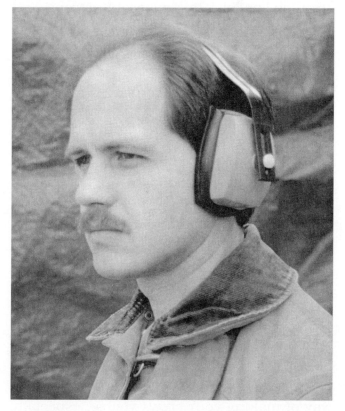

FIGURE 1.10 Earmuff-Style Hearing Protector

outer shell repels water and other liquids, and serves as the first layer of protection against objects that can abrade, lacerate, or penetrate.

A vapor barrier prevents or at least inhibits the transfer of water, steam, vapors, and some chemicals to the wearer. It also serves as the second layer of protection from mechanisms of injury.

The vapor barrier liner prevents the vapor barrier from coming into direct contact with the wearer's body. It also serves as the third layer of protection against heat and injury-producing mechanisms.

The thermal liner is the fourth layer of protection. Contrary to popular opinion, the liner is not included just to keep the wearer warm. While it does keep body warmth in, it also keeps radiant heat and cold out. Because of its thickness, the thermal liner affords good protection against objects that can pass through the other layers of protection—objects that can lacerate or penetrate the body. For that reason alone, the liner of a turnout coat should be worn year-round, not just during cold-weather months.

If you elect to wear a turnout coat for upper-body protection, pick one that just covers your hips. A longer coat may be difficult to work in when carrying out rescue operations in close quarters. Select a light-colored coat for high visibility as well as heat reflectivity. There should be reflective letters and stripes sewn onto the coat for maximum visibility at night and in inclement weather.

If you find the bulk and weight of a conventional turnout coat objectionable, consider wearing an **EMS** or **Rescue Jacket.** While these jackets may not offer the four levels of protection afforded by conventional turnout coats, they do have attractive features. An EMS jacket has a windproof, waterproof, lightweight, coated shell. It has a detachable liner, knitted wristlets, reinforced cuffs, a stand-up collar, a storm flap, and roomy pockets. It comes in several sizes and colors with reflective trim.

Hand Protection

Thick leather gauntlets and some so-called "firefighters' gloves" are so bulky that they prevent the manual dexterity that is so important to some rescue operations. On the other hand, most fabric "garden" gloves are so thin that they offer no protection from objects that can lacerate and puncture the wearer's hands.

Shop around for gloves. Try on different ones including supple leather work gloves that are supposed to be cut resistant. Try to pick up small items while wearing the gloves, and try handling the tools you would normally use during rescue operations. Then select gloves that seem to provide both protection and comfort.

Lower-Body Protection

Nomex Trousers or **Coveralls,** while they are expensive when compared to the cost of similar conventional garments, will provide a degree of protection from radiant heat. However, trousers and coveralls alone do not protect the wearer from injury resulting from forceful contact with sharp-edged or sharp-pointed mechanisms of injury.

Firefighter's Turnout Pants afford the greatest protection against both radiant heat and mechanisms of injury but, like a turnout coat, they sometimes make maneuvering in tight places difficult. If you choose to wear turnout pants, select a pair with cuffs wide enough to allow you to put them on without having to remove your shoes.

Foot Protection

While rubber firefighter's boots are easy to put on, and they keep the wearer's feet dry, they are heavy and bulky. Unless they are the correct size, they offer little of the foot and ankle support that is important when working on uneven ground or debris.

High-Top Leather Work Shoes are far better for rescue operations than rubber boots or low-quarter shoes. High-top shoes have several advantages. They can be worn all the time as part of a uniform. The extended tops support the ankles. Steel inserts support the soles of the feet from sharp-pointed objects, and steel caps protect the toes when a heavy object is dropped. Leather work shoes can be made water resistant with any of a number of silicone preparations available in shoe stores, shoe repair shops, and sporting goods stores.

If you elect to wear three-quarter-length firefighter's boots during rescue operations, be sure to wear them with the tops pulled all the way up. The "cuffs" that result when boots are worn only partially pulled up make great repositories for glass fragments and other small bits of debris. When you pull the tops up during the next rescue operation, the debris will fall into the foot compartments. Just a few steps may result in severe, if not incapacitating, foot injuries.

Ice Cleats, while not items for personal protection in the strictest sense of the word, can prevent dangerous falls when a rescuer must work on ice-covered roads. Several types are available. One model is made of an elastic material studded with small steel spikes; it is simply pulled over the shoes. A strap-on model has replaceable straps and spikes. Still another model can be worn attached to the shoes while driving.

Equipment for Increased Visibility on the Highway

The light-colored fabric and the reflective stripes and letters of a turnout coat make rescue personnel highly visible both day and night. However, rescuers who are not directly involved in extrication activities do not always wear turnout gear, and if they are wearing dark clothing, they may be difficult to see.

A **Traffic Vest** can be worn over a uniform, street clothing, or a light jacket. The fluorescent orange color and the reflective stripes make the wearer visible at all hours. Traffic vests are available from a number of safety equipment manufacturers and distributors. It is good procedure to have all personnel at the rescue site clearly visible. Traffic vests are an inexpensive and effective way of making your crews visible, especially to approaching vehicles.

Respiratory Protection

Every rescue vehicle should be equipped with respiratory protection whenever crew members may have to work in:

- Oxygen-deficient structures such as manholes, reaction vessels, storage tanks, tank trucks, ship compartments, cesspools and septic tanks, silos, manure storage facilities, or other confined spaces
- Smoke-filled structures such as buildings on fire and structures into which smoke is blowing from a fire in another location
- Smoke-filled areas such as those in close proximity to accident vehicles that are on fire
- High-temperature environments such as boiler and heater rooms, steel mills, manufacturing facilities, and structures exposed to open flames
- Toxic atmospheres such as chemical laboratories, manufacturing facilities, and accident locations where dangerous chemicals, commonly called hazardous materials, have been spilled or where toxic or noxious gases have been released

Following are some items for respiratory protection that are very effective in these environments:

Self-Contained Breathing Apparatus should be carried for every crew member. If storage space is limited, at least two self-contained units should be carried so that at least one pair of rescuers can work protected. At no time should a rescuer work in a hazardous environment alone.

A **Dust Respirator** or **Dust Mask** should be carried for the protection of each crew member from *nontoxic* dust particles that sometimes contaminate the atmosphere as the result of a truck accident, building collapse, or dust explosion.

A **Thermal Mask** will afford protection against the inhalation of extremely cold air during cold-weather rescue operations.

Personal "Pocket" Equipment

Rescue personnel carry all sorts of things in the deep, roomy pockets of turnout coats. It's not unusual to find candy bars, dry socks, or even a change of underwear! Among the other, slightly more utilitarian items that might be carried are:

A **Personal Flashlight** reduces the potential for injury when it is used to illuminate dangerous work areas. A number of small, bright, battery-powered flashlights are available, some with accessories. A helmet-mounted light clips onto most helmets and will illuminate work areas when both hands are needed for tool operations. The Universal Clip-On Light Bracket, available from W. S. Darley and Company, holds either a Mini-Mag or Streamlight, Jr. flashlight to any Cairns or Bullard helmet.

A **Cyalume® Lightstick** carried in your turnout coat pocket will provide emergency illumination when your flashlight or hand light fails, or when you suddenly find yourself in need of a safe light source while working in a flammable atmosphere.

A quality **Pocket Knife** should be carried by every rescuer, not so much for rescue operations as for survival measures.

A **Six-Foot Retractable Tape Measure** should be carried to measure openings for tool insertion.

Half-Inch-Wide Elastic Bands should be carried for use when it is necessary to close coat and pants cuffs tightly, as when working in the presence of a hazardous commodity or stinging insects. These big rubber bands can be cut from old inner tubes. Carry at least four in a turnout coat pocket. Do not keep them around your helmet, or they will become permanently stretched and will be virtually useless when you need them for personal protection.

*Supplies and Equipment for Protection
Against Infectious Agents*

Rescuers must consider infectious diseases such as HIV or HBV very seriously for two reasons: (1) They frequently work in the presence of blood and other body fluids, especially if they are part of a busy squad, and (2) they are subject to contact with sharp edges, pointed objects, and other mechanisms of injury. Rescuers are required to be trained to use body substance isolation (BSI) procedures under OSHA 1910.1030.

Every accident victim should be looked on as probably being infected with AIDS or Hepatitis B virus, and every rescuer should wear barrier protection when the likelihood of percutaneous (through the skin) or mucocutaneous (in the mouth, nose, or eyes) exposure to a victim's blood or other body fluids is present. In addition to the leather gloves that should be worn during all extrication operations, two other types of gloves should be available to rescuers.

Midweight Rubber or **Plastic Gloves** (such as household gloves) should be worn for non-patient care activities that may involve handling equipment contaminated with blood or body secretions, and when cleaning equipment that may be contaminated.

Medical-Grade Latex or **Rubber Gloves** should be worn for all patient care procedures that may result in contamination of the rescuer's hands with blood and/or body fluids, as when bandaging and dressing wounds and splinting open fractures.

Also, a **Medical-Grade Combination Face Mask with Eyeshield** should be worn in situations where blood and/or body fluids could be splashed in a rescuer's eyes, nose, or mouth.

Protection against the HIV or HBV virus should not be limited to wearing barrier devices at the location of accidents where blood and body fluids are present. Rescue personnel—indeed, all emergency service personnel who come in contact with injured people—should have cuts, abrasions, insect bites, and other breaks in the skin covered with adhesive compresses or other small dressings before reporting for work.

Supplies and Equipment for Victim Protection

It's bad enough when people's bodies are lacerated, incised, punctured, abraded, twisted, bent, broken, or crushed as the result of an accident. Shielding *patients* with some inexpensive devices and exercising care during rescue operations will minimize the chance that they will suffer additional injuries.

*Items That Can Be Used to Shield Patients
from Contact with Tools and Debris*

Patients, especially those who have been involved in motor vehicle accidents, are usually exposed to a variety of mechanisms of injury during rescue operations. They can be cut by a sharp-edged tool, for example, or can be injured when struck by a blunt object such as a hammer. And they can be hurt by flying pieces of debris generated during the rescue effort—debris such as particles of metal and glass, and bits of metal that break off when one steel tool is struck by another steel tool. Injuries such as these can be prevented by placing some sort of rigid barrier between patient and rescue tools.

The **Short Wood Spine Board** that is usually carried on a rescue vehicle is the rigid device most often used to shield patients from contact by tools and debris.

A **Plywood** or **Particle Board Panel** can be carried on a rescue unit just for patient protection. The size of the board depends on the dimensions of the storage compartment. Simple rope handles facilitate carrying wood panels.

A **Two-** or **Three-Part Hinged Plywood Panel** or **Shield Made of Particle Board** can be carried in a relatively small space in a rescue vehicle and can be inserted in small spaces in vehicles.

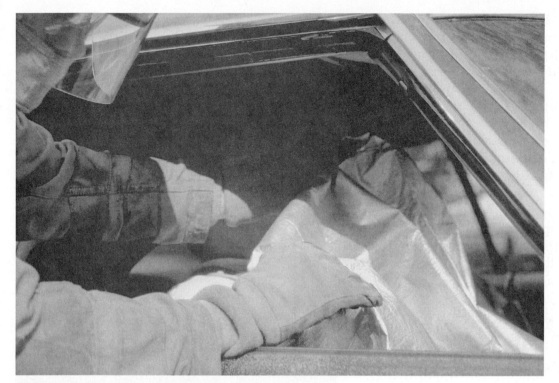

FIGURE 1.11 Aluminized Blanket

Items That Can Be Used to Protect Patients from Flames and Radiant Heat

Emergency service personnel must often work in the presence of spilled fuel at the scene of a vehicle accident or even close to a vehicle that is on fire. While rescuers, firefighters, EMTs, and paramedics have their turnout gear to protect them from radiant heat, seldom is anything available for protecting persons in the wrecked vehicles.

An **Aluminized Fabric Rescue Blanket** will provide trapped patients with a degree of protection from radiant heat while firefighting operations are underway, whereas a fabric or paper blanket is likely to catch fire. An aluminized blanket (Figure 1.11) should be used *only* for the purpose intended, however, and not for routinely protecting a person from contact with tools and flying particles. Reflectivity is sharply reduced when the aluminized coating flakes away or becomes dirty. Special Service and Supply, Inc., offers a 76-inch by 82-inch aluminized blanket designed specially for rescue operations.

An Important Point: An asbestos blanket should *never* be used to protect someone from radiant heat, for a reason other than the obvious danger of the person inhaling asbestos fibers. An asbestos blanket will absorb a great deal of heat, and if it becomes wet with water from a hose line, the resulting steam may scald the person underneath.

Items That Can Be Used to Protect Patients from the Elements

Inclement weather does a great deal more than just make things miserable for everyone during a vehicle rescue effort. Cold, rain, snow, sleet, and even heat can contribute to an injured person's quick deterioration and even death by lowering or raising his body temperature to a dangerous level.

A **Golf Umbrella** or a **Doorman's Umbrella** held by a rescuer, a firefighter, or even a spectator will protect an injured person from rain or snow during a short-term rescue effort. The width of the canopy makes a golf umbrella or a doorman's umbrella more suitable than a conventional umbrella. Both types of umbrella can be obtained from sporting goods, department, and discount stores (Figure 1.12).

A **Lightweight Tarpaulin** can be held by several people to shield a patient from the elements during a lengthy rescue procedure. Or, a lightweight tarp can be held over an accident vehicle with pike poles supported by ropes. The tarpaulin need not be an expensive coated-fabric fire service salvage cover; an inexpensive coated-paper tarp available in hardware and discount stores will work well.

A **Disposable Blanket** can be used to conserve the body heat of an individual trapped in a wrecked vehicle. If it becomes torn or soiled or impregnated with glass particles, it can be thrown away after use. The wool or synthetic fiber blankets usually carried on the ambulance for use on the stretcher should *not* be used to protect patients during window removal operations. It is virtually impossible to remove glass particles that become tangled in the fibers. Disposable blankets can be purchased from most emergency medical service equipment suppliers.

An **Aluminized Blanket** is an excellent device for conserving body heat. It comes folded to the size of a cigarette pack and can be easily carried in a jump kit or trauma box. A 50-inch by 86-inch aluminized blanket can be purchased from Dyna-Med (a Model Y12158 Aluminized Rescue Blanket). Similar aluminized blankets (called survival blankets) can be obtained at many sporting goods stores.

Items That Can Be Used to Protect a Patient's Head, Eyes, and Ears

Every effort must be taken to protect a patient's head from flying glass particles generated during the rescue operation, especially the eyes. Finely divided glass particles can be carried for a considerable distance by a breeze and deposited on eye surfaces. Even though they are only powder size, the particles can damage the corneas.

A **Construction-Style Hard Hat** can be used to protect a person's head during roof removal or other overhead rescue operations and from flying debris.

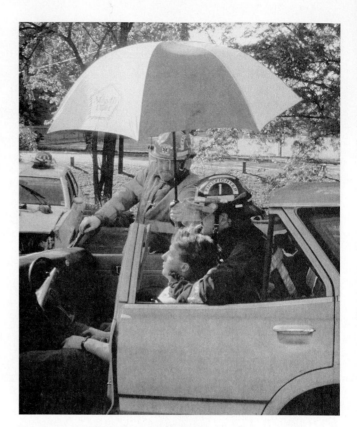

FIGURE 1.12   Golf Umbrella

Coverall-Type, Soft-Side Safety Goggles will protect a patient's eyes from the flying particles of glass and metal chips that are often generated during rescue operations, especially when power tools are used.

Earmuff-Style Hearing Protectors serve not only to shield the patient's ears from frightening noises but also to protect his ears from contact with tools and flying particles. One particular hearing protector, the Fibre-Metal Model 2011, covers both the ears and the noise-transmitting mastoid bones.

Items That Can Be Used to Protect a Patient's Respiratory Passages

Smoke, toxic gases, noxious fumes, dust, and finely divided particles of all sorts of granular materials can swirl around accident vehicles and threaten rescuers and patients alike. Rescuers can protect themselves with a breathing apparatus, but if there are not enough units for rescuers *and* patients or if a mask cannot be properly fitted to a trapped person's face, patients are likely to remain unprotected until they are placed in an ambulance.

Short exposures to smoke and nontoxic fumes may not constitute a health hazard; they may be nothing more than a minor nuisance that causes a little discomfort. On the other hand, continued exposure during a lengthy extrication operation may cause a trapped person to become nauseous. Retching, vomiting, or movement in an attempt to get away from the source of irritation may cause an injured person to aggravate his injuries.

An **Approved Disposable Dust Mask** will protect a patient's respiratory passages and lungs from dust and airborne particles of debris generated during rescue efforts. A dust mask is an important patient protection device in areas where dust storms are common or when finely divided materials such as grain have been spilled from a truck at the scene of an accident.

A **Thermal Mask** can be placed on a patient during cold-weather rescue operations. Remember that body heat is lost through normal respirations. Fibre-Metal, Erb Safety Equipment Company, and Bullard are some of the companies that manufacture disposable face masks.

Tools and Appliances for Vehicle Rescue Operations

It's an unfortunate commentary on our times when a rescuer throws up his hands and cries in despair that he cannot carry out a rescue operation. There are at least two reasons why a supposedly trained individual may act in this irrational manner:

- Basic training may not have trained the rescuer to cope with the particular accident situation.
- Exposures to printed materials and television pictures that show other rescue squads in service may have left the rescuer with a feeling of inadequacy—a feeling that accident

victims cannot be rescued without sophisticated tools and the knowledge of special techniques.

It may be too obvious to require mentioning, but when you think of your roles and responsibilities at the scene of a vehicle rescue operation, think positively! Experience shows that in the majority of accident situations examined, access to trapped persons was gained quickly with nothing more than hand tools. If your rescue unit is one that arrives first at the location with some pretty basic equipment, don't be discouraged. Remember that you can do a great deal with those tools, basic techniques, and an "I can make do with what I have" attitude.

Supplies and Equipment for Hazard Management Operations

Any of a number of hazards can be found at the location of an accident, including fire, smoke, noxious fumes, toxic gases, darkness, slippery surfaces, electrical conductors, water, unstable vehicles or other mechanisms of entrapment, threat of an explosion, spectators, traffic, and more. These hazards threaten not only accident victims but also the people who respond to help them. All rescue vehicles should carry supplies and equipment for a variety of hazard management operations.

Equipment for Fire Suppression and Prevention

A rescue vehicle, even one that has a pump, water supply, and hose, should be equipped with at least two fire extinguishers: a dry chemical extinguisher and a pressurized water extinguisher.

A **20-Pound Class A:B:C Portable Fire Extinguisher** can be used to extinguish fires involving ordinary combustible materials (seat cushions and paper and cloth products in the trunk, for example), spilled fuel, and electrical components. There are several makes and models of A:B:C extinguishers available from fire equipment suppliers (Figure 1.13).

A **2-1/2-Gallon Pressurized Water Fire Extinguisher** can be used to extinguish burning ordinary combustibles and to flush unignited fuel from under an accident vehicle when the response of an engine company will be delayed and the rescue unit does not have a pump and water supply.

A **Hand-Pump Water Fire Extinguisher** can also be used to combat fires involving ordinary combustibles and to flush small amounts of unignited fuel from under accident vehicles. The principal advantages of this type of extinguisher are that it does not have to be repressurized after use, and there is no problem with pressure loss during long storage periods. W. S. Darley and Company offers a variety of 2-1/2- and 5-gallon hand-pump extinguishers with steel, brass, or plastic tanks.

A **Class D Extinguisher** might be carried when there is room on the rescue unit. The special agent can be used to extinguish the magnesium components found on some vehicles.

A variety of extinguishing agents and sealants might be carried if the rescue truck has a pump and water supply.

Equipment That Can Be Used to Stabilize Vehicles

An unstable vehicle can cause injuries to occupants and rescuers alike. A vehicle that is on its wheels must be prevented from moving forward or backward. Moreover, injury-aggravating motion must be prevented. A vehicle that is on its side must be prevented from dropping back on its wheels or rolling onto its top. A vehicle that is on its roof must be stabilized in such a way that roof pillars will not collapse during rescue operations.

Unstable vehicles can be stabilized in dozens of ways, from using manpower to support the vehicle in position, to using complex pneumatic and hydraulic devices. The equipment suggested here can be easily stored on an ambulance and used by two crew members.

Wheel Chocks, such as the high tensile strength aluminum alloy models made by

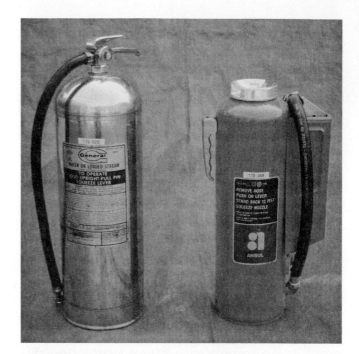

FIGURE 1.13 Fire Extinguishers—Dry Chemical and Pressurized Water

Ziamatic, are generally carried on an ambulance and used when the unit must be parked on a hill. The same wheel chocks can also be used to prevent the forward or rearward movement of an accident vehicle.

Eighteen-Inch Lengths of 2-Inch by 4-Inch and 4-Inch by 4-Inch Wood Cribbing can be used to support vehicles and other mechanisms of injury and entrapment during rescue operations. These lengths of wood enable rescuers to follow the important rule: Lift an inch, crib an inch. The pieces of cribbing that can be stored in a large plastic milk jug container are usually sufficient to stabilize a full-size passenger car. Lengths of rope attached to the cribs (Figure 1.14) serve as convenient carrying handles. The ropes enable rescuers to remove cribs quickly from under previously supported loads during equipment recovery operations.

While some rescue officials advocate the use of a hard wood, purchasing oak for use as cribbing is an unnecessary expense. There are few, if any, rescue situations when pine or fir cribbing would not be able to withstand the downward forces exerted by a load that has been lifted and supported.

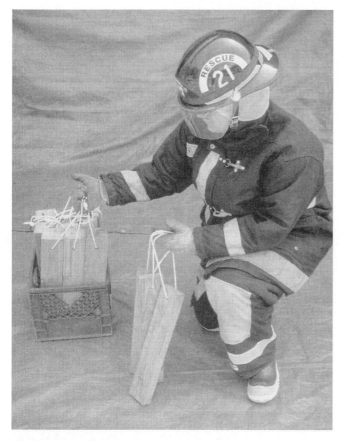

FIGURE 1.14   2-Inch × 4-Inch Cribbing with Ropes

Moreover, because it is so dense, oak tends to be somewhat slippery when wet.

While it may look nicer, cribbing should never be painted. Paint makes cribbing slippery when wet with water, and paint hides cracks that warn of a length of cribbing's un-

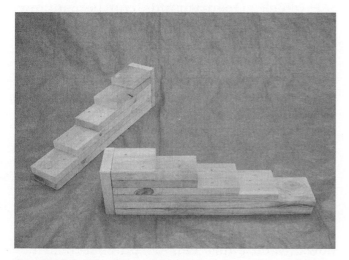

FIGURE 1.15   Step Cribbing

suitability for a rescue operation. If you wish to use paint to identify cribbing, paint only the ends.

Step Cribbing can be used in some situations to stabilize an accident quicker than with loose cribbing (Figure 1.15).

Cribbing Ladders come in handy during steering column, door, and seat displacement operations when the crushing of sheet-metal components is likely to be a problem.

Lengths of 4-Inch by 4-Inch Wood Cribbing Longer Than 18-Inches might be carried for a variety of stabilization operations when there is sufficient storage space on the rescue unit. Five- and six-foot lengths are essential for some steering column displacement operations.

Two-Inch by 4-Inch and 4-Inch by 4-Inch 12-Inch Wedges can be used to support a variety of mechanisms of injury and entrapment during gaining access and disentanglement operations; for filling voids that may result when cribs are built under objects that must be supported; and for supporting objects that are not parallel to supporting wood cribs. Like cribbing, wood wedges should not be painted.

Hard Rubber Wedges are superior to wood wedges in that they are less likely to slip or split while supporting a load.

Pneumatic Jacks, such as the Airshore™ Trench Jack, for trench shoring operations are excellent devices for stabilizing accident vehicles, especially trucks, and heavy loads that have shifted as the result of an accident. While the jacks can be pressurized by compressed air, nitrogen, or carbon dioxide, they can also be adjusted by hand, and when properly positioned can support a load of up to 32,000 pounds.

Items That Can Be Used to Stop the Flow of Flammable Fuel

Under-the-trunk fuel tanks of passenger cars are often damaged as the result of vehicle accidents, especially rear-end collisions.

If a seam fails or if a large opening is made in the tank shell, fuel is likely to be lost quickly, and there is little for first-arriving emergency service personnel to do other than to cope with the spilled flammable liquid. If only a small hole results, however, it may be possible to seal the tank and thus reduce the fire danger.

While a number of devices can be used to plug leaking tanks, few are really suitable for sealing the jagged, irregular holes that are usually produced when a vehicle's fuel tank is punctured. Expandable plugs must be inserted into the opening and then tightened with a screwdriver or wrench, a time-consuming procedure that must be accomplished by someone possibly standing in spilled fuel. Magnetic seals will not usually adhere to tank surfaces that are under-coated or crusted over with dirt.

A **Pliable Sealant** should be carried on the rescue unit for sealing irregularly shaped holes in vehicle fuel tanks. Plug and Dike Pre-Mix® is a nontoxic, high-absorption polymer that forms an immediate seal. Duct Seal® is a compound used to seal openings in heating, ventilation, and air-conditioning ducts. These products are available at most auto supply stores. Either can be quickly molded in the hand and pressed into a hole in a fuel tank. Duct sealant can be stored in its original foil wrapper or in a tightly sealable plastic food container. In cold-weather areas, sealant should be kept in a warm place on the rescue vehicle so it is ready for immediate use.

The rubber hoses that carry fuel from a vehicle's tank to the fuel pump are sometimes ruptured or severed as the result of an accident and thus contribute to the problem of leaking fuel. Hoses can be quickly plugged with a wood pencil, a ball-point pen, or an inexpensive stopper that many rescue squads carry just for this purpose.

Wooden Golf Tees are good sealing devices. The narrow shank slips easily into severed fuel lines, and the tapered heads make effective seals. A dozen golf tees can be stored along with duct sealant in its plastic container; thus the container becomes a handy, albeit minimal leak seal kit (Figure 1.16).

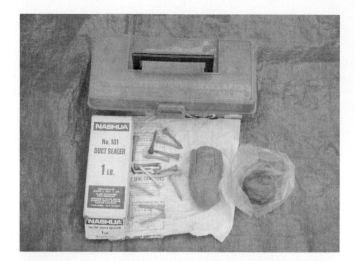

FIGURE 1.16   Gasoline Leak Seal Kit

A **Granular Absorbent Material** or **Absorbent Pads** can be used to stop the flow of flammable fuel away from accident vehicles.

Supplies That Can Be Used to Minimize the Spread of Glass Debris

It is often necessary for rescuers to break a vehicle's tempered glass rear window or side windows and cut or break out laminated windshields when injured occupants require immediate care and doors cannot be opened quickly. Regardless of how careful rescuers may try to be during window breaking and removal operations, glass fragments can be a serious problem both inside and outside the vehicle. Open wounds can be contaminated, and finely divided glass particles can find their way into the unprotected eyes of patients, rescuers, and bystanders.

Adhesive-Backed Shelf Paper can be quickly applied to a dry window when it is deemed necessary to minimize the spread of tempered glass particles to the interior of a vehicle. A roll of paper can be stored in a compartment, or, better yet, pieces of shelf paper just larger than the side windows of a full-sized passenger car can be folded or rolled, secured with a rubber band, and carried in the tool kit along with the tools used to break windows. Shelf paper can be purchased in department, hardware, and variety stores.

Two-Inch Fabric-Backed Tape can also be used to minimize the spread of glass particles. Aluminized duct tape, or a better quality (and, thus, more expensive!) fabric tape known as "gaffer's" tape are excellent choices. The same tape can be used for other tasks during a vehicle rescue operation, such as shielding jagged metal edges and the sharp ends of severed roof pillars.

Whether to use shelf paper or tape to cover windows is usually a matter of choice. Both are somewhat troublesome and time-consuming. Shelf paper is often difficult to separate from its backing, especially in a wind, and if it is to be effective, tape must be applied to windows in two layers, one at a right angle to the other. While both of these methods work, do not waste valuable time if you can break a window in an area away from the patient.

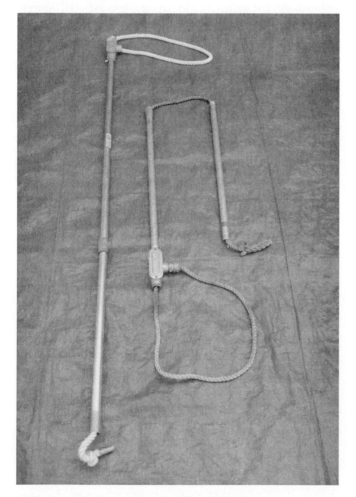

FIGURE 1.17 Animal Control Noose

Equipment for Animal Control

While it is not an everyday occurrence, rescue personnel sometimes respond to accident locations and discover that an injured person is guarded by a big dog that appears to have one thought in mind: to chew into little pieces anyone who so much as approaches its master!

Other than to call for help, there is little that rescue personnel can do when confronted with a guard dog. The response of a police officer may be delayed, and it may take a representative of a humane society or animal control agency quite a while to reach the scene—time that a severely injured person may not have. Some people argue that a guard dog can be driven off with an irritating agent such as tear gas or with water from a hose stream, but animal handlers maintain that these actions only make an already excited animal more aggressive and more likely to attack.

An **Animal Control Noose** should be carried on a rescue vehicle in areas where guard dogs routinely patrol offices, businesses, and industrial occupancies and where many homeowners keep guard dogs as pets. A manufactured noose can be purchased in 4-. 6-, 8-, and 10-foot lengths from W. S. Darley and Company, or one can be easily made from items available in a hardware store (Figure 1.17). Local SPCA branches, humane societies, animal control agencies, and animal handlers employed by security companies will often train emergency service personnel in the use of an animal control noose.

Equipment for Moving Downed Wires

The decision to equip a rescue unit with equipment for moving downed wires is not an easy one. Many officials argue that the procedures subject rescuers to unacceptable risks. But when the decision is made that rescue personnel can move downed wires at the scene of a motor vehicle accident in certain situations, only the equipment that is designed for the job should be placed on the unit. Ordinary firefighting gloves do not provide protection against electrocution, and wood-handled tools and manila rope cannot be safely used to move downed wires.

The **A/C Hotstick** manufactured by Delsar®, Inc., has gained acclaim for its life-saving capabilities. This electronic device alerts rescuers of the presence of electric current. In a vehicle accident situation where a power pole has been struck causing downed wires, or a pad mount transformer incident which has possibly charged the vehicles, the A/C Hotstick (Figure 1.18) will signal with a beeper and light that a problem exists.

A **Lineman's Glove Set** provides the basis for personal protection from current flow up to 40,000 volts. Glove sets typically consist of natural gum rubber inserts and leather gauntlets that protect the gloves from abrasion and laceration and, to a much lesser degree, from puncturing. Some gloves have a bright yellow inner layer bonded to a black outer layer. A spot of yellow showing through the black outer layer during a field examination of the gloves warns that the glove is damaged and should not be worn. Two glove sets should be carried on every unit, because moving a downed wire is necessarily a team effort (Figure 1.19).

Lineman's glove sets should be stored in a clearly marked metal box or canvas bag. Thus operating personnel will be less likely to use the gloves for firefighting or other activities during which the gloves might be damaged.

A **Can of Talcum Powder** should be included in the glove box or bag. Powdering the hands makes donning the gloves easier during hot or wet weather. An alternative to using powder is to keep several pairs of white cotton gloves (such as "parade" gloves) with the lineman's glove sets. The cotton gloves will absorb perspiration on the hands.

A **Spare Set of Rubber Glove Inserts** should be available for every set of lineman's gloves carried on the unit. Thus there will still be a glove set available if a glove appears defective during a field examination or while a set of inserts is away being tested.

A **Lineman's Clampstick** enables a rescuer to firmly grip a downed wire. A clampstick is often called a "shotgun" stick be-

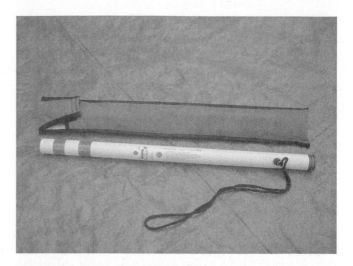

FIGURE 1.18   A/C Hotstick

cause of the slide action of the operating handle. Clampsticks are available in several fixed lengths. Kits are also available with sections that can be quickly and easily assembled to make clampsticks of different lengths. An example of a clampstick kit is the Hastings Model 81-544 kit (Figure 1.20).

A **Telescoping Hotstick** with an S-hook at the working end should also be carried. While one rescuer uses the clampstick to move a downed wire, the second rescuer can use the hotstick to unsnag the wire if necessary and lift it from the vehicle. Hastings also makes a telescoping hotstick, the Model SH-216 (Figure 1.21).

The principal advantage of extendable and telescoping sticks is that their length af-

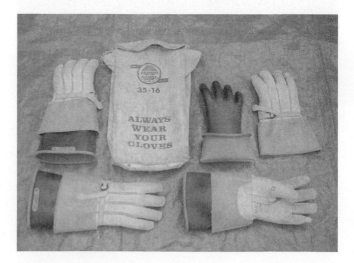

FIGURE 1.19   Lineman's Gloves

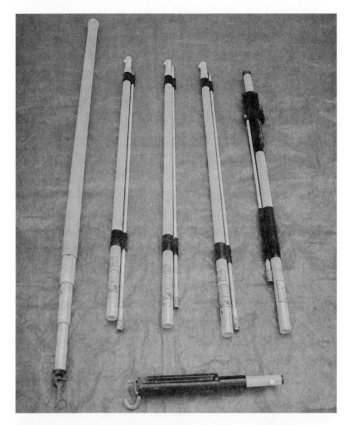

FIGURE 1.20 Clampstick

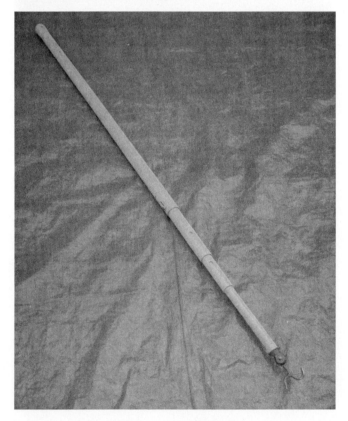

FIGURE 1.21 Telescoping Hotstick

fords rescuers a greater degree of safety when they must stand on wet ground or when they must move arcing wires.

Further information and training for rescuers in dealing with electrical hazards is usually available from the local power company.

Items That Can Be Used to Identify Hazardous Material Transport Vehicles

No effort will be made here to list supplies and equipment that rescue personnel should use in the presence of hazardous materials. The decision to equip rescuers with acid suits and other highly specialized equipment should be made after a thorough evaluation of hazards within the service area, consideration for available community resources, and participation in training programs.

Even though they may not be able to work around them, rescuers should be able to recognize hazardous materials. To that end, every rescue vehicle should have at least the following items.

A **Pair of 7 × 50 "Armored" Binoculars** will allow a rescuer to identify hazardous material placards from a safe distance. Armored binoculars have a rubber or plastic coating to protect the somewhat delicate mechanisms and lenses from rough rides and damage from dropping and contact with other tools. Armored binoculars can be purchased from better department and discount stores.

A **Hazardous Materials Action Guide** can be consulted for suggestions as to appropriate actions. Two especially useful guides are the U.S. Department of Transportation (DOT), *Hazardous Materials: The Emergency Response Handbook*, available from the Government Printing Office; and *Emergency Handling of Hazardous Materials in Surface Transportation*, available from the Bureau of Explosives, Association of American Railroads.

Binoculars, guides, and local protocols should be kept in an inexpensive attaché case along with lists of local hazardous material storage sites, standard operating procedures, community resource directories, and other pertinent information. Clearly marked as a "Hazardous Material Identification Kit," the case should be stored behind the driver's seat or in an easily accessible compartment where it will be available for immediate use.

Miscellaneous Items for Hazard Management

Several other items can be carried to make operations safer for rescuers and victims.

A **Plastic Jug Filled with Cat Litter** comes in handy when rescuers need to work on icy roads or roads covered with a slippery substance such as fuel oil. Sprinkling this sharp-edged granular material on the roadway assures a safe footing. Large laundry detergent jugs make excellent containers for cat litter (Figure 1.22).

A **Folding Pointed-Blade Shovel** is valuable to have when it is necessary to reach a person who has been buried under a spill of dirt, grain, gravel, or other granular material. While it cannot move as much material as a larger, long-handled model, a folding shovel can be better controlled; thus the likelihood of the buried person being injured by the shovel is reduced. Folding shovels are available in surplus outlets and the garden departments of hardware and department stores (Figure 1.23).

A **Folding Tree Saw** comes in handy whenever brush and/or trees must be removed from atop or around an accident vehicle. Axes and power saws can be used to clear large limbs and branches from the wreckage, but when vegetation must be cut close to a trapped person, the folding saw should be the tool of choice. Tree saws can be purchased in most large hardware stores.

Several Lengths of Split 1-1/2- to 5-Inch Fire Hose might be carried to protect rescuers, patients, and equipment from the razor-sharp edges that often result when openings are made in sheet-metal panels (Figure 1.24).

Several Unsplit Lengths of 2-1/2- or 3-Inch Fire Hose might be carried in addition to the split lengths of hose. The larger diameter unsplit sections can be slipped over sev-

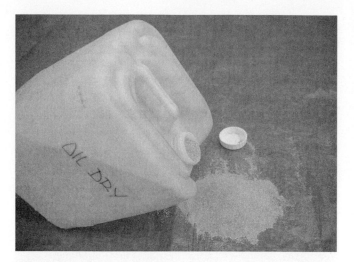

FIGURE 1.22   Cat Litter

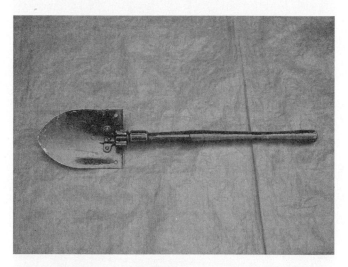

FIGURE 1.23   Folding Shovel

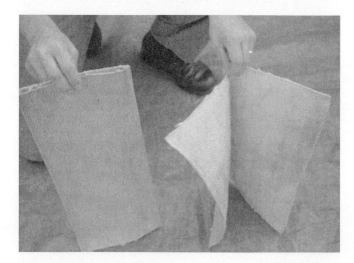

FIGURE 1.24   Split Fire Hose

ered roof pillars and other sharp projections that can injure emergency service personnel and patients during rescue and patient care activities.

Twelve-Inch and 36-Inch Heavy-Duty Shock Cords with S-Hooks at Both Ends can have a number of uses during vehicle rescue operations. They can be used to secure folded roof sections in place, to hold doors open, and to hold tarpaulins in place during lengthy inclement-weather operations. Shock cords can be purchased at truck-stop stores, hardware stores, and wherever supplies for recreational vehicles are sold.

A **Smoke Ejector** can be used for tasks other than ventilating smoke-filled buildings. During vehicle rescue operations, one of these powerful fans can be used to deliver fresh air to trapped persons exposed to smoke from a nearby burning vehicle or toxic or noxious fumes coming from a damaged hazardous cargo container.

The most popular smoke ejector has a 16-inch fan driven by an electric motor. A 10-foot flexible duct can be attached to the fan housing so that the unit can be situated at a distance from the work site.

Supplies and Equipment for Warning and Signaling

A rescue unit should be equipped with warning and signaling devices even when squad members seldom become involved in traffic control activities. There may be times when police officers are not able to reach an accident location quickly. If all squad personnel must be committed to the rescue operation, the warning and signaling devices can be given to other emergency service members or even apparently responsible bystanders with a few simple instructions as to what to do.

Remember that oncoming traffic may present a major hazard to rescuers. Drivers often have their attention distracted and are looking at the accident scene. Those directing traffic should be alert for the dangers that traffic may present. Each year many rescuers are hit by vehicles at accident scenes.

Items That Can Be Used for Traffic Control

Some people argue that pyrotechnic flares are too dangerous for use at vehicle accident locations and that the battery-operated warning lights commonly used at road construction locations are better. In their argument, these people fail to consider such factors as the differences in storage requirements, the cost of replacement batteries, and the maintenance problems. Moreover, flares can be seen for a far greater distance than flashing lights, especially in bad weather.

Pyrotechnic Flares are most commonly used to control the movement of vehicles past accident locations; traffic experts recommend that they be used at all hours of the day and night. Flares are available with 15-, 20-, and 30-minute burning times and with a wire stand, spike, or plain end. Flares with spike ends are designed to be driven into the ground or roadway for support. After they are used, they leave behind a sharp nail that could present a hazard if not disposed of properly. Flares with wire stands are preferred for rescue operations because they can be more easily set out in an upright position and leave no dangerous spikes.

Fifteen-Inch 12-Hour Cyalume® Lightsticks especially designed for traffic control can be used in place of flares when spilled fuel or another flammable material is present at an accident location. The Lightsticks can be hand-held, or held upright in special wire stands. Cyalume® Lightsticks are manufactured by American Cyanamid Company and are available from most fire and EMS equipment suppliers.

Red or Fluorescent Red Warning Flags with Staffs should be available for rescuers who have the responsibility of channeling vehicles from one lane to another during daylight periods. **Traffic Control Flashlights** should be available for traffic control duties during nighttime operations. A traffic control flashlight is far superior to a conventional flashlight; the large surface area of the illuminated wand or paddle makes the light visible for a considerable distance. A **Set of**

Replacement Batteries should be kept on the rescue unit for each traffic control light to assure that they are always operable.

Traffic Cones might be carried for extended traffic control activities when there is sufficient storage space on the rescue unit. There are four sizes of traffic cones: 12 inches, 18 inches, 28 inches, and 36 inches high. Accessories that are available for cones are reflective collars, flag holders and flags, and battery-operated flashing lights. When ordered in sufficient quantities, cones can be imprinted with the name of the fire department or rescue squad.

Flares, warning flags, traffic control flashlights, and traffic cones can be obtained from suppliers of emergency service equipment.

Equipment for Controlling the Movement of Spectators

Several items can be used to exclude spectators from the danger zones at accident locations when there are not enough rescuers, firefighters, or police officers for the job.

Three-Inch Barrier Banners are available in 1000-foot and 1200-foot rolls. The high-visibility yellow polyethylene tape can be purchased with the captions such as "Caution" or "Police [or Fire] Line—Do Not Cross" imprinted in black letters. Barrier barricade tape can also be custom imprinted.

Safety Barrier Rope can also be used to cordon off accident locations. The yellow and black 1/2-inch polypropylene rope can be used over and over; it will not absorb water and it is not affected by petroleum products. Barrier rope is available in 600-foot coils that weigh only 6 pounds.

Barricade Tape is yet another device for identifying danger zones at accident locations. The reusable 3/4-inch fluorescent red, vinyl-coated nylon tape is available in 150-foot rolls. It is not harmed by petroleum products and will not crack, peel, or stick.

All of the above items are available from W. S. Darley and Company.

Equipment for Audible Warning and Signaling

Portable transceivers enable rescue officers to communicate with rescue vehicles and the local communication centers, and vehicle-mounted public address systems can be used to relay orders and warnings to emergency service personnel and spectators. These are not the only devices that can be used for warning and signaling, however.

A **Powered Megaphone** (or loud-hailer or bull horn) can be used by a rescue officer to amplify orders and warnings when the ambient noise level is high at an accident location.

A **Freon-Powered Horn** can be used to warn rescuers of approaching traffic or, when an accident has occurred on a grade crossing, of an approaching train. A horn can also be used to sound a recall signal during the termination phase of a vehicle rescue operation.

A **Police Officer's or Referee's Whistle** is handy for rescuers assigned to traffic control operations. Use a quality metal whistle, not a cheap plastic toy.

Regardless of what device is used for audible warning and signaling, it's important that a list of signals be created by squad officers and that every squad member learn the signals.

Items That Can Be Used to Designate Priorities for Gaining Access

Confusion is a problem at multiple-vehicle accident locations when squad members do not understand what doors or windows are to be opened first in the effort to reach seriously injured persons. Unproductive efforts can be minimized when the assessing officer uses highly visible markers to establish priorities for gaining access.

Fluorescent Surveyor's Tapes (red, orange, yellow, and green) can be used during daylight hours to designate the order in which doors should be opened or windows removed. Surveyor's tapes are available from construction equipment suppliers and stores that sell drafting equipment.

Cyalume® Lightsticks can be used at night for the same purpose as the fluorescent tape mentioned above, because of their high visibility in low light or dark areas. These chemical light sticks are available in the same colors as surveyor's tapes.

Colored String Tags and even **Triage Tags** can also be used to designate priorities for gaining access.

Equipment for Power Generation, Distribution and Illumination

Every rescue vehicle should have a 110-volt power supply sufficient for the lights and electrically powered tools that are likely to be used during rescue operations.

Too small a power supply can be a real problem. Let's say that a rescue truck has a 2500-watt generator. During a nighttime operation, the officer-in-charge orders squad members to set up four floodlights. Since the lights have 500-watt incandescent bulbs, lighting alone will demand 2000 watts of available power. If the officer orders the use of electrically powered tools, there may not be a sufficient reserve of power for their use.

You can easily calculate how many electric appliances may be operated from your squad vehicle's generator if you know (1) the generator's power output and (2) the power requirements for the lights and the electrically operated tools. The following formula applies:

$$P = I \times E$$

where P is power in watts, I is amperage, and E is voltage. Observe how the formula works in the following example.

The rescue unit's generator is rated at 3500 watts at 110 volts. During a rescue operation at night, rescuers might connect two 500-watt floodlights, one 300-watt floodlight, and two 110-volt, 7-amp reciprocating

saws to the power supply. When all the lights are lit and both saws are operating simultaneously, the current draw will be about 2900 watts. By subtracting, we can determine that the current reserve will be about 600 watts, enough for another floodlight, if needed.

Many rescue officers calculate the power requirements for all their lights and electrically powered tools and appliances and mark the current ratings on the devices with paint, stamped metal tags, or embossed vinyl tapes. Then, when the tool or appliance is plugged into the generator panel or power distribution box, the driver/tool officer can easily determine the demand on the generator. He will know how much current is being supplied and how much is in reserve. All power tools and accessories must be provided with ground fault interupters (G.F.I.) for the protection of the rescuers *and* patients.

One Hundred Ten-Volt, 500-, 1000- and 1500-Watt Floodlights with Stands are sources of bright light. Like any other light source, floodlights should be used in pairs for shadow-free illumination. Portable floodlights are available with incandescent, quartz, and quartz-halogen bulbs.

A **100-Foot (or Longer) Length of Three-Wire Extension Cord Terminating in a Four-Outlet Junction Box** should be available for distributing power to lights and tools. The cord should be rated for heavy duty. A power cord can be stored coiled or in a reel.

Battery-Powered Handlights are available as units with replaceable batteries or as units that are stored in charging units in the rescue unit. A **Set of Replacement Batteries** should be carried on the rescue unit for each handlight if the handlights are battery operated.

A **12-Volt Trouble Light with a 50-Foot Cord and Battery Clamps** is a useful tool for off-road rescue operations. The light can be carried to the wreckage and quickly connected to an accident vehicle's battery. Quick illumination allows first-in rescue personnel to initiate rescue and emergency care procedures while other rescuers are stringing power cords and lights.

Cyalume® Lightsticks can be used for illumination when other sources of light are not available or when a dangerous area must be illuminated as, for example, the work area over a gasoline spill. High-intensity lightsticks provide a bright red, green, yellow, or white light for 30 minutes. Eight-hour lightsticks are available in either white or blue, and 12-hour lightsticks are available in green, red, yellow, and orange.

Tools for Gaining Access and Disentanglement

The tools in the next two groups are intended for (1) gaining access to persons who are trapped in an accident vehicle and (2) disentangling those persons from mechanisms of entrapment. While they are grouped in categories, many of the tools can be used for more than one of these operations: distortion, displacement, severing, and disassembly.

Small Tools

Although many rescue squads are purchasing newer and more sophisticated extrication devices, common hand tools still play an important part in vehicle rescue operations. Each rescue vehicle should have an easily stored and easily carried hand-tool kit that can be used to accomplish gaining access and disentanglement tasks, or at least to carry on these tasks while other rescuers are preparing powered tools for use.

If you have the responsibility for purchasing hand tools for your rescue squad, remember that purchasing cheap tools is often an exercise in false economy. Tools that break or bend easily and those that do not perform smoothly or properly will be of little value when they are most needed. Exercise the same care and judgment that you would use if you were buying tools for your personal use.

Hand Tools Carried Primarily for Disassembly Operations

While the tools in this list are usually used to disassemble mechanisms of entrapment,

many can be used for other operations during a vehicle rescue effort.

Eight-Inch and Twelve-Inch Adjustable Wrenches, such as the Crescent AC-18 and AC-112 models, can be used for general disassembly operations.

A Folding Lug Wrench is a handy tool when it is necessary to remove the wheels of an accident vehicle. Such might be the case when wheels are needed to stabilize an overturned vehicle or a vehicle on its side or when working space is needed around a person trapped under a vehicle. Folding wrenches for both SAE and metric lug nuts can be purchased in automotive supply stores.

Pipe Wrenches (such as those made by Rigid) seem unlikely rescue tools, but when pipes must be disconnected or when a shaft must be rotated in order to free someone (such as the power takeoff shaft of a farm tractor), a pipe wrench may be the most valuable tool in the kit. Two or three pipe wrenches in the mid-size range should be carried.

Hex Key Wrenches can be used to disassemble mechanisms of entrapment that are joined with hex-head machine screws. Hex key wrenches can be purchased individually, in pouches that contain several sizes, in sets with T-handles for easier use, and in folding kits with wrenches that can be pivoted from a handle like the blades of a pocket knife. Both metric and SAE wrenches should be included in the hand-tool kit. General model 895 (SAE) and model 897 MM (metric) are examples of folding hex key wrench sets.

Eight-Inch Battery Pliers simplify the task of disconnecting the battery from a vehicle's electrical system, a task that might otherwise have to be accomplished with a bolt cutter, a hacksaw, or a difficult to use wrench. The Proto 218G is an example of quality battery pliers.

A **Battery Cable Puller** can be used to remove corroded or otherwise stuck cables from battery terminals.

Eight-Inch Needle-Nose Pliers (Klein D-203-7, for example) can be used to disassemble mechanisms of entrapment when blunt-nose pliers and wrenches are not practical because of the width or thickness of the gripping part.

Eight-Inch Side-Cutting Pliers (such as the Klein model D-201) facilitate grasp during disassembly operations. They can also be used to sever small-diameter wires and tubular metal and plastic components. Pulling valve stems is another important use.

Eight-Inch Slip-Joint Pliers facilitate a rescuer's grasp during disassembly operations. Use the Crescent H-28 or its equivalent.

Ten-Inch Locking-Type Pliers (such as the Vise-Grip model 10WR) provide grip and leverage. Locking pliers can also be used to break the plastic covering from around a steering wheel when the wheel must be severed with a bolt cutter.

Ten-Inch Water Pump Pliers (Channel Lock 430G pliers, for example) facilitate grasp and provide leverage during disassembly operations. Water pump pliers can also be used to break the plastic covering of a steering wheel.

Standard-Blade, Square Shank Screwdrivers, such as the 8-inch Stanley 66-178 and the 12-inch Stanley 66-172, can be used to disassemble mechanisms of entrapment that are held together with slotted screws. The square shank enables a rescuer to apply force with an adjustable wrench when removing a screw is difficult. A 12-inch standard-blade screwdriver can also be used effectively as an alternative sheet-metal cutting tool and as a prying tool.

Phillips-Type Screwdrivers enable rescuers to disassemble mechanisms of entrapment that are held together with Phillips-head screws. Stanley models 64-102, 64-104, and 64-172 are examples of 4-, 8-, and 10-inch Phillips screwdrivers.

A **10-Inch Cabinet-Blade Screwdriver with a 3/16-Inch Tip,** such as the Stanley 66-180 model, can be used for disassembly operations. A more important use, however, is for unlocking a passenger car's trunk lid when the key is not available.

A **Torx Screwdriver Set** is a must for disassembling vehicle components that are secured with Torx fasteners. Use the set manufactured by Stanley or an equivalent.

A **Combination Open-End and Box Wrench Set** can be used to disassemble mechanisms of entrapment. An excellent set of tools for a rescue vehicle is the Armstrong Combination Wrench Set No. 25-629. It contains 18 combination wrenches from 5/16 to 1-1/4 inches in a roll-up vinyl pouch. Also consider the increased use of metric bolts and nuts. You can only benefit by having both kinds. The most popular size body metric bolts are 13mm and 15mm.

A **1/2-Inch Socket Wrench Set, 1/4- to 1-1/4-Inch Capacity, with Ratchet Drive and Extensions,** can be used for a variety of disassembly operations, especially for removing doors during a vehicle rescue effort and when a combination wrench cannot be used because of space limitations. True Craft, Armstrong, and Craftsman socket wrench sets are quality products. Here again, consider adding a complete set of metric sizes to your arsenal.

Hand Tools Carried Primarily for Cutting Operations

An **8-Inch Combination Aircraft Snip** can be used to cut lightweight sheet-metal panels, metal cargo straps, web straps, and seat belts. Snips can also be used to make openings in the roofs of many late-model lightweight passenger cars. The Wiss Model M3R is an example of a quality combination aircraft snip.

A **1-Inch by 12-Inch Cold Chisel** can be used for destructive disassembly or severing operations, as when it is necessary to cut a cast iron pipe to free a child's trapped foot. A cold chisel can also be used to make openings in sheet-metal panels. Select a Stanley 18-311 or an equivalent.

A **Hacksaw Frame** (such as the Lenox Hackmaster) fitted with a 12-inch, 18-teeth-per-inch high-speed shatterproof blade is one of the most widely used tools in a rescue tool kit. A hacksaw can be used for jobs such as severing an accident vehicle's roof pillars, breaking the edges of a vehicle's roof so it can be folded back, severing steering wheel rims and even steering columns, and severing rods, pipes, bars, and other mechanisms of injury and entrapment. Gradually replace your hacksaws with the one piece hacksaw frame, thereby eliminating the need for spare parts.

A **Hacksaw Frame Fitted with a Carbide Rod Saw or a Carbide-Tipped Blade,** such as that manufactured by Remington, can be used to cut hardened steel components like the shackles of padlocks used to lock the doors of large trucks.

A **Low-Profile Hacksaw,** such as the one manufactured by Klein, is handy for severing trim or other metal or plastic components that may be impaled in an accident victim or so close that the use of a conventional hacksaw is impossible or impractical.

A **Glas-Master®** glass removal tool (Figure 1.25) manufactured by Wehr Engineering has proven itself to be the number one windshield removal tool in the business. As shown in Phase six, it is fast and efficient.

A **2-Inch by 18-Inch Ripping Chisel** is an excellent multipurpose rescue tool. The sharp edge can be used to sever metal components, and the long shank serves as a lever when severed components must be separated. A ripping chisel can be used to destroy a vehicle's door lock, for example, or as an alternative sheet-metal cutting tool.

A **Utility Knife with a Retractable Blade (Razor Knife)** can be used to cut seat belts, a vehicle's headliner or upholstery, soft dash components, or an injured person's clothing. Use the Stanley 10-099 knife or an equivalent.

A **Carpenter's Hand Saw** may be useful when it is necessary to cut through wood debris, as when wooden crates have splintered or a load of lumber has been spilled. A hand saw can often be used when a powered saw cannot.

A **Spray Container Filled with Soap Solution** can be used to lubricate hacksaw blades during metal-cutting operations. A number of cutting fluids are available from tool and plumbing suppliers. Most are petro-

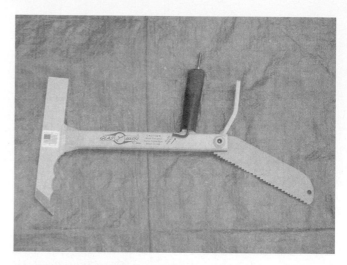

FIGURE 1.25   Glas-Master

leum products, however, and if oil is inadvertently sprayed into an open wound (as is often the case when a mechanism of entrapment must be cut near an injured person), the oil may be difficult to remove; soap is not. Ordinary generic dishwashing liquid can be used. Mix 1 part soap with 6 parts water. The spray bottle can be one in which household cleaner comes or a spray bottle that is sold in the garden department of department and discount stores. Always put the water in the container first, then add the soap. This prevents the foaming action.

Hand Tools Carried Primarily for Striking and Applying Force

A **3- or 4-Pound Drilling Hammer** provides striking force sufficient to drive panel cutters and cold chisels, yet is short enough to fit in a tool box or bag. The Stanley model 56-703 is an example of a quality 3-pound drilling hammer.

A **16-Inch, 4-Pound Engineer's Hammer** can be used when more striking force is needed, but there is not sufficient working space for a rescuer to use a sledgehammer. The Stanley model 850H-4 is an example of an engineer's hammer.

A **Rubber Mallet,** while it does not have the striking force of a drilling hammer, can be used to drive and tighten wedges, distort sheet metal, and so on. A distinct advantage is that a rubber mallet can be used as a source striking force near flammable materials.

Hand Tools Carried Primarily for Prying Operations

A **12- to 15-Inch Multipurpose Pry Bar** (Stanley 55-515 or equivalent) is probably the most useful prying tool in a rescue tool kit. As examples, the pry bar can be used to move a vehicle's window frame away from the body so that a noose tool can be used to unlock the door, or it can be used to remove the trim from around a windshield, or to force a vehicle's damaged door open after it has been unlocked and unlatched.

A **12-Inch Ripping Bar** is also useful for vehicle rescue operations.

Hand Tools Carried Primarily for Opening Vehicle Doors

A **Steel Shank Awl,** such as the Stanley model 69-007A awl, can often be used to unlock the front doors of a passenger car when non-destructive techniques are either impossible or unsuccessful.

A **Noose Tool** can be used to unlock vehicle doors that have accessible mushroom-head or straight-shank (anti-theft) lock knobs. A noose can be purchased from a locksmith or a locksmith supplier, or one can be easily made.

A **Panel Cutter** is designed to make openings in sheet metal and should be the tool of choice for making an opening in a vehicle's door to reach the lock mechanism or for making an opening in the roof of a vehicle. The panel cutter most often used for vehicle rescue operations is the model 10 cutter made by the Schild Manufacturing Company.

A **Dent Puller** can be used to pull lock cylinders from door panels and is especially useful for opening trunk lids when a key is not available. Dent pullers are available in different sizes and weights from automotive supply stores.

A **Slide Lock Tool** can be used to unlock the doors of some cars that have sliding bar locks.

A **Locksmith's Tool,** such as a Slim Jim, Skinnie Minnie, or Loc-Joc, can be used to unlock the doors of some cars.

Hand Tools Carried Primarily for Removing Vehicle Windows

A **Prick Punch,** such as the Stanley 18-376, is the tool of choice for breaking tempered glass windows.

A **Spring-Loaded Center Punch** (also called an **Automatic Center Punch**) can also be used to break tempered glass windows. The advantage of this tool is that it can be used without a hammer. The Starrett model 818 is an excellent center punch for vehicle rescue operations.

A **Linoleum Knife,** such as the Russell Linoleum/Roofing Knife, is the tool of choice for removing channel-mounted vehicle windows. This inexpensive tool can also be used to cut a vehicle's headliner or upholstery.

A **Windshield Knife** enables rescuers to remove mastic-mounted windshields and rear windows intact. Removing a windshield rather than breaking it will reduce the likelihood that open wounds will be contaminated with glass particles. An example of a windshield knife is the RK-160 knife made by the Reid Manufacturing Company. Two blades are available for the RK-160 knife: the RKB-141 blade for most mastic-mounted windows, and the 1-1/2-inch-long RKB-142 blade made especially for windows with extra-wide mastic strips.

Replacement Parts for Hand Tools

It's not unlikely for blades to break and small parts to be lost from hand tools during aggressive rescue operations. Accordingly, every rescue unit should have a kit that contains:

- Replacement blades for the hacksaw frames, windshield knives, panel cutters, and utility knives
- A spare carbide rod saw that fits a hacksaw frame
- Pins for the panel cutter

An important point about hacksaw blades: The inexpensive blades that are available from neighborhood hardware stores and shopping mall discount houses should *not* be used for rescue operations; they are likely to break during the first few cuts. Instead, use high-speed, shatterproof, 18-teeth-per-inch blades such as the Lenox Hackmaster II blades that can withstand rough use, even bending. Top-quality hacksaw blades can be purchased from tool suppliers and welding supply firms.

Homemade Hand Tools

In addition to the hand tools that can be purchased from fire department suppliers, hardware stores, and other outlets, many rescue squads use certain homemade devices to advantage. No rescuer should be ashamed to use homemade equipment for rescue operations. It is far better to have and use homemade equipment than not to have any equipment at all. The ability to develop makeshift tools when economy dictates is a credit to any rescue squad.

Can openers are among the most useful homemade devices. These tools can be fashioned from rotary lawn mower blades and pieces of leaf spring. Some can openers are operated with a rocking motion, much like the old kitchen utensil; some are struck with a hammer to achieve a cutting action. Crude as they may be, homemade can openers cut through automotive sheet metal quickly (Figure 1.26).

Long-Handled Tools

Long-handled tools afford increased leverage that is not available with tools that have short handles.

The first tool ever to be used for a vehicle rescue operation was probably a long tree limb used in conjunction with a rock! Picture two or three men using the tree limb as a lever and the rock as a fulcrum, trying to lift a gasoline buggy off of its driver, who is lying under the vehicle as a result of turning a corner at the breakneck speed of 10 miles an hour. Picture, too, the onlookers muttering something like, "Dangerous contraption that

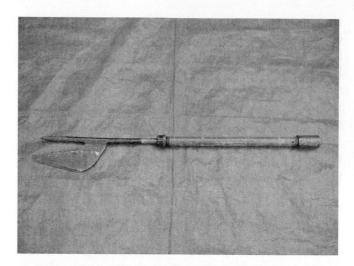

FIGURE 1.26 Homemade Can Opener

scares the horses and kids. Will never last!" Rescuers don't use tree limbs and rocks anymore, but they still use leverage during rescue operations.

A simple formula can be used to determine the amount of force needed to lift an object with a lever when the weight of the object and the length of the lever are known:

$$\frac{\text{Load}}{\text{Force}} = \frac{BC}{AB}$$

where BC is the distance from the end of the lever to the fulcrum, and AB is the length of the lever between the end of the lever under the load to the fulcrum.

Say the load is 400 pounds, the length of the lever under the load from the load-bearing end of the lever to the fulcrum is 10 inches, and the length of the lever between the fulcrum point and the distant end is 50 inches. By substitution you can determine that the mechanical advantage is 5 to 1, and that the rescuer will have to exert 80 pounds of downward force on the end of the lever to lift the load.

Following are long-handled tools that might be carried on a rescue unit. Some provide leverage, some provide increased striking force, and some provide both leverage and striking force.

An **Ax-Style Combination Forcible Entry Tool** can be easily carried in a tool box or bag and used for a variety of rescue operations. At the scene of a vehicle accident, for example, a rescuer can use a tool such as the Pry-Ax (from Partner) or the Biehl Tool (from Paratech) to break tempered glass, cut away a section of laminated glass, make an opening in sheet metal, open damaged doors after they have been unlocked and unlatched, and separate mechanisms of entrapment. An extendable handle provides increased leverage; for that reason it is included in this category.

A **36- or 42-Inch Combination Forcible Entry Tool,** such as the Partner Hooligan Tool or the Ziamatic Quic-Bar, is another useful multipurpose tool that provides the user with considerable leverage. The tool is useful for a number of tasks other than commonplace prying operations. For example, the spade edge of the tool can be used to make openings between vehicle doors and frames so that the tips of a hydraulic tool can be inserted. When the pike is driven into the fender of a passenger car, the tool will prevent the creep of a hand winch when a door is being moved beyond its normal range of motion.

A **36- or 42-Inch Bolt Cutter with Hardened Steel Jaws,** such as either the H. K. Porter model 36-0390-MCX or the Porter model 42-0590-MCX, can be used to cut hard or soft metal rods, bolts, cold-drawn spring wire, tempered spring wire, concrete reinforcing rods, steering wheel rims, chain-link fencing, and padlocks. When storage is no problem, selection of the longer cutter assures the largest possible jaw opening.

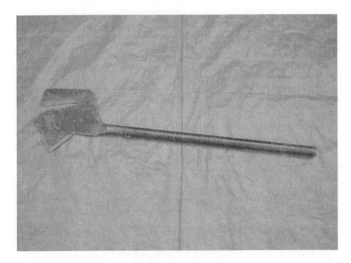

FIGURE 1.27   Topper Rescue Axe

A **Can-Opener Style Tool** can be used to make openings in vehicle roofs. The Topper Rescue Axe®, manufactured by Traco Distributors, is an example of a lightweight (8 pounds) can-opener tool (Figure 1.27).

A **36-Inch, 6-Pound Flat Head Fire Ax** can be used for a number of rescue activities, including clearing vegetation, cutting through wood debris, making openings in wood floors and roofs, and opening locked doors in structures. When driven by a sledgehammer, a flat head ax can also be used to make openings in sheet-metal panels. Use the Sager Ax manufactured by the Warren Ax and Tool Company or an equivalent.

A **36-Inch, 6-Pound Pick Head Fire Ax** can be used for a number of cutting operations. The pick can be used to make holes in sheet-metal surfaces, as when it is necessary to make an opening for the lifting toe of a jack.

A **51- or 60-Inch Pinch Point Crow Bar** gives a rescuer considerable leverage when it is necessary to separate mechanisms of entrapment during gaining access and disentanglement operations. For example, a pinch bar can be used to pull down a passenger car's B-pillar, a B-pillar and rear door assembly, or, for that matter, the entire side of the car in one operation. The Leetonia Tool Company models 51-00977 and 60-00980 have proved to be excellent tools for rescue operations.

A **32-Inch, 8-Pound Sledgehammer,** such as the Stanley 56-808, provides a rescuer with striking force not available with a short hammer.

Eight-Foot (or longer) Pike Poles can be used to move debris and vegetation and to hold a lightweight tarp over an accident vehicle to protect the occupants from rain, snow, and sunlight, among other tasks. At least one pike pole should have a fiberglass handle if the rescue unit has a weighted throwing line for moving downed wires.

Equipment for Lifting, Lowering, and Pulling

A simple lever may not be sufficient to lift or displace mechanisms of entrapment at vehicle accident locations. Rescuers often need the mechanical advantages offered by hand winches, jacks, ropes, and block and tackle.

Hand Winches

A **2-Ton Chain or Cable Hand Winch** (often called a come-along) is especially useful when pulling force is needed during rescue operations. A hand winch can be used to move a door beyond its normal range of motion, for example, or to displace a vehicle's seat or steering column. A hand winch can also be used to stabilize accident vehicles and to move debris and other mechanisms of entrapment.

Hand winches are available from a number of sources at widely varying prices. Two-ton cable winches, usually called come-alongs, can be purchased for as little as $10.00 at department stores and discount tool outlets. While they may be suitable for stretching fence wires and other farm and home tasks, these cheap hand winches should never be used for rescue operations. Handles may break, other parts may fail, and cables may part at loads far less than those for which the winch is rated. As with other tools, only hand winches that are offered by reputable tool manufacturers should be carried on a rescue unit.

CHAINS, STRAPS, AND SLINGS

Hand winches can seldom be used alone. A chain or web strap must be used to secure the winch to an anchor point, and a second chain or strap must be used to secure the winch hook to the object that must be moved. Not all chains and straps are suitable for rescue operations. They must be able to withstand at least the pulling force of the hand winch that they will be used with, and they must have ends that make them useful in a number of situations.

A **Rescue Chain Set** might include one 6-foot chain and one 12-foot chain, or two 12-foot chains, each with 1/4-inch links having a working strength of 4100 pounds and a breaking strength of 13,000 pounds. For maximum usefulness, one end of each chain should be fitted with a running hook, while the other end should have a ring or oval and a grab hook. J & B Equipment Company, Inc., New Castle, Delaware, is a source for rescue chain sets.

A **Rescue Strap Set** might be carried in place of chains. One such set, marketed by Rescue Training Consultants, consists of three straps. One end of each strap has a steel triangle, while the other end has a steel choker triangle. The straps are rated for 5600 pounds when used with a straight pull, 4200 pounds when formed into a choker, and 11,200 pounds when used as a basket sling. Straps have three major advantages over chains: They are stronger, they are less likely to become snagged in debris, and if they break, they are less likely to cause injury (Figure 1.28).

A **J-Hook Set** is handy for stabilizing accident vehicles. A typical set consists of two 20-foot chains, each with a hook at one end and a ring and grab hook at the other end. J-hook sets can be purchased from companies that supply wrecker and recovery services, or they can be fabricated with chains and hooks made from truck spring U-bolts. J-hook sets should not be used with hand winches unless the components are rated for at least the pull exerted by the winch.

Synthetic Fiber Web Straps, Wire Mesh, and Wire Rope Slings can be used as anchor points for hand winches. Moreover, slings are necessary when a crane or an A-

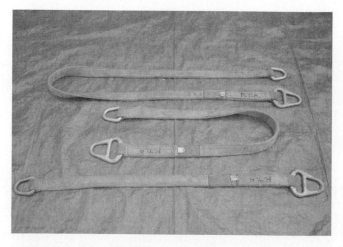

FIGURE 1.28   Rescue Strap Set

frame must be used to lift a load from an accident vehicle. A wide variety of slings are available from specialty manufacturers and larger hardware supply firms.

Jacks

Three types of hand-operated jacks can be used by rescue personnel to lift heavy-load mechanisms of entrapment: hydraulic jacks, ratchet jacks, and screw jacks.

Hydraulic Hand Jacks have a reservoir for oil and two different-size cylinders, each with a tight-fitting piston. The smaller of the pistons is attached to a lever and serves as a pump. When the lever is operated, oil from the reservoir is pumped under pressure from the smaller cylinder to the larger one. Lift is achieved when the larger cylinder fills with oil and pressure forces the piston upward. How much lift is achieved depends on the areas of the two piston faces. If the face of the small piston is 1 square inch and the face of the larger piston has an area of 100 square inches, the mechanical advantage is 100 to 1. Oil pumped from the smaller cylinder at 100 psi exerts 10,000 pounds of force on the face of the larger piston and thus provides 10,000 pounds of lift. Hydraulic hand jacks are available with lifting capacities ranging from 1-1/2 to 100 tons. Enerpac and Hein-Werner are two manufacturers of hydraulic hand jacks.

Ratchet Jacks are often used in vehicle rescue operations. A lever works against a ratchet to lift the load, and the ratchet supports the load between strokes of the lever. TK Simplex jacks are available in 5-, 10-, and 15-ton models. An advantage of this particular make of ratchet jack is that lifting can be accomplished with the toe, when the load is close to the ground, or with the cap.

The **Hi-Lift® Jack** is a mechanical ratchet jack well suited for a variety of vehicle rescue operations. It can lift 7000 pounds almost 48 inches and can be used with a chain set as a powerful come-along. Hi-Lift jacks are available in most farm equipment stores.

Screw Jacks are also used when heavy loads must be raised during rescue operations. A lever positioned horizontal to the ground turns the screw, which in turn raises the load. The screw jack is an especially safe lifting device since there is no chance for slipback. TK Simplex screw jacks will lift and support 12 tons. A swiveling cap automatically levels and centers load forces. Ratchet jacks and screw jacks will lift and continually support a load. A load should not be allowed to remain supported solely by a hydraulic jack, however; if fluid leaks from the cylinder the load will drop.

Jack Plates, also known as ground plates, should be carried when a rescue vehicle is equipped with jacks; these plates prevent jack bases from sinking into soft ground. Usually constructed of 3/4- or 1-inch plywood, jack plates can be as large as 24 inches square, depending on the size of the compartment in which they will be stored.

Rope for Rescue Operations

There is no one rope perfect for every use. Before acquiring a new rope, you must first determine what the rope will be used for: vehicle rescue, high angle or confined space rescue, rappelling, water rescue, crowd control, moving equipment from one level to another, and so on. Next consider the environment(s) in which the rope will be used: around gritty rocks, on sandy soil, in salt water, in mud, over sharp edges, and so on. Then match your requirements to the various types of rope and make an educated decision as to what to purchase.

ROPE CHARACTERISTICS

Ropes are made in a number of ways. Strength is a factor of construction.

Laid Ropes are made by twisting together bundles of fibers, the oldest form of rope making. Fibers are twisted together one way into yarns. Then a number of yarns are twisted in the opposite direction to form strands. Finally, three strands are twisted in the same direction as the fibers to form the finished rope. While they will not become completely undone, most laid ropes will untwist somewhat when suspending a load in midair. Un-twisting also causes hockles and kinks to form in laid rope.

All of the load-bearing fibers appear at the surface a number of times throughout the length of twisted rope. Thus abrasions and other surface damage have an immediate and direct effect on a laid rope's strength. Laid ropes tend to be stretchy, a characteristic that can be a disadvantage in rescue operations. Even though they were once used as lifelines, laid ropes should be used for noncritical applications such as crowd control.

Eight-Strand Plaited Rope is a soft, supple rope that is very easy to handle. Unfortunately, this type of rope is susceptible to abrasion and the "picking" of fiber bundles when snagged on equipment, rocks, and sharp building edges.

Braid on Braid Rope looks a lot like kernmantle rope. As the type name suggests, this rope has a braided core under a braided sheath.

Dynamic Kernmantle Rope is most often used for rock and ice climbing. Dynamic kernmantle ropes are very stretchy: 35% to 45% elongation at failure. Stretchiness is built into this type of rope; it absorbs some of the energy generated in a fall, thereby lessening the forces that would be transmitted throughout the rope system, especially to the person who has fallen. Dynamic rope must be used on rock and ice climbing and in any situation where a fall of greater than factor 1 might occur. A fall factor is a number that expresses the maximum distance a load can fall while secured to a given length of rope.

Rescue operations often involve lowering equipment or people, and the stretch built into dynamic ropes may cause a loss of control at critical times, thus increasing the danger to the people on the rope. This same stretchiness may cause a loss of control when lowering a litter, clearly a situation to be avoided. Dynamic ropes are manufactured with a thin sheath that will wear out quickly.

Static Kernmantle Rope has a braided sheath (the mantle) over a core (the kern) made of parallel untwisted fibers. Static ropes have low stretch (15% to 20% elongation at failure) when compared to dynamic kernmantle ropes. The core bundles contribute most to a static rope's strength; they are continuous in length and run parallel, and are protected from abrasion by the tightly woven sheath.

Static kernmantle construction is the preferred rope for most rescue operations because of its low stretch, high abrasion resistance, and no-spin qualities. However, a static rope should not be used as a dynamic belay line or as a safety line when the potential fall factor exceeds 1. A dynamic rope should be used for these applications. For fall factors (see pg. 35) of 1 or less, a static kernmantle rope should be satisfactory, assuming the wearer has an adequate harness, the entire rope system is properly rigged with good hardware, and the rope is protected from cutting and abrasion.

ROPE FIBERS

In addition to the manner of construction, rope strength also depends on the material used to construct the rope.

Natural Fibers have been used to make rope for as long as people have been using it. Today, however, they are not the best raw materials. Natural fibers lose strength, whether a length of rope is used or not. They are brittle and they lack the ability to absorb shock loads. They are attacked by molds, mildews, and fungi. Natural fibers are not continuous throughout the length of a rope; short lengths are combined into the yarns that form the basis for laid ropes. Temperatures as low as 180 degrees F. have been known to damage natural fiber ropes; this is not a high temperature to be experienced during firefighting operations. Because of the many shortcomings, natural fiber ropes should not be used for lifelines or for critical applications such as moving injured persons.

Polypropylene and **Polyethylene Fibers** are used primarily to make ropes that will be used in and around water. They are impervious to acids and will not conduct electricity when dry. An additional positive factor is that this rope will float. A problem is that polypropylene will melt at about 270 degrees F, and polyethylene will melt at about 225 degrees F. This makes them unacceptable for use during fire ground rescue operations. Another problem is that polyolefin ropes (the family name for polypropylene and polyethylene) have a very low resistance to abrasion; thus they wear out quickly. Other than for water rescue, ropes in this family are poor choices for rescue operations.

Kevlar is among the strongest of man-made fibers, and it can resist much higher heat than other synthetic fibers can. Nonetheless, Kevlar is not good for rescue ropes. It has a very low elongation (stretch) when pulled to the breaking point, which means that it cannot absorb energy generated in a fall. It is also very susceptible to abrasion, and the very brittle fibers tend to break when bent tightly (as in a knot).

Polyester fibers are used in many ropes; Du Pont's Dacron is an example. Polyester offers good resistance to heat and will not melt under 480 degrees F. Polyester fibers are strong and have a high tensile strength even when wet. Wet polyester will lose only about 1% of its dry strength. Its resistance to ultraviolet radiation makes polyester rope a good choice when the rope will be exposed to a great amount of sunlight. Because of these characteristics, polyester rope is often used for fire service ladder halyards. A negative characteristic is that polyester fibers do not elongate much, and because of this low dynamic energy absorption ability, the fibers cannot handle shock loading or repeated loading as well as nylon can.

Nylon is the most common fiber used in the construction of **rescue ropes**. Two types of nylon are used: type 6 and type 6.6. Both are similar, with the major difference being that 6.6 nylon has a slightly higher melting point and is a little tougher than type 6. Moreover, ropes made of type 6.6 nylon will stand up to abrasion better and will wear better than ropes made of type 6 nylon. New dry nylon is about 10% stronger than poly-ester, but nylon can lose 10% to 15% of its strength when wet. Nylon can absorb approximately 15,000 pounds of force per pound of rope, so nylon can cope with about twice the shock loading than polyester can, wet or dry. Nylon is an inert material that is impervious to most chemicals, although some acids will degrade nylon ropes. Strength, its ability to absorb energy, and resistance to heat and chemicals makes nylon an excellent material for rescue ropes.

FALL FACTORS

The term "fall factor" has been used several times thus far. A fall factor is a number that expresses the maximum distance a load can fall while secured to a given length of rope. To compute fall factor, divide the distance that a load attached to the rope could fall by the length of rope between the anchor and the load.

Consider these three scenarios:

In the first scenario, the rescuer is standing on the balcony of a building. The 10-foot safety line that is attached to the rescuer is attached to the railing of the balcony on which he is standing. If the rescuer falls from the balcony, he can fall for only the length of the rope; the fall factor is 1. Thus the length of the rope does not affect the outcome. In a situation like this, the fall factor will be 1 regardless of whether the rope is 10 feet, 100 feet, or 1000 feet long.

In the second scenario, the rescuer is secured to a 25-foot rope that is attached to the railing of the balcony above him—a distance of 12 feet. If the rescuer falls from the balcony, he will fall for only 13 feet. Using the equation stated above, we can determine that the fall factor is less than 1, just over .5, in fact.

In the third scenario, the rescuer is two floors above the railing to which his rope is anchored. His 25-foot rope has very little slack. If he falls, the fall factor will be 2 since he will travel for a distance twice the length of his rope. Fall factors cannot exceed 2 since it is impossible to fall more than twice the length of the rope (and have the rope remain intact, that is).

Again, it is proper to use a static kernmantle rope when the fall factor is 1 or less, and a dynamic kernmantle rope when the fall factor is greater than 1.

ROPE STRENGTH

Just as no one rope is perfect for every use, no one rope size or strength is perfect for every need. Rope strength is usually expressed as tensile strength at break, or the number of pounds of force needed to break a particular size of rope. While this seems quite straightforward, it is not. There are as many ways to measure and describe rope strength as there are manufacturers of rope. Many factors come into play in rope testing, any of which can increase or decrease test scores. For examples, the rate at which pull is applied, the temperature of the rope at the time of testing, and the diameter of the rope used in the pull can all influence test results. Descriptions can be just as bad. "Maximum," "average," and "minimum" are terms commonly used to describe the tensile strength of rope, and some rope manufacturers list only nebulous safe working loads for their products, not tensile strengths.

Keep in mind that a laboratory test that is repeatable anytime, anywhere cannot accurately reflect conditions experienced in the field. A laboratory test does not take into account such things as knots, bends, hitches, sharp building edges, rough rocks, and shock loading, all things that have a direct effect on the strength of a length of rope.

Before you select a rope for rescue operations, you should first determine the greatest working load you will expect the rope to support during its lifetime. Will it be used to lift or lower an injured person in a stretcher? Or will it serve as a lifeline for two rescuers who must make an emergency exit from a burning building? Or will it be used only for moving equipment? Then select a rope that has a minimum tensile strength several

times greater than the load it will be expected to support. The difference between the two figures is called the safety factor and is expressed as a ratio. The higher the ratio, the higher the safety margin. A rope that will be used only for lifting and lowering equipment should have a safety factor of 7:1; that is, the minimum tensile strength of the rope should be at least 7 times greater than the load it will be expected to bear. The National Fire Protection Association recommends that a rope that will be used for live rescues have a much more conservative safety factor of 15:1. Additionally, it recommends that a rope be "downgraded" after each use.

The current NFPA Standard states that a rope for a one-person rescue should be not less than 3/8 inch nor more than 1/2 inch in diameter, with a minimum tensile strength of 4500 pounds and a working strength of 300 pounds (15:1). A two-person rescue rope should be no less that 1/2 inch nor more than 5/8 inch in diameter, with a minimum tensile strength of 9000 pounds and a working strength of 600 pounds (15:1).

Again, the decision as to what kind of ropes and how many ropes to carry on a rescue vehicle should be made only after a thorough analysis of how the ropes will be used.

Blocks and Tackle

While too many people seem to think that they belong to an era of rescue that is long gone, blocks and tackle still have a place in today's rescue operations. When a rescue unit does not have a winch, and when a wrecker or mobile crane cannot respond immediately, an arrangement of blocks and a rope can be used to lift or move heavy objects.

The most often used arrangement has two 6-inch, double-sheave wood shell blocks and 3/4-inch manila rope. The working load for these components is 3800 pounds. Block and tackle sets can also be made with static kernmantle rope and the steel pulleys used in technical climbing operations.

The standing block of a block and tackle set is that which is secured to an anchor point. The fall line, the rope that will be pulled on, extends from the standing block. The running block is attached to the load by means of a strap, sling, or chain. A leading block, usually a snatch block, is put into the system to change the direction of pull when rescuers might otherwise be required to work in a tight or dangerous space. A drop link on the snatch block enables rescuers to attach the block to the rope instead of threading the entire standing part of the line through the opening between the sheave and the shell.

The rule of thumb for determining the mechanical advantage of a block and tackle arrangement is that when friction is ignored, the weight that can be lifted is equal to the applied force times the number of parts of rope that are leaving the movable block. A block and tackle set should be carried rigged so it can be placed in service immediately in an emergency situation.

Equipment That Can Be Used to Move Patients Away from or from Underneath Mechanisms of Entrapment

The following devices enable rescuers to move persons who may have spine injuries with a minimum of twisting and bending.

A **Long Spine Board,** such as the Reeves Sleeve® with the Reeves spine board slipped inside, is a truly versatile patient-carrying device. The board can be used to move an in-

jured person from within or under a mechanism of entrapment. It rigidly supports an injured person during transportation to a medical facility. It can be used to facilitate the entry of EMS personnel into wrecked vehicles. It can even be used to shield patients from contact with tools and debris during rescue efforts.

Nine-Foot by 2-Inch Nylon Web Straps with Aircraft-Style Quick-Release Buckles should be available to secure injured persons to long boards and other patient-carrying devices not equipped with straps.

A **6-Foot Diameter, 1-Inch Nylon Rope Sling with a Sliding Steel Closure** (such as the Rescue Training Consultants Endless Rope Sling™) can be used in an emergency situation by a single rescuer to pull an injured person onto a long spine board with little or no movement of the person's spine (Figure 1.29).

A **Disaster Pouch** (such as the Dyna-Med Model Y27101) is an essential piece of equipment for rescue vehicles; accidents produce fatalities. Disaster pouches, or "body bags," are usually vinyl- or rubber-covered fabric containers with four or six handholds and a full-length zipper. Some pouches have disposable liners. Many squads keep disposable rubber gloves in disaster pouches so rescuers will not have to search for gloves when they must handle human remains.

Equipment That Can Be Used for Off-Road Vehicle Rescue Operations

The equipment in this category should be carried on rescue vehicles in areas where off-road vehicle accidents are likely.

One-Inch Tubular Nylon Webbing can be fashioned into a seat or a harness and used with a rope and descent device to descend a steep hill.

A **Full-Body Harness** should be available for hoisting or lowering a rescuer or a sick or injured person.

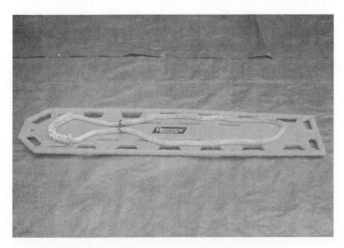

FIGURE 1.29 One-Inch Nylon Rope Sling

Locking Steel "D" Carabiners are used in the making of lowering systems.

A **Figure-Eight Descent Device with Ears** can be used to reach vehicles at the bottom of steep hills and to form patient lowering systems.

Locking-Type Ascent Devices can be used to facilitate the transfer of stretcher patients up steep hills. An example of an ascent device is the Jumar Ascender.

A suggestion for including the items just listed in an off-road rescue kit is made later in this phase (see pg. 39).

Miscellaneous Equipment for Vehicle Rescue Operations

Following are additional items that can be carried on a rescue unit for accident scene support operations.

A **Step-to-Straight Ladder** is a handy device for a rescue vehicle that has room to store it. Often fire apparatus that accompanies ambulances and rescue units to accident locations will not have a ladder shorter than a 10-foot folding ladder or a 12-foot roof ladder. Either of these may be too cumbersome to use around vehicle wreckage. A step-to-straight ladder locks into one position as a stepladder and into another position as a straight ladder. Some models are available with fiberglass beams, nonskid feet, and a strap that helps support the ladder against a tree or utility pole.

Safety Cans for Gasoline Storage should not be overlooked on a rescue vehicle. If the unit is equipped with a generator and gasoline-powered rescue tools, it should have gas for refueling.

Gas and Oil Mixtures should be carried in safety cans when gasoline-powered tools have two-cycle engines.

Stiff Brooms enable rescuers to move glass fragments and other small bits of debris from the roadway at accident locations.

Square Point and Scoop Shovels enable rescuers to dispose of debris once it has been swept up.

Preparing Useful Kits of Supplies and Equipment

Small hand tools are often carried in metal or plastic tool boxes, in open-top canvas book bags, or in hinged canvas mason's bags. Regardless of the container, when a particular hand tool is needed for a vehicle rescue operation, it is usually necessary for the potential user to dump the entire contents of the container to find the tool. A much-needed tool is never at the top of a tool box or bag!

Time can be saved by putting the hand tools necessary to accomplish certain tasks in separate, clearly marked containers. Then when it is necessary to use the tools during a rescue effort, they can be quickly acquired, carried to the damaged vehicle, and used by one or two rescuers while other squad members are locating and staging other equipment.

A **Leak Seal Kit** might include a container of a commercial leak-sealing preparation or ordinary duct sealant, and a dozen golf tees (as discussed earlier in this phase).

A **Window Removal Kit** might include a Glas-Master Glass Removal Tool, a 3-pound drilling hammer, a manual center punch, a spring-loaded center punch, two short pry bars, two linoleum knives, two windshield knives, a small ax or ax-style forcible-entry tool, precut pieces of adhesive-backed shelf paper, a roll of shelf paper, and a roll of fabric-backed duct or gaffer's tape. With this equipment, two rescuers can work together or independently to remove a vehicle's windshield that cannot be removed intact, and break tempered glass windows with a minimal spread of fragments to the interior of the vehicle. Lengths of adhesive-backed shelf paper slightly larger than full-sized windshields and rear windows can be cut from the roll, folded or rolled, secured with a rubber band, and stored in the kit box. Thus they are ready for immediate use during a rescue operation.

A window kit might also contain 33-gallon trash bags that have been laid out flat, slit across the bottom and down one side, then rolled and secured with a rubber band. The resulting pieces of plastic can be unrolled at the time of a rescue operation and used either to provide initial protection for trapped persons or to catch fragments of broken glass as side or rear windows are broken.

An **Off-Road Rescue Kit** might include a length of static kernmantle rope, two rope pads, two locking D carabiners, a large figure-eight descender with ears, and several lengths of 1-inch tubular nylon webbing, all kept in a combination rope and equipment bag. Two such bags of equipment will provide the means for two rescuers to descend a hill while supporting a stretcher full of equipment between them. Other rescuers can descend via the same ropes with equipment taken from the truck inventory.

A **Victim Protection Kit** might include helmets, eye protection, lightweight tarps, aluminized blankets, and other items that are suggested for keeping patients from harm during rescue operations. The round nylon fabric bags that firefighters and medics keep their personal gear in will hold enough protective equipment for several victims.

Powered Equipment That Can Be Used for a Variety of Rescue Operations

Hydraulic-, electric-, gasoline-, and air-powered rescue tools give rescuers pushing, pulling, and cutting forces they would not otherwise have with hand tools. All sorts of "kits" of powered equipment can be carried on a rescue vehicle.

Hydraulic Powered Tools and Accessories

Hydraulic rescue tools are available in two forms: those operated by hand and those powered by an electric motor or a gasoline engine.

HAND-POWERED HYDRAULIC TOOLS AND ACCESSORIES

Hydraulic "rescue" kits have been carried on squad vehicles for years. They are seldom used, however, because few rescuers have been trained to assemble the components. When the tools are used, they are often used without success, since few users really know what they can and cannot do. These problems not withstanding, hydraulic jack and spreader units and hydraulic jack and ram assemblies can be used to open jammed doors, displace steering columns, spread B-pillars, displace seats, and lift or separate mechanisms of entrapment.

Enerpac makes two especially good kits of industrial-quality equipment that can be used for a variety of pushing, pulling, spreading, and clamping operations often needed during a vehicle rescue operation. These 4-, 10-, and 20-ton kits have a hand-operated pump, one or more cylinders, wedge and duckbill spreaders, bases, toes, saddles, and connectors.

POWERED HYDRAULIC TOOLS

A powered hydraulic rescue tool set enables rescuers to separate and cut mechanisms of entrapment with considerable force. There are many such tools to choose from, coupled with either gasoline, electric, or hydraulic power units. Manual and electric rewind reels are available to enable tool operators to work up to 300 feet from the power unit.

Many different sizes of spreading tools are available with various spreading and pulling forces. Cutting tools with up to 75,000 pounds of cutting force and many different jaw widths are also marketed. Manifolds allow the use of several tools at the same time, and many accessories are constantly coming on the market.

The latest and perhaps, as time will tell, the most important development in the hydraulic tool industry is the Power-Take-Off (PTO) Operated Pump System introduced by **Amkus Rescue Systems.** The System addresses several problem areas when operating hydraulic rescue tools with extended hose lengths. These include speed of the tools under no load (simply opening and closing the tools); power reaction time (the longer the hose, the longer it takes to get power); safe pump controls (pump controls are always at the rescue vehicle, not at the point of use); multiple tool use (simultaneous operations); and system versatility. The System is designed to reduce wear on all drive line components as well as reducing heat in the tools.

Just a few of the advantages of the System: A 32-inch spreader will open in 9 seconds through 100 feet of hose; maximum pump pressure is obtained in 5 seconds or less; a pump control box operates the solenoid valves to charge and dump lines right where the tools are being used instead of back at the rescue vehicle. The System is very ingenious in that it can slow tools down, speed them up, adjust one line to operate faster than another, change the length of the hoses without losing performance, and control each line individually.

The "Add On" Solenoid Valve System would allow the initial installation of a one-, two-, or three-tool arrangement and add to it as needs increase, without replacing the existing system. On the surface, this would seem to be just another "better mousetrap," until you stop to realize the long-range implications of the layout. They now have a "Hydraulic Center" for *any* hydraulic powered tool regardless of PSI or GPM! This would include diamond-blade or standard-blade chainsaws; diamond-blade, carbide-tipped, or conventional blade circular saws; core drills; pumps; and all such small tools that use a circulatory system.

Imagine working in front of a collapsed structure with six different tools working up to 300 feet (a football field) away, all with various pressures and speeds. And then back to the everyday vehicle rescue problems. Quite an accomplishment!

A few of the hydraulic tool manufacturers are marketing hydraulic rams in various sizes. These rams have both pulling and pushing forces. Their uses will be discussed in later phases of this book.

A device that is well suited for use with hydraulic spreading tools is the Rescue Roller™, manufactured by Brandon Rescue Apparatus, Inc., of Vineland, New Jersey. It is a sturdy, steel-beam device that allows the use of a hydraulic rescue tool without fear of collapsing sheet-metal components.

Electric-Powered Tools and Accessories

Electric-powered tools are relatively inexpensive and they take up little compartment space; yet with the two tools listed below, rescuers can accomplish more than thirty vehicle rescue tasks.

A **Variable-Speed Reciprocating Saw** is one of the most useful tools that can be carried on a rescue unit; it can be used for jobs ranging from removing a section of a mastic-mounted windshield to removing a vehicle's roof. Black & Decker, Milwaukee, Porter Cable, and Makita all make reciprocating saws well suited to rescue operations. Disconnect the trigger lock button if the saw is so equipped. It can be dangerous to the inexperienced tool operator and serves no good purpose. Include a few long-handled "T" allen wrenches.

Four- and Six-Inch High-Speed, Shatterproof Metal-Cutting Blades, such as the Bi-metal Hackmaster Blades made by Lenox, should be included in the saw kit. Ordinary blades are likely to shatter if the saw bucks or if the point of the blade strikes a rigid object. A new bi-metal blade from Lenox is the 650R. It is a six-inch .050-gauge blade with 10/14 teeth per inch, which we find to be much stronger and longer lasting than the 618R (which has been the standard in the past). This new blade will handle pillars, hinges, steering wheels, and steering columns with ease.

The Lenox 960R nine-inch blade is excellent for deep reach work such as the safety (nadar) bolt and hinges.

The Lenox 966R nine-inch blade works well on plastic as the tooth set is quite wide. It is primarily a wood cutting blade.

Needless to say all of these blades work well on safety glass. Caution must be taken to cover the patient well, as the blades produce larger amounts of fine powder glass.

While some mechanisms of entrapment can be severed with a reciprocating saw, others can be disassembled with the following.

A **1/2-Inch Drive, Electric-Powered Impact Wrench** can be used to disassemble mechanisms of entrapment. Wheels can be removed quickly when they are needed for stabilization or when they interfere with the care of a person under a vehicle. Doors can be removed from a vehicle as quickly as the deep socket can be moved from one hinge bolt to another. Truck and farm machinery components can be easily disassembled with this high-torque tool. Use a Black & Decker, Porter Cable, or Skil electric impact wrench or an equivalent.

Half-Inch Power Drive Sockets, such as those made by Proto or Apex, must be used with impact tools; ordinary sockets will be destroyed by the high torque of the tool. The set carried on a rescue vehicle should include sockets with both SAE and metric openings, an adapter and power drive bits for No. 1 through No. 4 Phillips machine screws, a 5- and a 10-inch extension, and a universal joint.

A ready-for-use "system" results when the tools and accessories are stored with a power supply. If the unit has a 110-volt power supply, a **Live Reel with 100 Feet of Cord** can be installed in the tool storage compartment and connected to the vehicle's 110-volt system. The power cord should terminate in a four-receptacle junction box so that the saw, the impact wrench, and one or two floodlights can be operated without having to continually change cords. Power cords can be stored coiled or on a reel.

When the unit arrives on the scene of an accident, a rescuer need only carry the tools, accessories, and the end of the power cord to the wreckage to be ready for gaining access and disentanglement operations.

If the unit does not have a 110-volt power supply, or if it routinely responds to off-road locations where the wreckage is distant from the roadway, a **Compact Generator** can be mounted on a two-wheel cart along with the tools, accessories, and power cord. A rescuer can then transport the entire rescue system in one movement.

Gasoline-Powered Tools and Appliances

While they are considered to be "rescue" saws, the gasoline-powered saws with abrasive and carbide-tipped blades should not be used for vehicle rescue operations. The combination of high speeds, breakable blades, and a "rooster tail" of sparks makes them too dangerous for use near trapped persons and flammable fuels.

A **Chain Saw** can be used to advantage when it is necessary to clear fallen trees and brush away for accident vehicles during off-road rescue operations. Chain saws are also available with electric motors.

Air-Powered Tools and Accessories

Air-powered tools might be carried on a rescue vehicle if the unit has a number of spare breathing apparatus cylinders or a storage compartment tall enough for a 300-cubic-foot compressed air cylinder.

Many of the air-operated compact devices that are sold as rescue tools today are merely machine shop and body shop tools or modifications thereof. Two problems make these tools less than effective. Those that operate at low pressure (90 psi) can seldom do little more than drive cutting chisels through sheet metal, while those that operate with pressures in excess of 200 psi, and thus develop more force, consume air at the rate of up to 10 cubic feet per minute.

The **Airgun 40 Kit** has been developed by Paratech, Inc. specifically for rescue operations. With this kit, squad members can carry out a variety of vehicle rescue operations, from cutting sheet metal to breaking hinges and severing safety bolts (Figure 1.30).

A **1/2-Inch Drive Air-Operated Impact Wrench,** such as the Black & Decker No. 2298 Air Impact Wrench, can be used to disassemble others.

Power Sockets, Bits, and Accessories for the Air-Operated Impact Wrench should be carried; they are the same as those described for the electric impact wrench.

Air Bags

Since the 1970s, air bags have proven to be a valuable tool in vehicle rescue operations. These bags are designed to lift and move heavy tonnage, and they inflate in seconds from any of a number of compressed air sources. Air bags have become an integral part of rescue squad equipment inventories in over fifty countries around the world.

Available in a variety of sizes and lifting capacities, air bag uses range from prying away doors and steering columns in wrecked vehicles to lifting overturned trucks. Because no metal is exposed, there is no danger of sparking when the bags contact metal objects.

Three categories of air bags are available for rescue operations: high-pressure air bags, medium-pressure air bags, and low-pressure air bags. Each type has specific characteristics, advantages, and applications (Figure 1.31).

High-Pressure Air Bags

The construction of high-pressure air bags, which operate at between 115 and 150 psi, is comparable to a steel- or Kevlar-belted radial tire. Hot vulcanization, a heat and pressure molding process, is used to produce the tops and sides of the bags. These areas consist of several layers of neoprene/nitrile, with steel or Kevlar reinforcements. The inlet/discharge nipple of a high-pressure bag is always located in the corner of the bag. Other visible features indicative of the highest quality bags include double-locking safety nipples, double-locking hose couplings, a surface design that provides adhesion and abrasion protection, light-reflective labels for nighttime or other poorly lit working conditions, complete instruction guides that include tonnage and lifting stroke mea-

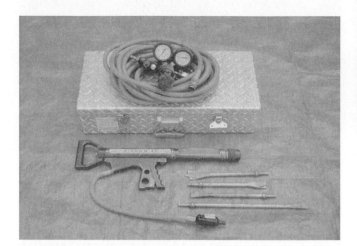

FIGURE 1.30   Airgun 40 Kit

surements, and the presence of permanently affixed operating pressures on one side of the bag.

High-pressure air bags offer the following advantages:

- They can lift heavy loads quickly; for example, 10 tons in 3.8 seconds and 74 tons in 66.3 seconds (inflation times depend on air-pressure supply).
- They need just 1 inch of insertion space for placement under a load.
- They operate on low air volumes, ranging from 2.7 cubic feet for a 10-ton bag to 51.2 cubic feet for a 74-ton bag, when each is inflated to maximum pressure for maximum tonnage.

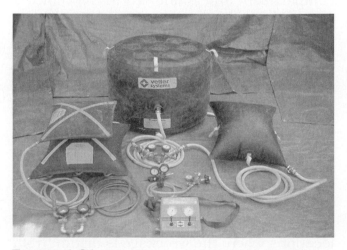

FIGURE 1.31   Hi-, Low-, and Medium-Pressure Air Bags

- They require minimal maintenance. Bags can be checked visually for exposed or broken steel/Kevlar cords and returned to the manufacturer for recertification or safety recommendations. After using bags with oil or hydraulic fluids, cleanup is a simple matter of washing the bag with mild soap and water. Every six months, the bag's proper operation should be confirmed by connecting it to a regulator, a controller, and hoses.

- They can be inflated from varied air sources, including air tanks, air ompressors, SCBA 2.2 or 4.5 air bottles, cascade systems, spare tires, hand pumps, foot pumps, train air brake systems (with the rail glad hand adapter).

- They are light in weight: A 10-ton bag weighs 9.9 pounds; a 74-ton bag weighs 85.8 pounds.

- They store easily because of their 1-inch thickness.

- They assure stability and traction through the neoprene/nitrile construction and a wide base. Most manufacturers put skid-resistant surfaces on bags.

- They are safe for use in situations where conventional jacks would be dangerous or unusable as, for example, in sand, mud, or snow, on rubble or debris, or in angle lifts.

- They achieve greater lifting heights when one bag is stacked on top of another. Two 74-ton bags, for example, will produce a 41-inch lift. While stacking two bags will increase the height that a load can be lifted, stacking will not increase the lifting capacity. A 10-ton bag stacked on top of a 26-ton bag will lift 10 tons, not 36 tons. However, when the two bags are placed side by side under a load, they will lift 36 tons.

- The danger of sparking is eliminated by the neoprene/nitrile construction.

- They work well with other extrication tools to accomplish more efficient rescue operations.

High-pressure bags also have some disadvantages:

- They have a low lifting height; the maximum height that a load can be lifted is 41 inches.

- They are not field repairable. If a repair is possible, a damaged bag must be returned to the manufacturer to undergo the hot vulcanization process.

- They will dent thin-skinned vehicles and lose lifting height. Bags must be positioned against the frame braces of thin-skinned vehicles, such as train cars, subway cars, fiberglass buses, and aluminum tank trailers, to avoid the loss of lifting height.

- The lifting ability of a high-pressure bag decreases as it inflates. For example, a 30-ton bag with a maximum lifting stroke of 10 inches will lift 30 tons 1 inch or 15 tons 10 inches.

- High-pressure air bags have a 1-inch sidewall that causes them to become convex when inflated. Thus the higher the lift, the lower the surface contact between the ground and the load, and the less weight the bag is able to lift.

High-pressure air bags can be used in a variety of ways. They are excellent for lifting and moving cylindrical and odd-shaped objects. They can be used to lift collapsed floors, beams, trees, and poles. During vehicle rescue operations, they can be used to move doors, door posts, pedals, and dash assemblies. They can be used to open elevator, subway and bus doors, and locked car trunks. Manufacturers of high-pressure air bags include Vetter Systems, Maxi-Force, Holmatro, Lampe, and Hurst.

MEDIUM-PRESSURE AIR BAGS

Medium-pressure air bags normally operate at 14.5 psi. Unlike high-pressure bags, they are made of fabric canvas or Aramid-Kevlar impregnated with rubber/neoprene. Each manufacturer uses different fabrics and coatings. The top-quality medium-pressure air bag has Kevlar fabric coated with a nitrile compound similar to neoprene. Average-quality bags have canvas fabric with a rubber coating. The lowest-quality bag is canvas with a vinyl coating. Bags manufactured with a cold vulcanization process are cut from sheets and glued together; the use of epoxy glue is "state of the art."

Other features of high-quality bags are seam overlap at the corners and inlet; internal support with nylon strapping, which prevents ballooning of the top and bottom plates; six-ply top and bottom layers for abrasion resistance; and carrying handles molded into the bag. The inflate/deflate nipple of medium-pressure bags is centered in the sidewall construction so that air can be released during deflation.

The specific advantages of medium-pressure air bags used for vehicle rescue are listed below.

- They will lift loads higher than high-pressure bags. The smallest bag will lift an object 14.4 inches, while the largest medium-pressure bags will lift a load 60 inches.
- The insertion space necessary for positioning medium-pressure bags under loads ranges from 3/8 of an inch to 6 inches.
- These bags do not lose surface contact at increased heights.
- Nitrile/neoprene bags do not require dusting; thus maintenance is easier and bags last longer.
- Medium-pressure bags are field repairable.
- Medium-pressure bags are lightweight. They range from 3.2 pounds for the 3.5-ton bag to 66 pounds for the 12.9-ton bag. Lifting heights for these two bags are 17.7 and 44 inches, respectively.
- These bags inflate quickly from a number of air sources.

- Stability is enhanced by having a larger surface area in contact with the ground and with the load being lifted.
- Medium-pressure bags are excellent for use with thin-skinned vehicles and objects.
- They are safe to use in situations where conventional jacks would be dangerous or unusable.

The disadvantages of medium-pressure air bags include:

- Inspection is necessary every three to four months. The inspection process includes complete inflation, sponge bathing to locate leaks and/or crazing of rubber, and thorough drying and powdering with talcum powder before returning to storage. Talcum powder absorbs moisture. Dusting is important for rubber-coated bags but is not necessary for neoprene bags.
- Due to their bulkiness, medium bags require more storage space.
- Large volumes of air are needed for inflation; for example, 3.4 cubic feet are needed for a 2.5-ton bag and 287 cubic feet are needed for a 3-cell, 17-ton bag.

Applications for medium-pressure air bags include recovery operations involving tank trucks, vans, buses, subway cars, vehicles, and aircraft; uprighting thin-skinned vehicles such as fiberglass buses; raising collapsed car roofs; lifting aircraft; rerailing subway cars in tunnels; and high lifts from overturned car hoods or trunks. Manufacturers of medium-pressure air bags are Vetter Systems, Lampe, and Hurst.

LOW-PRESSURE AIR BAGS

Low-pressure air bags operate at 7.5 psi. Low- and medium-pressure air bags have many of the same advantages, disadvantages, and construction features. One exception is that medium-pressure air bags have a thicker coating that permits operation at 14.5 psi. In fact, the basic difference between medium- and low-pressure air bags is that medium-pressure bags operate at 14.5 psi, while low-pressure bags operate at 7.5 psi. Another important difference is that medium-pressure bags have double the lifting capacity at a cost of only 50% more.

Both medium- and low-pressure air bags were developed specifically for rescue and recovery operations involving thin-skinned, light-wall vehicles such as aluminum tank trailers, subway cars, fiberglass buses, and aircraft. If a high-pressure bag were used with these vehicles, the lift would be lost through the breaking away of side walls.

Consider the problem of an overturned gasoline tanker with the driver trapped underneath. The tank has to be lifted to reach the driver. Using high-pressure bags risks denting and/or ripping the aluminum tank, probably with catastrophic results. Obviously, the safe way to lift the tank is with low-pressure bags designed for the task. The manufacturers of low-pressure air bags are Vetter Systems, Vepro, Goodyear Rubber, Lampe, MFC (London, England), and RFD (Surrey, England).

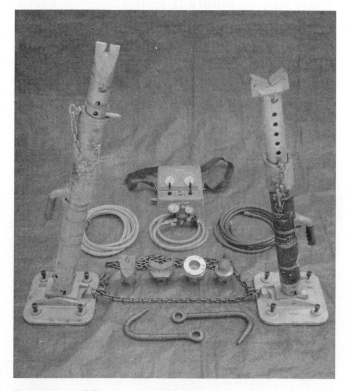

FIGURE 1.32 Jimmi-Jak System

Pneumatic Jacks

There are many devices that can be used to stabilize and support accident vehicles. However, many are ill suited for rescue operations because they were designed and constructed for other purposes. Mechanical and hydraulic jacks may be too short to be effective, or they may not be strong enough to support a vehicle or a heavy piece of machinery that is carried on a vehicle. Hand winches are excellent stabilizers, but they may be needed for lifting and pulling tasks, and hydraulic jack and ram assemblies and air bags may be needed for gaining access and disentanglement activities. A pneumatic jack system designed specially for rescue operations is the Jimmi-Jak® System, available from J & B Equipment Company, Inc., New Castle, Delaware.

THE JIMMI-JAK SYSTEM

The components of the Jimmi-Jak System were designed and constructed so that rescuers might have safe and efficient tools to work with in virtually every instability situation.

The Jimmi-Jak System pictured in Figure 1.32 includes the following components:

- Two "A" jacs that are 28 inches long when the piston is fully retracted (closed) and 38 inches long when the piston is fully extended (open). Each "A" jac weighs 20 pounds without attachments.
- Two "B" jacs that are 35 inches long when closed and 53 inches long when open. Each "B" jack weighs 25 pounds without attachments.
- Four hinged base plates.
- Four swivel attachments.
- Two slotted wedge attachments.
- Two steel point attachments.
- Two V-block attachments.
- One 6-foot rescue chain with a slip hook and a grab hook and oval.
- One 12-foot rescue chain with a slip hook and a grab hook and oval.

- Two J-hooks.
- One 3000/100 psi pressure regulator with a hose, air flow valve, and hand wheel.
- One deadman-style, dual safety control unit.
- Two color-coded air hoses with double-lock safety couplings.

Four jacs of two different lengths are the heart of the Jimmi-Jak System, but it is the matching components that give the system versatility and value in a variety of rescue situations.

Pivoting base plates allow for the jacs to be positioned at an angle to the load without reducing the area of contact with the ground. Rubber pads and pointed setscrews serve to make the base plates slip resistant.

A number of attachments can be locked into either end of each jac without tools. V-blocks are especially useful when the jac must be used to support round objects. Sharp-pointed attachments are handy when the piston must be worked into a tight place. Swivel ends are provided for times when the jacs must be used to support a load that is not parallel to the ground or another object. The slotted wedge attachments can be used directly to support a load, or with the chains. All of the attachments can be interchanged with the base plates, for times when it may be desired to separate one object from another.

The pistons of the Jimmi-Jaks can be extended manually or by the pressure of compressed air, nitrogen, or carbon dioxide. A dead-man controller allows fine control of the piston movement.

At the locations of vehicle accidents, Jimmi-Jaks can be used to stabilize unsteady vehicles, widen door openings, and prevent truck loads from shifting. Besides vehicle rescue operations, Jimmi-Jaks can be used for bracing machinery, shoring trench walls, supporting elevator cars, bracing subway cars, bracing weakened walls, strengthening weakened floors, supporting heavy rolling overhead doors, and other tasks. When used with air bags and an appropriate base plate, Jimmi-Jaks can break through doors that cannot be opened by more conventional means. The system is being changed so that airshore jacks can be equipped with ends that will adapt to the Jimmi-Jak accessories with a simple pin arrangement. This will allow support bolsters up to 12 feet for structural collapse situations, with tremendous strength.

The **Colum-Master**® (Figure 1.33) manufactured by Wehr Engineering provides the means for displacing steering columns safely and quickly.

Marking Equipment for High Visibility

Even when great pains are taken to set up and maintain an equipment staging area, rescue tools are often spread for a great distance at accident locations. The problem of recovering and sorting equipment can be minimized, especially at night, when every tool and appliance has a reflective marker that includes the rescue unit number or the squad name. Even greater visibility is possible when, in addition to the unit markers, tools also have strips of tape applied in such a way that they will reflect light regardless of the position of the tool. The sweep of a powerful hand light will usually locate properly marked rescue tools left on the ground or on accident vehicles.

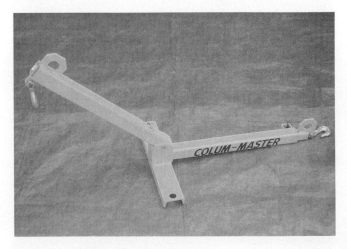

FIGURE 1.33 Colum-Master

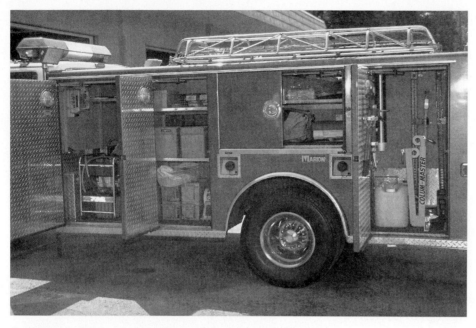

FIGURE 1.34   Compartment Storage

*Storing Supplies and Equipment
on the Rescue Vehicle*

Just what is stored in the compartments of a rescue truck depends on several factors, including the size, weight, and dimensions of tools, the size of the compartment, the number of shelves and their placement, the availability of hooks for hanging objects, and so on (Figure 1.34). Because a compartment is often a jumble of unrelated supplies and equipment, every compartment door should have an inventory prominently posted on the inside panel. The inventory sheets should be white with large black lettering for optimum visibility. A typewritten list is difficult to read in low-light situations. The inventory sheets should be sealed in a Mylar or acetate envelope to keep them dry.

A compartment door inventory form serves several purposes. It helps new squad personnel to learn where rescue supplies and equipment are stored. It allows experienced squad members to review the contents of the truck compartments without stripping them. It serves to remind squad members where tools go after a rescue operation. And it serves as a checklist to assure that what *should* be in the compartment *is* there.

The Inventory of a Limited Service Rescue Vehicle

Listed in Figure 1.35 are the supplies and equipment that might be carried on a limited service rescue unit, one that responds primarily to motor vehicle accidents.

FIGURE 1.35	A SUGGESTED INVENTORY OF RESCUE TOOLS AND EQUIPMENT FOR A LIMITED SERVICE RESCUE UNIT	
Category/Group Item		**Number**
Equipment for Safeguarding Accident Victims **Item to shield victims from contact with tools and debris generated during rescue operations**		
24- by 30-inch sheet of plywood or particle board		1
Item to shield victims from radiant heat and flames		
Aluminized rescue blanket		1

Continued

Figure 1.35	A Suggested Inventory of Rescue Tools and Equipment for a Limited Service Rescue Unit (con't.)	
Category/Group Item		**Number**

Items to protect victims from the elements

Disposable paper blankets	2
Aluminized survival blankets (in cold-weather areas)	2

Items to protect a victim's head, eyes, and ears

Construction hard hats	6
Soft-side, vented safety goggles	6
Earmuff-style hearing protectors	6

Items to protect a person's respiratory passages

Disposable dust masks	6
Thermal masks (in cold-weather areas)	6

Supplies and Equipment for Hazard Management
Equipment for fire suppression and prevention

5-pound A:B:C Fire Extinguisher	1
20-Pound A:B:C Fire Extinguisher	1
2-1/2-gallon pressurized water extinguisher (if the unit does not have a pump and water)	1

Equipment that can be used to stabilize accident vehicles and other mechanisms of entrapment

Wheel chocks	2
Lengths of 2- by 4- by 18-inch wood cribbing	24
2-inch by 4-inch by 12-inch wood wedges	6

Supplies that can be used to stop the flow of flammable fuel from damaged fuel tanks and fuel supply lines

Package of pliable sealant	1
Wooden golf tees	12

Supplies that can be used to minimize the spread of glass fragments

Roll of adhesive-backed paper	1
Roll of fabric-backed duct tape	1

Equipment for moving downed wires

Lineman's glove sets	2
Can of talcum powder	1
Spare sets of rubber glove inserts	2
Sectioned lineman's clampstick kit	1
Lineman's telescoping hotstick	1

Items that can be used to identify hazardous materials

7 × 50 armored binoculars	1
Hazardous materials identification guide	1

Miscellaneous items for hazard management operations

1-gallon (or larger) plastic jug filled with cat litter	1
Split sections of 1-1/2-inch fire hose of various lengths	12

FIGURE 1.35	A SUGGESTED INVENTORY OF RESCUE TOOLS AND EQUIPMENT FOR A LIMITED SERVICE RESCUE UNIT (CON'T.)	
Category/Group Item		**Number**
Short unsplit lengths of 2-1/2-inch or larger fire hose		12
24-inch heavy-duty shock cords		2
36-inch heavy-duty shock cords		2

Supplies and equipment for traffic control

30-minute road flares	24
Red warning flags with staff	2
Traffic control flashlights	2
Spare battery sets	2

Supplies and equipment for spectator control

Roll of 3-inch barrier tape	1

Equipment for power generation, distribution, and illumination

Built-in or portable generator	1
100-foot, 3-wire extension cord terminating in a 4-outlet junction box with a pilot light	1
110-volt, 500- or 1000-watt floodlights with stands	2
Battery-powered or rechargeable hand lights	2
12-volt trouble light with a 50-foot cord and battery clips	1
High-intensity Cyalume Chemical Lightsticks	12

Small tools for gaining access and disentanglement

8-inch adjustable wrench	1
12-inch adjustable wrench	1
Awl with a steel shank	1
8-inch combination aircraft snips	1
Manual or spring-loaded center punch	1
1- by 12-inch cold chisel	1
3-pound drilling hammers	2
Folding lug wrench, SAE	1
Folding lug wrench, metric	1
One-piece hacksaw frame with a 12-inch, 18 teeth-per-inch high-speed shatterproof blade	3
Replacement blades for the hacksaws	12
Hacksaw frame with a carbide rod saw	1
Linoleum knives	2
Noose tool for lock knobs	1
Mini-hacksaw	1
Replacement blades for the mini-hacksaw	2
12- to 15-inch multipurpose pry bars	2
Panel cutter	1
Replacement blades for the panel cutter	1
Battery pliers	1
10-inch slip joint pliers	1
8-inch locking-type pliers	1
10-inch water pump pliers (channel-lock)	1

Small tools for gaining access and disentanglement

8-inch standard-blade, square-shank screwdriver	1
12-inch standard-blade, square-shank screwdriver	1

Continued

| FIGURE 1.35 | A SUGGESTED INVENTORY OF RESCUE TOOLS AND EQUIPMENT FOR A LIMITED SERVICE RESCUE UNIT (CON'T.) |

Category/Group Item	Number
8-inch Phillips screwdriver	1
10-inch Phillips screwdriver	1
10-inch cabinet blade screwdriver with a 3/16-inch tip	1
Torx screwdriver set	1
Spray container filled with soap solution	2
Utility knife with retractable blade	1
Spare blades for the utility knife	5
Windshield knives, standard blade	2
Windshield knives, long blade	2
Spare blades for the windshield knives	8
Glas-Master	1
Long-handled tools for gaining access and disentanglement	
Ax-style forcible entry tool	1
36- or 42-inch combination forcible entry tool	2
51- or 60-inch steel pinch point crowbar	1
36-inch 8-pound sledgehammer	1
Equipment for lifting, lowering, and pulling	
2-ton chain or cable hand winch	1
Rescue chain or strap set	1
Hi-Lift jacks	2
1/2-inch static kernmantle rope (lengths as needed)	2
3/8-inch static kernmantle rope (for utility purposes)	2
Colum-Master	1
Equipment for moving accident victims away from or from underneath mechanisms of entrapment	
Long spine board	1
9-foot by 2-inch nylon web straps with quick-release buckles	3
6-foot diameter, 1-inch nylon rope sling with sliding choker	1
Scoop stretcher	1
Reeves Sleeve with spine board	1
Basket stretcher with bridle	1
Equipment for upper-body immobilization	
Short spine board	1
Vest-type immobilization device	1

Needless to say, all sorts of other supplies and equipment might be carried on the rescue unit: additional hand tools, powered tools, other devices for more sophisticated hazard management operations, equipment for off-road rescue, and other patient-carrying devices. The selection is limited only by the availability of storage space and the ability to purchase!

While the inventory just listed does not appear imposing, much can be accomplished with the minimal supplies and equipment suggested for a limited service rescue unit. Rescuers can:

• Identify hazardous materials carried in vehicles.

- Control the movement of vehicles around accident locations.
- Control the movement of spectators that might interfere with rescue operations.
- Move and anchor downed wires.
- Extinguish fuel burning under a vehicle.
- Extinguish a fire in the engine compartment.
- Extinguish a fire in the passenger compartment.
- Extinguish a fire in the trunk.
- Extinguish a tire fire.
- Stop the flow of fuel from a damaged tank.
- Stop the flow of fuel from severed fuel lines.
- Stop the flow of fuel away from a vehicle.
- Stabilize a vehicle on its wheels.
- Stabilize a vehicle on its side.
- Stabilize an overturned vehicle.
- Make oil- or ice-slick roadways slip resistant.
- Light work areas.
- Disable a vehicle's electrical system.
- Gain access to trapped patients through door openings.
- Gain access to trapped patients through window openings.
- Minimize the spread of glass particles.
- Gain access to trapped persons through openings made in the body of an accident vehicle.
- Force open doors that remain jammed after being unlocked and unlatched.
- Enter the trunk of a vehicle.
- Gain access to a person trapped under a vehicle.
- Protect patients from mechanisms of injury during disentanglement operations.
- Protect patients from the elements during disentanglement operations.
- Create working space and exitways through which injured persons can be removed from accident vehicles.
- Disentangle patients from mechanisms of entrapment.

- Package injured persons for removal.
- Remove injured persons from a vehicle that is on its wheels.
- Remove injured persons from a vehicle that is on its side.
- Remove injured persons from an overturned vehicle.
- Transfer injured persons to an ambulance.

Up to this point, we have considered the mechanical half of the people–machine relationship that we call a rescue squad. Now let's consider the human element.

THE RESCUE CREW

The need for human intervention has virtually been eliminated in many systems where there was once a strong people–machine relationship. Computers solve in milliseconds problems that might have taken mathematicians months to solve with slide rules, pencils, and paper. Automated machines do tasks that once took hundreds of workers to accomplish. Electronic devices can sense trouble and shut off machines before they are damaged.

The rescue service greatly differs from these automated systems. The finest rescue vehicle is useless without a human operator who must start it and drive it to and from accident locations. A person must decide how rescue forces are to be committed. Even the most sophisticated piece of rescue equipment needs a human operator.

How ready a rescue crew is to respond to an emergency depends a great deal upon its organization. In large cities, rescue squads are usually part of the fire department, although in some cities, rescue is a responsibility of the police department. A chief officer is usually responsible for rescue services, and junior officers are in charge of the squads. In many areas, rescue officers report to the fire commander or officer in charge of any given incident. Smaller cities may have only one rescue squad to service the entire city. The rescue crew may be made up of firefighters who are assigned to the squad under the supervision of a captain or lieutenant, who in turn reports to the next higher ranking fire officer.

Volunteer fire departments that provide rescue services generally have an elected or appointed rescue officer. Rescue crews are often comprised of volunteers who have responded to the alarm. In many locations throughout the country, organized rescue squads operate independently of the community's fire and police services. These squads are usually organized like volunteer fire departments, or third service EMS agencies.

Chain of Command

An effective chain of command is essential not only in rescue operations but also in all phases of emergency service operations. Successful emergency scene operations depend on the transmittal of orders from the officer-in-charge to the subordinate officers to the crew members who execute those orders. An effective chain of command works two ways: Every person within the chain knows to whom he reports and who reports to him.

During an emergency, failure to follow the established chain of command usually results in chaos. If the fire chief gives orders directly to the crew members, the rescue officer will be unaware of their missions, and he may give orders different from those given by the chief. If the rescue officer acts independently, the chief may be placed in the awkward position of not knowing what is happening. Thus failure to follow the chain of command may cause personality clashes as well as chaos.

In the paid rescue service, the chain of command is generally well established. Rescuers know to whom they report, and operating procedures are followed as a matter of course.

In the volunteer services, however, the chain of command is much more flexible. Different officers take command at different times. Officer and crew combinations are seldom fixed until the time of a response. Each officer and crew member must be ready and able to accept varying degrees of responsibility at different times.

PHASE TWO

Responding to the Location of the Accident

INTRODUCTION

The second phase of a vehicle rescue operation includes three stages of activity that are undertaken in order: (1) acquiring information, (2) traveling to the location of the incident, and (3) parking at the scene.

These are not steps to be taken lightly, although they often are. The acquisition and transmission of incorrect or incomplete information about a call to which you are responding can delay the response of emergency service units, and selecting a congested route instead of a clear one can delay their arrival. Parking in an unsafe place at the scene can result in injuries to EMS and rescue personnel and the loss of equipment.

ACQUIRING AND TRANSMITTING INFORMATION ABOUT A MOTOR VEHICLE ACCIDENT

There are several ways in which a citizen can call for emergency service assistance. In most areas of the country, a person need only dial 9-1-1 to access the emergency services dispatch center. Elsewhere you may be dealing with a direct line to the ambulance or rescue squad, and speaking with an untrained person.

Can a dispatcher elicit any more information about a vehicle accident? Surely! Let's see how you might do a better job of gathering and transmitting information.

- First, identify the emergency reporting center that the caller has reached.
- Then identify yourself and ask whether the person is reporting an emergency situation.

This opening should be routine for all calls because it lets the caller know that he has reached the proper agency.

- Ask the caller's name and the number of the telephone he is using.
- Determine the exact location of the incident.
- Determine the number and types of vehicles involved.

- Determine the approximate number of people injured.
- Ask whether any of the vehicle occupants appear trapped.
- Ask about hazards that might have been produced by the accident.
- Determine whether traffic is moving past the scene.

If you can inform responding units that the main road leading to the scene is blocked, drivers can select alternate routes and thus shorten the response time.

It takes a little time to gather this information, to be sure, and there is always the chance that a caller will overestimate the seriousness of the situation. However, the more you can learn from the caller and pass on to rescue personnel, the easier it is for them to plan effective responses.

TRAVELING TO THE LOCATION OF THE INCIDENT

While the dispatcher plays the key role during the first few minutes of response (the information-gathering period) and the rescue officer plays the pivotal role during the last few minutes of the response (parking the rescue unit at the scene), it is the unit's driver who is most important during the response itself. If the squad members and the equipment carried in the unit are to be of any value to trapped and injured persons, the driver of a rescue vehicle must be able to get them to the scene safely and quickly. The best-trained rescue squad in the world, traveling in the finest vehicle with the most sophisticated equipment, is of no value if it does not reach the scene of an accident when needed.

Consider the responsibilities of the driver of a rescue truck:

- He must know much more than the route that will take him from quarters to the location of an accident.
- He must understand the local and state laws that regulate the operation of his emergency vehicle.

- He must have basic defensive driving skills in addition to being able to handle his vehicle.
- He must be aware of the proper use of the audible and visible warning devices that are provided on his rig.
- He must be able to put all of this knowledge to use in times of stress.

Understanding the Laws

Every state has statutes that regulate the operation of emergency service vehicles. While the wording of the various statutes may be somewhat different, the intent of the laws is essentially the same. Emergency vehicles are generally granted certain privileges with regard to speed, parking, passage through traffic signals, and direction of travel. But the laws also clearly state that an emergency vehicle operator who does not drive with regard for others must be prepared to pay for the consequences of improper actions. Every person who drives a fire apparatus, rescue unit, or ambulance, regardless of whether he is paid or a volunteer, must fully understand the state laws. He must know the privileges granted and the protection afforded by law, and he must be aware of the penalties for willful disregard of the law.

The Driving Task

Successful completion of the driving task—the safe movement of a vehicle from one place to another—depends on the interaction of three components: the driver, the vehicle, and the road.

The Driver

The most important of the three components is the driver. He must be physically and mentally capable of controlling the movement of his vehicle at all times. No emergency service vehicle should be operated by a person with defective vision. Nor should an emergency vehicle operator have a heart condition, seizure disorders, or other medical problem that might impair his actions while responding to an emergency. An emergency vehicle operator should not drive while taking certain medications. Some cold remedies, for example, cause drowsiness, and manufacturers specifically warn against their use when it is necessary to drive or operate machinery. Pep pills (amphetamines) induce temporary euphoria and interfere with concentration. Painkillers and tranquilizers can dull the senses, cause inattention, and bring on sleep. An emergency vehicle operator should never drive within six hours after drinking. Alcoholic beverages work to dull reflexes and impair judgment. Alcohol combined with certain drugs can cause death. Altitude can make a driver weak, sleepy, or dizzy. Needless to say, the operator of an emergency vehicle should not have any physical disability that might prevent him from properly steering, shifting gears, or operating the foot pedals.

Mental condition is also an important consideration in emergency vehicle operation. The driver of a rescue vehicle should be able to devote his full attention to the driving task. He should not be preoccupied with personal problems, and he should certainly not drive when he is upset about something. He should have a healthy attitude toward his own driving abilities, and the abilities of other drivers using the road. He must not think that he is the best driver in the world. Every emergency vehicle operator should have confidence in his own driving ability, but a feeling of superiority is dangerous. It is crucial that he be able to accept and tolerate the imperfections of other drivers.

An emergency vehicle operator must appreciate the importance of cooperation. He and the rescue officer need to be able to work together. There should be no argument as to where the unit will be parked at the location of an accident, for example, or how squad members will be initially deployed. The driver of a rescue unit and the rescue officer should be able to think alike in certain situations, a condition that results from comprehensive cross-training.

An eight-year study of emergency vehicle accidents shows that most accidents occur in daylight hours on dry roads at intersections. This is a point that all emergency drivers should remember.

The Vehicle

Like its driver, an emergency vehicle must be in optimum operating condition at all times. Preventive maintenance and formal inspection programs are vitally important, as are the informal walk-around inspections that should be conducted at the start of each shift or, in the case of a volunteer organization, once daily.

The Road

While drivers can be trained and vehicles can be tuned for peak performance, little can be done by rescue squad personnel to assure that road conditions are always the best.

Inclement weather can be a severe problem for emergency vehicle operators. Rain, ice, and snow can cause road conditions that tax even the most experienced and proficient drivers. Studded tires and chains help a driver keep his vehicle under control on an ice-covered roadway, but these devices should not be substituted for special driving skills and a good measure of common sense. For example, when slowing on ice, as on all slippery surfaces, a driver should avoid locking the wheels of his vehicle. When wheels are locked but a vehicle continues its forward motion, no amount of steering effort will cause the vehicle to turn. If brakes are pumped, however, rolling friction will be retained between the wheels and the road, and the driver will be able to steer and brake simultaneously.

The first few minutes of a rainfall are an especially dangerous time to drive. Oil residue from vehicles floats on the road surface for a while, and during that period the road can be as slippery as if coated with ice.

Hydroplaning is another danger associated with wet roads—one that results from a combination of speed, wet pavement, and tires with little tread. When a vehicle reaches higher speeds, there is a tendency for a film of water to develop between the tires and the road surface. The tires ride on the water rather than the road, and steering is virtually impossible. The solution to hydroplaning is to slow down gradually, not to jam on the brakes.

Even dry roads can present hazards to unsuspecting drivers. Gravel or dirt roads, newly surfaced tar and chip roads, and high-crowned roads all call for special driving skills. Curves that are flat or banked in the wrong direction necessitate low speeds. A thorough knowledge of all roads within the response district is necessary for successful completion of any driving task.

Planning Alternate Routes

Knowing that a variety of changing conditions *can* affect an emergency response is not enough. It is important to have a plan for times when changing conditions *do* affect response.

Obtain detailed maps of your response district. Use a colored marker to indicate on the maps the usually troublesome traffic spots such as schools, bridges, tunnels, railroad crossings, and other heavily congested areas. Also show the temporary problem areas such as road and building construction sites. Mark in both short- and long-term detours. Using another color, show alternate routes around bridges and tunnels, industrial complexes, and areas that might be isolated by trains. Indicate snow routes and so on.

Hang one map in quarters and place another map in the rescue unit. Then when you must travel past a problem area in response to an urgent call for help, you will be able to select an alternate route to get to your destination quickly and safely.

PARKING AT THE ACCIDENT SCENE

Far too many emergency vehicles are parked at accident locations according to this formula: The closer the unit is to the wreckage, the shorter the distance that supplies and equipment must be carried. This is not parking: This is merely stopping! Worse yet, it is stopping without regard for other vehicles that must use the roadway (including other emergency vehicles) and any of a number of hazards that can threaten the safety of the unit.

Establishing the Danger Zone

A "danger zone" exists around the wreckage at the site of every accident. It may contain the damaged vehicles, debris, spilled fuel, and other hazards. The size of the zone depends on the nature and severity of any hazards that may have been produced by the accident. In any case, a rescue unit or ambulance should never be parked within a danger zone.

When there are no apparent hazards:

- Consider the danger zone to extend for 50 feet in all directions from the wreckage even when there are no apparent hazards.

The unit will be away from broken glass and other debris, and it will not be in the way of rescuers who must work around the accident vehicles. At night, the headlights will be close enough to illuminate the wreckage until other lights can be set up.

When wires are down:

- Consider the danger zone as the area in which persons and vehicles might be contacted by energized wires if they pivot around their points of attachment.

Even though you may have to carry equipment and stretchers for a considerable distance, the rescue unit should be parked at least one full span from the utility poles to which the broken wires are attached.

When fuel has been spilled:

- Consider the danger zone to extend 100 feet from the wreckage.

In addition to parking outside the danger zone, park upwind if possible. The unit will be out of the way of the dense smoke that will be produced if the fuel ignites. If fuel is flowing away from the wreckage, park uphill as well as upwind, if possible.

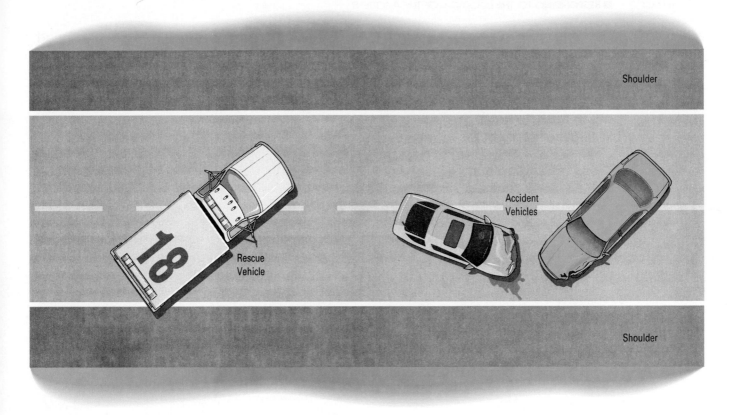

Shoulder

Accident
Vehicles

Rescue
Vehicle

Shoulder

FIGURE 2.01   Parking the Rescue Unit on the Scene

When a vehicle is on fire:

• Consider the danger zone to extend for
100 feet in all directions even if the fire
is small and limited to the engine
compartment.

If leaking fuel is ignited, an explosion could
easily damage the rescue unit if it is parked
closer than 100 feet.

When a hazardous commodity has been
released or spilled:

• Check your hazardous material guide
for suggestions as to parking, or request
advice from Chemtrec or a local
advisory agency.

In some cases you may be able to park 50
feet from the scene, as when no hazard is
present, while in other cases you may be
warned to park 2000 feet or more from the
site, as when there is the possibility that
high explosives may detonate. In all cases,
park uphill and upwind from the wreckage
and behind a manmade or natural barrier, if
possible.

Parking the Rescue Truck

The only way to assure the safety of a rescue
vehicle is to park it completely off the roadway, as on a service road or in a driveway. To
do so, however, will severely reduce or even
destroy the ability of the lights to warn approaching drivers of the hazardous condition
before traffic control measures are effective.

There are two schools of thought about positioning an emergency vehicle on the roadway at an accident site. Some officials argue
that the unit should be located beyond the
wreckage (relative to the direction of traffic
flow). However, most officials favor placing the
unit at the edge of the danger zone between
the wreckage and approaching vehicles. This
is the best position for the vehicle's warning
lights to warn oncoming drivers, although it
does not reduce the need for other warning
devices. Moreover, the unit's headlights will
serve to illuminate the wreckage at night until

other lights can be set up. And, although everyone shudders at the thought of this happening, the unit will help to stop a vehicle that does not change lanes and cannot stop by the time it reaches the danger zone (Figure 2.01). Once the rescue vehicle is parked, its emergency brake should be set and wheel chocks wedged firmly against the tires.

An important point: The truck's headlights should be turned off if the unit is facing oncoming traffic. Even low beams can cancel the effectiveness of flashing and revolving warning lights. Headlights may also blind or confuse approaching motorists.

PHASE THREE

Assessing the Situation

INTRODUCTION

The scene of a motor vehicle accident is often a nightmare that can tax the emotional stability of even the most experienced rescuers. When one considers the sights of twisted wreckage and broken bodies, the sounds of sputtering electric wires and the cries of the injured, and the odors of spilled gas, it is quite easy to understand why rescue and EMS personnel often jump from their rigs and rush headlong to the assistance of the injured persons without regard for their own safety. Unfortunately, this very basic desire to help may result in disaster.

Let's not talk in nebulous terms about what may happen to *someone else* when the urge to help overcomes common sense at the location of an accident. Let's talk about what might happen to *you* in your role as an officer or member of a rescue squad.

- You may be electrocuted if you contact a downed wire that you overlooked in your rush to aid injured persons.
- You may be severely burned if spilled gasoline bursts into flames from one of the many sources of ignition present at accident scenes.
- You may be contaminated by a hazardous material.
- You may be crushed if an unstable vehicle—such as one that has come to rest on its side—suddenly drops on you.
- You may spend valuable minutes gaining access to, disentangling, and removing slightly injured persons while persons with life-threatening problems are left unattended. Remember that slightly injured people often scream louder than individuals who are seriously injured, and that loudly screaming people are often mistakenly cared for first.
- You may aggravate injuries or cause death by attempting to pull from the wreckage those persons who require manual stabilization of the head and neck before being moved.
- You may injure yourself while trying to accomplish difficult extrication procedures while in a highly charged emotional state.

- You may expose yourself to bloodborne pathogens by failing to take Body Substance Isolation precautions.

Difficult as it may be, resist the urge to grab a tool and run to the damaged vehicles as soon as you arrive at the location. Put on your protective gear, assess the situation, decide on a course of action, then start the rescue operation.

The Problem of Tunnel Vision

There is a peculiar eye defect commonly known as tunnel vision. An afflicted person has no peripheral vision; that is, he can see only what he has his eyes fixed on, not to the side. He views the world much as a person with normal vision would while looking from one end of a tunnel to the other. Hence the term "tunnel vision."

Spectators at the locations of vehicle accidents often suffer from tunnel vision. They see only something highly visible like a severely injured person or fire blossoming from under the hood of a car. Because they are not trained for rescue work, spectators are unable to understand why the activities of emergency service personnel are not immediately concentrated on firefighting or extrication efforts. Accordingly, spectators may become quite agitated and vehemently express their displeasure with the apparent slowness of the operation.

Unfortunately, even well-trained and otherwise disciplined rescuers are subject to attacks of tunnel vision. This temporary defect, coupled with a strong desire to help, often prods emergency service personnel into frenzied activity at the time of an emergency. This can lead to loss of the planned approach, and an effort that doesn't take into consideration the "big picture." Some things don't get done, time and effort are spent doing things that don't need to be done, and things that need doing are overlooked. Resources aren't used in the most effective manner. Tunnel vision can lead to an approach that often is less effective, wastes time, and is many times danger-

ous. However, rigorous and continuous training, experience, and an appreciation of the value of a proper assessment do much to prevent tunnel vision.

THE ON-SCENE ASSESSMENT

Assessment does not begin when an emergency service unit arrives on the scene. It begins when someone at the communications center receives the first bit of information about the incident. It continues during the response to the scene, and doesn't end until the person in charge (up to that point, that is) has made a walk-around inspection of the entire scene.

If your dispatcher does a good job acquiring and transmitting information, you will know before you leave quarters, or before you are very far from quarters:

- The exact location of the accident
- The number and types of vehicles involved
- The number of people that appear injured
- Whether anyone appears trapped
- Whether any of the vehicles is on its side or top
- Whether any of the vehicles is on fire
- If a truck is involved, whether something is leaking from the cargo compartment
- Whether traffic is moving past the scene, and if not, how far traffic is backed up

If you are alert while en route, you will hear status reports from other responding emergency service units, and you will see such things as:

- Evidence of a power outage, perhaps caused by the accident.
- A lack of opposing traffic—a signal that the roadway at the accident location may be completely blocked.

If you are observant as you approach the scene, you will be alert for dangers such as:

- Visible fumes or vapor clouds—perhaps an indicator that a dangerous commodity has been released
- Accident victims lying on or near the roadway
- Broken utility poles and downed wires
- Persons walking along the road toward the wreckage—people who will become victims if they—and you—are not careful
- The signals of a police officer or other emergency service worker already on the scene
- Odors that warn of spilled fuel or another hazardous material
- Developing fire
- Fuel flowing in a gutter or ditch adjacent to the roadway

While information from the dispatcher and the observations that you make while responding should give you a pretty good idea of what to expect when you reach the scene, you won't be able to formulate a plan of action until you make a thorough on-scene assessment that includes consideration of hazards, mechanisms of entrapment, and injuries.

It takes a minute or two to make a proper walk-around assessment or size-up, even at the scene of a single-vehicle accident. In that time, firefighters can have hose lines ready to stretch and extinguishers pooled in a staging area near the apparatus. EMS personnel can have trauma boxes and other patient care supplies and immobilization equipment strapped to the stretcher and ready to be moved as a unit. Squad personnel can pool equipment kits, cribbing, lights, cords, and other equipment at a central location. They can start the power unit and purge hydraulic rescue tools. They can assemble lineman's equipment if wires are down at the scene, and so on. Once the firefighting, rescue, and emergency care equipment is staged at a convenient place near the units, there is no need for personnel to rush from compartment to compartment for needed tools after the officer has completed his assessment and ordered them

into service. Nor is there any need for this sort of frenzied and time-consuming activity during the subsequent rescue operation.

Before you leave the location of the rescue unit:

- Put on your full set of protective gear. Remember that you may come close to some life-threatening hazards during the size-up—spilled fuel, for example.
- Then put on a vest, helmet, or something else that clearly identifies you as the rescue officer. Other emergency service personnel will be able to keep you in sight, and spectators will see (and better react to) someone who is obviously an authority, not just another firefighter or rescuer.
- Carry a portable radio so that you will be able to give orders to rescue personnel as soon as you discover a hazard that needs immediate attention, and then the orders that will put the entire rescue team in motion as soon as you have finished the size-up. Use of the radio will eliminate the need for a lot of shouting and walking back and forth between the rescue scene and the emergency service units.

If you have a power megaphone:

- Carry it to give directions to spectators without having to deviate from the size-up path, and to the occupants of accident vehicles without shouting and without having to approach dangerous areas too closely.

At night:

- Be sure to take a bright, dependable flashlight or hand light with you.

Rather than just walking from vehicle to vehicle without a real plan:

- Make your walk-around size-up in a spiral fashion, closing the spiral until you have reached the most serious hazard.

- Continually sweep your head from side to side making observations as you walk, and when you see a hazard that warrants immediate attention, order the appropriate personnel into action without delay.

As the result of this walk-around size-up, you will know:

- The number and types of vehicles involved
- The number of vehicle occupants, although you may not know the exact number of injured because you are not actually able to see all of the occupants
- The hazards that have been produced in addition to the broken glass, sharp metal edges, and pointed objects normally associated with a motor vehicle accident (downed wires, leaking fuel, instability, and spectators)

Moreover, by the time you complete the assessment, you will have been able to reduce the overall level of danger at the accident scene substantially before the extrication effort begins.

What you have just read are suggestions for conducting a basic walk-around size-up of an accident situation. Please don't think these steps are "chiseled in stone" and applicable in every instance. Each accident will require a different assessment procedure because of variables such as the number and types of vehicles involved, the number and nature of hazards, the nature of the roadway and surrounding terrain, the number of people injured, the nature and extent of their injuries, and so on.

It's not important whether you carry out the steps of a size-up in a spiral manner as described in the preceding scenario, or by walking in a circle, or by following the outline of a square or rectangle. What is important is that you:

- Get an overall picture of the scene;
- Examine the vehicles closely for hazards that you may not have seen at a distance; and

- Examine the vehicles for mechanisms of entrapment and the occupants for injuries. If you do so, by the time you complete the size-up, you will have sufficient information for developing an effective plan of action.

A walk-around size-up need not be made by a rescue (or other) officer alone. If both a chief fire officer and the district EMS supervisor respond to scenes in their cars, there is no reason for them not to accompany the rescue officer on the walk-around size-up. When a hazard is discovered that requires the immediate attention of firefighters, the fire officer can radio orders directly to engine company personnel. The EMS supervisor can transmit information on the nature of injuries directly to ambulance personnel, and the rescue officer can give orders directly to squad members. It's vitally important that all three officers work in concert, however. The independent and uncoordinated actions of officers can be confusing to members of the rescue team, and as nonproductive and dangerous as the independent and uncoordinated actions of rescuers.

Note that there were no suggestions to rap on windows to gain the attention of occupants or to pull on door handles to see if any of the doors could be opened easily. Rapping on a window can cause a person in a vehicle to turn his head sharply to the side. Any damage to the cervical spine could be aggravated by the movement. If the occupants can see you, it is a good idea to tell them to not move and that you'll be there quickly. Pulling on a door handle first gently and then increasingly harder to see if it can be opened can cause rocking motions that are easily transmitted to a person's injured spine. The rule "Try before you pry" should be exercised only *after* a vehicle is stabilized, not before.

Assessing the Potential for Injuries

The schedule for gaining access to injured individuals trapped in vehicles is usually based on the seriousness of their injuries. Patients with one or more of these life-threatening problems should be reached first:

- Respiratory arrest
- Difficult breathing
- Severe bleeding
- Severe open head injuries with unconsciousness
- Open chest, crushed chest, or obvious flail chest
- Open abdomen
- Burns of the face that probably involve the respiratory tract
- Obvious cervical spine injury
- Obviously painful, swollen, deformed thigh-fractured femur (because of the potential for massive blood loss)

Any person who is obviously unconscious should be placed in this high-priority category since the cause of his unconsciousness is not known. So should a person who apparently goes into cardiac arrest.

Patients with one or more of the following problems should be reached next:

- Severe burns to parts of the body other than the face
- Moderate bleeding
- Obvious head injuries, but conscious
- Obvious multiple painful, swollen, deformed extremities (fractures)

Persons with one or more of the following problems can remain in place until more seriously injured persons have been reached and cared for unless they are threatened by fire, the chance of an explosion, or exposure to a toxic material:

- Minor soft tissue injuries
- Minor painful, swollen, deformed extremities (fractures)
- Minor burns
- Obviously mortal injuries

The job of assessing injuries and establishing priorities for gaining access and disentanglement would be much easier if all the rescue or EMS officer had to worry about were these obvious injuries. But accidents produce injuries that are not obvi-ous—injuries that can be fatal if they are not discovered and cared for quickly—injuries like those to the brain, heart, lungs, and other internal organs. While patient assessment procedures can be used to discover such injuries, the assessment procedures are often too involved for multiple-vehicle, multiple-casualty incidents (MCI), and in some cases they cannot be used because of the nature and degree of entrapment. Thus it is vitally important that rescue officers and EMS personnel be able to assume that hidden injuries are present in patients by observing such things as the nature and extent of damage to vehicles, and whether the patients have shoulder and lap belts in place.

Four separate collisions are possible during a motor vehicle collision:

- The first collision occurs when the vehicle impacts with another vehicle or other object.
- The second collision occurs when the still-moving occupants impact with parts of the vehicle.
- The third collision occurs when still-moving internal organs impact with other organs or the cavity wall, or are suddenly restrained by ligaments or muscles.
- The fourth collision occurs when occupants are struck by unrestrained items or passengers set into motion by the collision forces.

Especially dangerous are items being carried on the package deck under the rear window. Those items are directly in line with occupants' heads.

Indicating Priorities for Gaining Access

A rescue officer who has only one vehicle to deal with usually has no difficulty in making squad personnel aware of his plans for gaining access and disentanglement. He simply points to the door or window that he wants opened first and says, "Open it" (or words to that effect).

The officer responsible for extricating many injured persons from several vehicles has a much greater problem. With all there is to demand his attention—especially in the area of hazard management—by the time he finishes the size-up he may have forgotten the order in which he would have squad members open the vehicles. A simple tagging procedure can eliminate a great deal of confusion.

Highly visible, vinyl surveyor's tapes and Cyalume Lightsticks are available in a number of colors. The eye-catching qualities of surveyor's tapes makes them especially suitable for marking vehicles. The fluorescent colors can be easily distinguished at a distance, even in low-light situations, and because the tapes are so thin, they flutter in even a light breeze.

- A length of red surveyor's tape secured to the radio antenna, a windshield wiper, or another easily seen part of a vehicle signals rescuers to open that vehicle first; it contains the most seriously injured people.
- A length of yellow tape tells rescuers to open that vehicle after all of the vehicles tagged with red tapes have been opened.
- A length of green tape signals rescuers to open that vehicle after those marked with red and yellow tapes have been opened.
- A length of blue tape attached to a prominent point on a vehicle tells rescuers to open that vehicle after opening those tagged with a length of red, yellow, or green tape.

At night, same-color Lightsticks can be used in place of surveyor's tapes.

Twenty-four-inch to 30-inch lengths of each color tape can be rolled or folded flat and secured with a rubber band or piece of sticky tape and carried in the pocket of a turnout coat. Or, the rolls of tape, several pre-cut lengths of each color tape, and several Lightsticks of each color can be stored in the rescue truck in a specially marked,

immediately accessible box. Moisture will not affect either the tapes or the Lightsticks.

If you elect to use a priority marking system such as the one just described, be sure to train squad members in its use. The color scheme is easy to remember. Priorities run from hot (red) to cold (blue).

Getting Help

There are two major sources of assistance: emergency service organizations and local businesses. Your first request should be for specially trained personnel and equipment designed for rescue operations.

Calling for Help from Emergency Service Organizations

Don't just pick up the radio and holler, "Help," or transmit some vague message such as "Send me all available ambulances and rescue trucks." You know what must be done, and you know what you have to work with. You should know what you need, so call for help, but be specific. Indicate the number of ambulances you need, and remember to specify if you need advanced life support (ALS) or basic life support (BLS) units.

AMBULANCES

One of the reasons that ambulances evolved from those built on a hearse chassis to modern, modular units was the need for working space. Depending on the exact configuration of the patient compartment, today's medics can work at the head, on either side, or over the stretcher patient—that is, if the remainder of the patient compartment is not packed with walking wounded!

Many EMS services have adopted the policy of transporting only one critically ill or seriously injured person per ambulance except in the most extreme emergencies. This is a good policy that assures optimum patient care. But it also creates delays in transporting injured persons from multiple-vehicle, multiple-casualty accident locations. A thorough assessment with efficient triaging and a quick request for additional ambulances, can minimize delays.

The procedure for calling in additional ambulances varies according to local protocols. In communities with limited local dispatch facilities, a medic must specify the communities from which he wishes additional ambulances to respond. Where countywide or regional communications centers operate, a medic need only tell the dispatcher how many ambulances he needs, and the dispatcher will choose from available units. This assures continuous coverage for the rest of the dispatch area.

Whatever the procedure in your EMS area, resist the urge to call for "all available ambulances" when faced with an accident situation involving multiple vehicles. Large areas might be left unprotected. Instead, calculate the need for additional ambulances and call for them according to that need.

RESCUE UNITS

Depending on where you live, you may or may not get the rescue unit that you need so badly at the scene. You may get a truck loaded with every tool and appliance designed for rescue operations and manned by trained rescuers. Or, you may get a truck loaded with equipment but manned by people who have not the foggiest idea of how it all works. You might get a truck that is more coffee wagon or salvage unit than rescue unit. Unlike that which walks like a duck and squawks like a duck, therefore it must be a duck, just because a truck looks like a rescue unit and has the word "RESCUE" painted on the side, doesn't mean it is necessarily a rescue unit.

If your EMS response district has an emergency service communications center that maintains inventories of rescue units, you may be able to get exactly what you need in the way of specialized equipment by asking for it. If you need two hydraulic rescue tools, for example, and ask for them specifically, the dispatcher will consult his files and have units that carry the tools respond.

If you live in an area that does not have a communications facility that keeps inventories, you would do well to visit local rescue squads, learn what they have, and keep a list of specialized equipment in the ambulance. Then when you need a piece of special equipment you can request the response of a certain unit.

FIRE APPARATUS

While in many parts of the country a fire apparatus is dispatched to the locations of accidents at the same time as an ambulance, in some areas an automatic response is not the policy. If the latter is the case in your EMS response area, be sure to request a fire apparatus as soon as you feel there is a potential for fire to develop in or around the wrecked vehicles. The ideal situation is the automatic dispatch of an engine company on any entrapment.

If fire districts within your EMS area do not have rescue units, and rescue units from other districts may be a while reaching accident locations, consider calling in a fire apparatus even though the fire potential is low. Engines have a variety of tools and support equipment that can be used for rescue operations, and personnel that can be used for many tasks even though they are not specifically trained for rescue operations.

Even aerial apparatus have important roles in vehicle rescue operations. When stretchers must be raised or lowered, as from one level of roadway to another, an aerial ladder or elevating platform can be a very useful crane.

HELICOPTERS

State police agencies, large city fire departments, forestry services, utility companies, and many hospitals and private organizations operate either helicopter ambulances or helicopters that can be used for medical evacuation. In addition, many fire departments and EMS organizations have made arrangements with local military units to provide helicopter service when sick or injured people have to be removed from otherwise inaccessible locations or when they have to be transported to regional trauma centers.

EMS and rescue personnel who have a helicopter service available should meet with the appropriate officials to discuss policies. Helicopter pilots have certain procedures they would like followed prior to landing at an accident scene. It may be necessary for someone on the ground to locate a landing zone which is free of hazards and to control the movement of vehicles and spectators. In many locales, certain individuals within emergency service organizations are trained to assist the pilot in safely setting the craft down. The procedures for creating a safe landing area and signaling helicopter pilots are included in Phase Eleven.

Calling for Help from Local Businesses and Agencies of Local Government

When your rescue unit is not equipped and staffed for every type of emergency, you may be able to get the supplies and equipment and the specially trained personnel you need from local businesses or agencies of the local government. Thus as a rescue officer, you should be aware of what local businesses and agencies can provide.

Wrecker Services, Large Garages, Truck Service Centers, and Vehicle Recovery Companies can provide heavy-duty wreckers with equipment that can be used for rescue operations, ranging from hand tools to powered tools. Some recovery service vehicles have air bags, generators, and lights. Moreover, wreckers and recovery vehicles are usually operated by people who are completely familiar with vehicle construction features—knowledge that is important during difficult disentanglement operations. A wrecker (Figure 3.01) can be used to (Figure 3.02):

- Stabilize vehicles, especially those that are upside down on the roof, and those that are situated off the road on a hillside

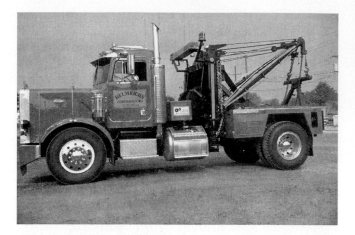

FIGURE 3.01   Wrecker

- Move doors beyond their normal range of motion
- Displace steering columns
- Displace seats
- Move one vehicle from another when separation is necessary in order to reach trapped persons
- Move large pieces of debris away from accident vehicles.

Yet wrecker operators are often seen standing by their rigs with one foot on the bumper while ambulance crews toil feverishly to reach and free trapped persons. Don't hesitate to use a wrecker operator if you are short of equipment and manpower. Be aware of the kid who responds to the

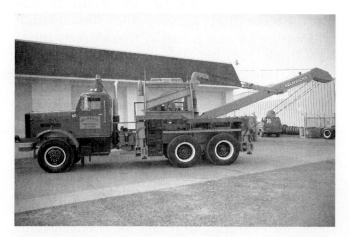

FIGURE 3.02   Recovery Company

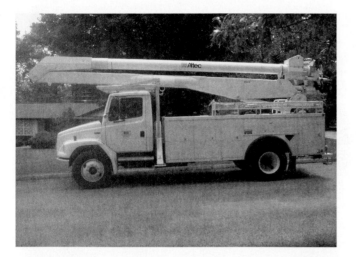

FIGURE 3.03   Tennessee Valley Authority Line Truck

scene with a pickup truck that has a hydraulic sling. His experience may be limited to changing tires, jumping batteries, and pulling in disabled cars.

Utility Companies send crews to accident locations to deal with downed wires and broken utility poles. The crews bring to accident scenes vehicles similar to a heavy-duty rescue truck. They have equipment such as hand tools, chain and cable hand winches, powered cutting devices, chains and slings, and warning and signaling devices, and the crew members are trained to use the equipment (Figure 3.03).

Like power and light company trucks, large telephone company line trucks are

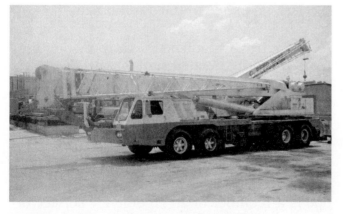

FIGURE 3.04   Hydraulic Truck Crane

stocked with equipment that can be used for vehicle rescue operations, especially warning and signaling devices. Water department trucks and highway department trucks also have equipment and personnel that can be used to advantage during extensive rescue operations. If you see any of these units stopped by the side of the road at an accident location, don't hesitate to ask the person in charge for assistance.

Crane Rental Companies can supply lifting power when one vehicle must be removed from atop another vehicle, or when a piece of heavy machinery must be moved in order to reach trapped persons. Many emergency service organizations have plans in effect whereby a crane can be dispatched quickly to the scene of a serious accident at any time of the day or night (Figure 3.04).

Large Medical Facilities usually have teams of doctors and nurses who can respond quickly to accident scenes and provide advanced life support to seriously injured persons when disentanglement will take a while.

Scuba Clubs will send divers and equipment to locations where a vehicle is in a body of water. Many fire and police departments have dive teams available for vehicle rescue operations (Figure 3.05).

The **Local Humane Society** will send officers to locations where animals are a problem.

Farm Equipment Service and Supply Firms will send mechanics to locations when someone is trapped in a farm implement, or when a machine rolls off of a transport vehicle onto a car.

State or Local Highway Departments and **Barricade Service Companies** can be contacted for warning and signaling equipment when rescue operations will be lengthy, or when a road must remain closed for a while as the result of an accident.

Churches and Religious Institutions can send clergymen who are extensively trained in crisis intervention and in techniques of dealing with emotionally distraught persons. The mental comfort that can be offered by a minister, priest, or rabbi may be

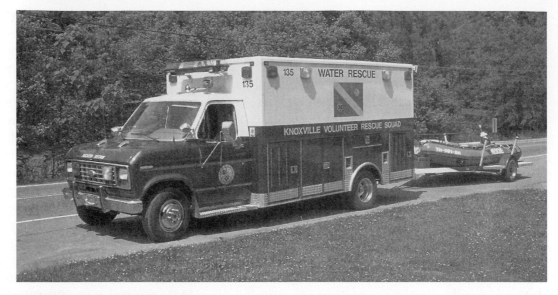

FIGURE 3.05   Dive Truck

just what a severely injured person needs during a long and painful disentanglement procedure. Death is not a pleasant thought for anyone, and the prospect of dying while trapped in twisted wreckage is especially terrifying. The soothing words of a clergyman may prevent a trapped and injured person from a complete emotional breakdown during a rescue effort.

Recruiting Temporary Assistants from the Ranks of Spectators

One radio call may be all that is necessary to get an army of trained and equipped personnel on their way to an accident scene. What you will do in the interval between the call for help and the moment that help arrives will depend on how well the on-scene units are equipped and how well you can utilize spectators.

While you would not call upon them to operate tools or carry out emergency care measures (unless they are trained to do so), you can call upon onlookers to:

• Place flares or other warning devices.
• Either stop the flow of vehicles or keep them moving past the danger zone.
• Keep other spectators a safe distance from the wreckage.

• Carry supplies and equipment from the staging area near the ambulance to the accident vehicles.
• Guard the emergency service units when all hands are needed for rescue operations.
• Hold lights while rescuers operate tools.
• Hold doors steady while rescuers are removing them.
• Hold devices that will protect victims during disentanglement operations.
• Support injured persons (physically and emotionally) during rescue operations.
• Assist with the removal of packaged patients from the wrecked vehicles.
• Assist with the transfer of patients from the wreckage to the ambulance.

As you can see, onlookers can provide many pairs of badly needed hands when you and your partner must work alone at accident locations. However, you must be able to recruit the right people. Not everyone is suited for the job.

Before either pointing to individuals and asking for their help, or simply asking for volunteers, ask the onlookers whether anyone is a member of an emergency service organization. It's not unusual for a firefighter, rescue squad member, or medic to be in the crowd, especially in an area served predominantly by volunteer organizations. Some are reluctant to volunteer, but will help when asked.

If you can't find any trained people to help, recruit truck drivers, especially the drivers of long-haul trucks. These are usually stable individuals who have a pretty good idea of what goes on at accident scenes because they have witnessed a number of rescue operations. Moreover, truck drivers have a great appreciation for what EMS and rescue people do for their fellow drivers.

If there are no emergency service personnel or truck drivers in the group of onlookers, ask for volunteers, but choose from among them carefully. Avoid selecting someone who has volunteered, but appears distressed by the sights and sounds of the accident scene. Chances are that person won't hold up well, especially if there is a lot of blood.

Also, avoid recruiting someone who is obviously excited by the sights and sounds at the scene. This individual probably has been quite noticeably running around pointing out this to someone and that to someone else and maybe even volunteering to help before you've asked. While he may sincerely want to help, this person may be hard to control. If you don't watch him closely, he may undertake efforts that *he* thinks are best for the trapped persons.

Whatever you do, don't put your temporary assistants in dangerous positions without protection. Give them eye protection if they are likely to be exposed to flying debris, gloves if you expect them to handle sharp objects, and a helmet if they must stand close to tools in operation. If you are responsible for equipping a rescue unit in a response area where onlookers are often used as helpers at accident locations, you would do well to consider equipping the unit with extra protective gear.

When assigning your temporary assistants to jobs, make sure your instructions are clear and concise. Don't tell someone to "go down the road and put out some flares," tell him where to go and exactly where to place the flares. Don't tell someone else to "hold the light." Tell him exactly where to hold the light so it will best illuminate the work area. Keep in mind that when people turn out to be more of a hindrance than a help at an accident scene, the fault can usually be laid at the door of the person giving instructions.

The assessment phase of operations is over. You know what has to be done. Now assign the people to do it.

ASSURING THAT ALL VICTIMS ARE ACCOUNTED FOR

When all of the doors of vehicle are closed and all of the windows are rolled up, you really have no reason to suspect that the vehicle does not contain all of the persons who were traveling in it at the time of the accident. But when you see that a door is open but no one is either on the seat next to the door or just outside the vehicle near the door opening, you should suspect that at least one person is missing from the vehicle. An injured person may have walked away from the wreckage to seek help, especially if the accident has occurred at night on a little-used road. Or, spectators may have helped an injured person into a car or a nearby building, or even taken the person to a hospital.

If after your size-up, you suspect that not all of the victims are present at the scene:

• Ask conscious and coherent occupants how many people were in the vehicle when the accident occurred.

Do not ask questions or make statements in a way that suggests some of the victims are not accounted for, however. Learning that a family member or friend is missing may cause an injured person to become emotionally unstable or even slip into deep shock.

If all of the people in the vehicle are unconscious or have altered mental status:

• Ask witnesses to the accident whether they saw someone walk away from the wreckage, or whether someone helped a victim to a car or nearby building.

If neither the occupants of a wrecked vehicle nor witnesses can provide information about the number of victims or their location:

- Look for clues that will tend to confirm your suspicion that someone else was in the vehicle.

Coats, jackets, briefcases, schoolbooks, lunch boxes, toys, luggage, and a multitude of other items may be tossed about in a vehicle at the time of impact. To an untrained observer, these may appear to be nothing more than debris common to any accident location. To the trained rescuer, however, such items will be clues that will help him to determine whether all of the victims are present at the scene.

- Three briefcases—each with different initials—in a car that has two occupants suggests that three people were in the vehicle at the time of the crash.
- A child's lunch box in a car that is occupied by only a young woman suggests that a child was in the vehicle when it crashed. The fact that the accident occurred at 7:30 A.M. on a road leading to an elementary school lends credence to the theory.
- Women's clothes in a wrecked vehicle occupied by a lone male suggests that the man had a female companion in the car at the time of the accident.

Distinctive objects, time of day, and the location of the accident may all have significance.

Now then . . . what can you do when you suspect that not all of the victims of a vehicle accident are in or near the wreckage? Needless to say, neither you nor members of the immediate rescue team can search for missing persons when a number of trapped and injured persons must be reached and cared for. However, you can have other emergency service personnel initiate a search. Call for another rescue squad or engine company. As soon as they arrive on the scene, have them check a number of locations.

Roadways. When a car careens out of control while traveling at a high speed, it is not unlikely for the vehicle to continue for several hundred feet before coming to a stop. At any time, a door may pop open and an occupant may be thrown out some distance from where the car finally stops. During daylight hours, it will be easy to spot a person who has been thrown from a vehicle if he is still on the roadway. At night, sighting this person may be difficult, especially if the road is not lit, or if emergency vehicles have approached the accident scene from the opposite direction.

When it is evident that a vehicle has traveled out of control for a considerable distance, rescuers should always look for an ejected occupant along the entire path that the careening vehicle took.

Ditches and Gullies. When a vehicle accident occurs on a road bordered by a deep ditch or gully, the possibility always exists that an occupant of a vehicle has crawled away from the site in the ditch. He may have been strong enough to crawl for some distance, but he may not have had the strength needed to climb from the ditch. Heavy weeds, mud, and water in the ditch might also be concealing the person. When it seems likely that someone has crawled away, rescuers should search the side of the road in both directions, looking especially in high weeds and other natural covering that would make spotting someone in a ditch difficult.

Hillsides and Ravines. When a vehicle leaves the road and plunges down a hillside or into a ravine, the situation will tax even the most proficient rescuer. The degree of the slope and the depth of the ravine may make it extremely difficult for rescuers to reach and remove patients. At any point during the travel of the vehicle a door may open, allowing an occupant to be thrown out. Whenever a vehicle leaves the road and plunges down a hill, it is necessary for rescuers to search not only along the path that the vehicle took on its way to the bottom but also for a considerable distance on each side of that path.

Tall Grass and Crops. On rural roads, tall grass and crops often grow within a few feet of the road. Therefore, a person who crawls just a few feet from a wrecked vehicle may be concealed from view. When confronted with this possibility, rescuers should look for clues such as bent stalks or perhaps a blood trail leading from the scene.

Nearby Buildings and Vehicles. As a rule, spectators do not become involved with injured persons. On occasions, however, a good Samaritan may help an injured person to his own car to await the arrival of an ambulance. When victims seem to be missing, rescuers should not dismiss this possibility. They should make a quick check of the cars that are stopped at the scene.

Good Samaritans might also be inclined to take slightly injured persons into nearby homes and businesses, especially if the weather is bad. If an accident occurs in a residential area, rescuers should check houses and apartment buildings on both sides of the street when there is a possibility that not all victims are accounted for.

Hospitals. When rescuers have checked all logical locations—and those that are not so logical—and still have reason to believe that not all of the victims have been found, consideration should be given to the possibility that someone has taken a missing person to a hospital. This is especially true when an accident occurs on a rural road where an ambulance may take a long time reaching the scene. A radio or telephone call to local hospitals can usually quickly confirm the arrival of a patient in a vehicle other than an ambulance. Don't forget to check the many neighborhood emergency care centers that are being built all over the country.

Remember: Accident victims may be found anywhere—in the wreckage, along the road, in natural cover, or in nearby buildings and vehicles.

Finally: Always check the trunk of every vehicle involved in an accident.

Reaching Off-Road Rescue Sites

INTRODUCTION

Not all vehicle rescue operations are carried out on pavement or level ground. Sometimes cars and trucks come to rest at the bottom of a hill or ravine following a collision. When this happens, reaching the wreckage may be more difficult than all of the rest of the rescue operations.

Descending to a car that is at the bottom of a near-vertical cliff is a procedure that requires special equipment and techniques that should be learned under the close supervision of a technical rope rescue instructor. However, descending a hill that is just a bit too steep to walk down can be accomplished by any rescuer with minimal training and equipment.

DESCENDING A HILL BY MEANS OF ROPES

The easily stored, easily carried, easily used descent kit described in Phase One includes the following items:

A Combination Rope and Equipment Bag. The bag holds everything necessary for a hillside descent and is easy to pack and use. Packing a rope bag involves nothing more than poking one end of the rope through the grommet in the bottom of the bag, forming a figure-eight stopper knot in the end of the rope that is through the grommet, and randomly stuffing the rest of the rope into the bag. When you have all but a few feet of rope stuffed in the bag, form a figure-eight knot on a bight in the end. The rope will then be ready for immediate use at the location of an off-road rescue.

Static Kernmantle 1/2-Inch Rope. Three-eights-inch diameter rope can be used when the line will be used only for descending hills. However, when 1/2-inch rope is included in a rope kit, the line can be used for lowering stretchers and people from elevated structures as well as for descending hills. Static kernmantle rope is light enough to be easily handled, yet strong enough to meet the NFPA standard for a two-person rescue rope. Whatever the diameter, the rope should be long enough to reach the bottom of most hills within the rescue response area.

Two Rope Pads. Static kernmantle rope is very strong and has excellent abrasion resistance; nonetheless, it will abrade and it can be cut by sharp edges. A bare rope must never be allowed to pass over an unprotected edge or rub against any surface harder than the nylon that makes up the rope. Abrasions and cuts destroy the rope's integrity and shorten its life. Rope rollers can be used to protect ropes from the sharp edges common to structures, but they are often difficult to use in off-road rescue operations.

Canvas-duck rope pads can be folded into small packages and stored in the rope bag. Lengths of static accessory cord fastened to the rope pad grommets make securing the 24- by 18-inch pads to trees and guardrails an easy task.

Two Locking D Carabiners. One carabiner is used to secure the end of the rope to an anchor point; the other is used to secure a figure-eight descender to the rescuer's web seat or harness.

A Large Figure-Eight Descender with Ears. A figure-eight descender allows a rescuer to travel down a hill securely and in complete control of his descent. Figure-eight descen-ders are available in aluminum and steel. The aluminum figure-eight is lighter and develops more friction than the steel model, but the steel figure-eight will not wear out as quickly. The strength of both models is in excess of 10,000 pounds. The ears of a figure-eight descender prevent the rope from slipping to the top of the descender and forming a girth hitch that will effectively strand a rescuer until he can remove his weight from the device. Ears also make it easier for a rescuer to lock off his rope when it is necessary to stop and remain in place during a descent.

One-Inch Tubular Nylon Webbing. When the ends are joined to form a continuous loop, a 14-foot length of webbing will make a harness suitable for an average-size adult male. More or less webbing may be necessary, depending on the size of the rescuer. Various-size continuous loop slings can also be purchased from rope equipment suppliers. Having a personal continuous loop sling eliminates the need for a rescuer to form one at an accident location (Figure 4.01). Approved specially designed seat harnesses and full-body harnesses are also commercially available.

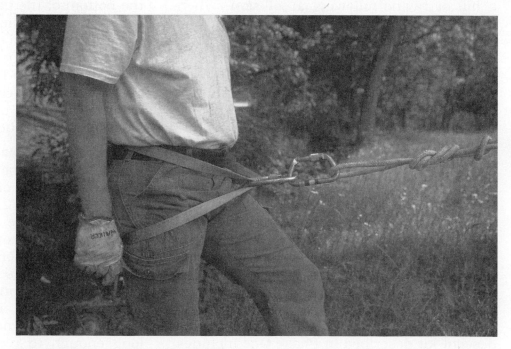

FIGURE 4.01   Diaper Harness

There are distinct advantages to having two such descent-assist kits. When two lines are deployed side-by-side, two rescuers can save time and effort by descending together while holding a stretcher full of equipment between them. Moreover, the parallel lines can be used as handholds by a stretcher-handling team when they are ready to move an injured person up the hill.

A rope kit can be as simple as the one pictured and described, or it can be expanded with additional equipment. For example, another length of webbing, a figure-eight descender, and a carabiner can be included so that another rescuer can descend each line. Additional lengths of webbing can be included for anchor points when the kit will be used to move stretchers from buildings. A pulley or two can be included so that the direction of pull can be changed when a stretcher must be pulled, rather than carried, up a hill.

Let's say that you have to reach a vehicle at the bottom of a 50-foot hill that is too steep to walk down without some sort of support. The rescue truck has two of the rope kits just described. Three operations will get you to the bottom of the hill: deploying the descent lines, putting on or rigging a seat or body harness, and descending the hill.

Deploying the Descent Lines

Trees make excellent anchor points for ropes. If you decide to use a tree, make sure that it is a big live one with an extensive and deep root system. Some trees—even large ones—have root systems so shallow that the trees can be pulled over by one or two people with a rope. Remember that the higher you tie the line, the greater potential you have for pulling the tree over.

To deploy the descent lines:

- Situate the rope high enough on the anchor point that it will be about waist level over the entire length of the slope when pulled taut by someone standing at the bottom of the hill. Use a ladder, if necessary.

- Wrap the end of the rope several times around the anchor point, and secure the loop formed by the figure-eight knot to the standing part with a carabiner.

- Adjust the loops around the anchor point as necessary for an even pull. This will minimize pressure on the knot.

- Visualize the path that the rope will take from the anchor point over the brow of the hill.

- Secure a pad where the rope will pass over a sharp edge or rough surface.

- Stand at the brow of the hill and toss the rope bag to the bottom. Use an underhand toss and loft the bag to get maximum distance. Use caution to not knock loose debris or hit the patient with the bag.

- Repeat the procedure with the second rope bag at an anchor point about 10 feet distant.

The distance between the two parallel lines is somewhat critical. If the interval is a great deal more or less than 10 feet, you and your partner will have trouble starting your descent with a stretcher full of equipment between you. Moreover, rescuers who are bringing the stretcher up the hill may not be able to maintain a grip on the rope as they near the top of the hill.

Rigging a Seat Harness with Webbing

If you do not have a seat or full-body harness or a personal continuous loop sling, you can make one with a 14-foot length of webbing. The resulting 6-foot sling should be suitable if you are of average size. Make a smaller loop if you are small, or a larger loop if you are large.

To join the ends of the length of webbing:

- Form a loose overhand knot 12 to 15 inches from one end.

- Pass the other end around the parts of the overhand knot from the opposite direction until you have a tail that is about 12 inches long. Make sure that the webbing parts lie flat against each other.

- Pull the resulting knot—a water knot—tight. The tails should be about the same length when the knot is formed.
- Tie a "keeper" on each side of the water knot by forming overhand knots around the sling with the loose tails of webbing.

To form a seat with the sling that you have made with the webbing:

- Hold the sling behind you with one hand.
- Reach behind with your other hand and draw a portion of the sling taut against your back at waist level.
- Pass your arms through the sling from outside and allow the webbing to rest on the back of each wrist.

With both hands:

- Reach down between your legs and grasp the loose part of the sling that is draped behind them.
- Pull this part of the sling forward and up between your legs.

As you do:

- Allow the part of the sling that is resting on each wrist to slide down your hands.
- Join the part of the sling that you have in each hand with a locking carabiner.
- Adjust the leg loops so they rest in the crease of each buttock, not behind the calf of each leg.
- Tuck the carabiner behind your belt, or catch your belt with the open carabiner to hold the sling in place while you complete preparations for the descent.

The seat must fit you snugly. If it is so loose that it is likely to slide down when you walk or work, retie it.

Descending the Hill

Following is a procedure that you and another rescuer might use to descend a hill while carrying a plastic basket or stokes stretcher full of equipment between you. Before you start the descent, be sure that the equipment is lashed securely to the stretcher with web straps.

- Position the stretcher on level ground at the top of the hill between the anchor points. You stand at one end of the stretcher facing one anchor point while your partner stands at the other end of the stretcher facing the other anchor point.
- Each form a bight in your rope.
- Pass the bight through the large eye of the figure-eight, and then around the neck of the device.
- Join the small end of the figure-eight to the carabiner that is clipped to your seat harness. Run the knurled coupling up snugly.

An Important Point: It was once suggested that the threaded coupling be run up snugly and then backed off a half-turn to prevent the threads from binding if considerable force is applied to the carabiner. This is no longer recommended. Many new carabiners lock on the gate. Backing the threaded coupling a half-turn may unlock it.

- Put on your gloves.

With your outboard hand (the one that will not be holding the stretcher):

- Pull taut the rope from the anchor point.
- Position your hand against your buttock. That hand will be the brake hand.
- Together, pick up the stretcher with the free hand.

When you are both ready:

- Loosen the grip of your brake hand slightly, walk over the brow of the hill, and start down.

As you descend:

- Do not try to balance yourself and walk upright; let the rope support your weight.
- Tighten or loosen the grip of your brake hand as necessary to slow down or speed up your descent, but do not let go of the rope.

When you get to the bottom of the hill:

- Put the stretcher down. Unclip the figure-eight from the carabiner, but leave the carabiner clipped to your seat harness.
- Remove the figure-eight from the rope and put it in your pocket or belt pouch.
- Either get out of the sling or tuck the carabiner behind your belt to hold the sling in place while you work.

Rescuers who are not experienced in the procedure often feel uncomfortable making a descent while trying to hold on to an equipment-laden stretcher. They prefer to keep their free hand on the taut section of rope while using the other hand to control the speed of descent. If this is your preference, have other rescuers slide the basket stretcher full of equipment down the hill at the end of the rope.

DESCENDING A HILL BY MEANS OF LADDERS

While sliding down a rope is a fast way to reach an accident vehicle at the bottom of a hill, manhandling a stretcher between two ropes may not be the easiest way to move an injured person from the wreckage back to the roadway.

When you have to get down and then back up a hill that is no deeper than 50 feet—especially a fairly steep hill—consider using a ladder or a combination of ladders instead of ropes. Moving up and down a ladder that is placed against the side of a hill is no different than moving up and down a ladder that is placed against the side of a building, as long as the climbing angle is nearly correct.

Engine companies usually have a 35-foot extension ladder and a 12- or 14-foot roof ladder. Truck companies carry a variety of ladders ranging from stepladders to 50-foot extension ladders. Large rescue units often have at least a 10-foot roof ladder. All are suitable for off-road vehicle rescue operations.

Following are several procedures that you might employ if you are a rescuer charged with the responsibility of having squad members or firefighters rig ladders to reach the bottom of a hill.

Using a Roof Ladder

A roof ladder can be used to descend hills up to a foot or so deeper than the ladder is long. If the hill is no deeper than the length of the ladder:

- Have two rescuers—one alongside each beam—simply lift the ladder and ease the butt over the brow and down the hill.
- Direct one rescuer to stand by the tip of the ladder and hold it securely while other rescuers are climbing down and up the hill.

If manpower is limited:

- Have the rescuers secure the tip in place with two ropes leading to suitable anchor points.
- Direct them to keep the ropes at ground level, if possible, to prevent them from becoming tripping hazards or interfering with the movement of rescuers to and from the ladder.

The portion of the tip of the ladder that remains above the brow of the hill will serve as a convenient handhold. Rescuers can hold on to the tip and swing onto the ladder much as they would when descending from the roof of a building to the ground.

The next procedure might be used when the depth of the hill and the length of the ladder are just about the same. A length of 1/2-inch rope is required.

- Direct two rescuers to position the ladder at a right angle to the slope with the butt at the brow of the hill.

When the ladder is in position:

- Lay the coil of the rope (or the rope bag) on the ground a few feet beyond the tip.
- Form a loop in the end of the rope large enough to slip over the tip of the ladder.
- Secure the loop with a bowline and a safety.
- Have the rescuers support the ladder at an angle so the tip is a few feet off the ground.

From underneath:

- Pass the loop through the space between the third and fourth rungs from the tip.
- Carry the loop back and over the tip.

While you pull the standing part of the rope with one hand:

- Work the loop down to the third rung with your other hand.
- Continue to pull on the standing part of the rope until the two resulting loops are locked around the beams. This will be the main working line. Assign a rescuer to it.
- Direct the rescuers with the ladder to ease the butt of the ladder over the brow of the hill.

As they do:

- Have the rescuer who is manning the lowering line maintain tension on the rope.

While the other rescuers guide the ladder by the beams:

- Direct the rescuer who is manning the line to lower the ladder.

When the butt of the ladder is in place at the bottom of the hill:

- Direct the rescuer to secure the lowering line to a tree, a utility pole, the rescue unit, or another suitable anchor point.

As you can imagine, getting onto the ladder will be difficult since there is no tip to grasp while boarding. Someone will have to remain in position at the brow of the hill near the tip of the ladder to assist rescuers on and off of it throughout the rescue operation. Supplies and equipment should be lowered down the hill by rope so rescuers can move down the ladder unencumbered.

The following technique might be used when a hillside is covered with heavy brush that might be caught by the heel plates while the ladder is being slid down the hill.

- Direct two rescuers to secure the end of a rope with a clove hitch and a safety to each of the ladder beams between the heel and the first rung.
- Have them push the hitches tight against the rung.
- Then direct the rescuers to lay the ropes out on each side of the ladder and take a position on the brow of the hill a few feet from the ladder.

While the rescuers with the ropes hold the ladder horizontal:

- Have other rescuers slide the ladder out over the brow of the hill until the tip is close to the edge.

While the rescuers at the beams of the ladder support and maneuver the tip as necessary:

- Have the rescuers with the ropes lower the heel of the ladder to flat ground.

When the ladder is in place:

- Have the rescuers with the ropes secure them to suitable anchor points.

- Have them keep the ropes at ground level if the tip of the ladder projects over the brow of the hill.

Using an Extension Ladder

What happens when the slope of a hill is too long for a roof ladder? Use a longer ladder! Three-section fire service extension ladders are available in lengths up to 50 feet.

Following is a procedure that you might use when an accident vehicle is 30 feet below the surface of the roadway and the engine company that has responded to the scene with your rescue unit has a 35-foot, three-section extension ladder. Three firefighters have carried the ladder from the engine to the brow of the hill.

- Have the firefighters lay the ladder on the ground at a right angle to the slope, with the bed section down and the heel of the ladder close to the brow of the hill.

While two firefighters hold the bed section in place:

- Direct the third firefighter to grasp the top rung of the ladder and pull the fly sections to their fully extended positions.

Be sure that one of the firefighters who is holding the bed section in place maintains tension on the halyard as the fly sections move. Otherwise the halyard may bunch and foul the sheaves. When the fly sections are fully extended:

- Check to see that rungs are resting in the curved portion of the pawls. Make adjustments as necessary.
- Secure the top section to the middle section, and the middle section to the bed section with short pieces of 1/2-inch rope (6 feet long) using clove hitches and safeties tied around the overlapping rungs near the pawls (a total of four hitches). Push the clove hitches snugly against the beams.

This important step should be done with all extension ladders used in this way. When it is in position, the ladder may not be resting on its heel plates, but suspended by the ropes. If the rungs of each section are not tied tightly together, they will separate. The weight of the ladder will be borne by the stops and tripping hazards will be created by the offset rungs.

The next step is to rig ropes for lowering the ladder. Needless to say, the ladder could be lowered by hand; that is, rescuers could simply push the heel over the brow of the hill, tilt the tip up, and manhandle the ladder until the heel is resting on level ground at the bottom of the slope. However, if one or two of the rescuers at the very edge of the hill lose their footing and slip while they are handling the ladder, they and the 185-pound ladder can slide down the slope with disastrous results. Once the ladder begins to slide, it's unlikely that rescuers standing at the top of the hill will be able to stop it without being pulled down the hill themselves. Use ropes and prevent an accident!

- Direct two rescuers to secure a 1/2-inch rope with a clove hitch and safety to the beam of the bed section on both sides of the ladder between the first and second rungs.
- Have each rescuer position the remainder of the coil or the rope bag so the rope will pay out freely while the ladder is being lowered.
- Have each rescuer stand at the brow of the hill with his rope.

When everyone is in position:

- Direct the firefighters to slide the ladder toward the slope until about half of the bed section is over the brow of the hill.
- Have the rescuers who are manning the support lines keep a strain on their ropes.

Next:

- Have the firefighters tilt the tip of the ladder up until the weight of the ladder starts it moving down the hill.

- Direct the rescuers who are handling the support lines to simply keep the ladder moving in a straight line; warn them not to attempt to control the descent.

When the heel plates of the ladder are on level ground:

- Instruct a rescuer or firefighter to support the tip while other rescuers climb down the ladder.

If there is not sufficient manpower for this task:

- Secure the tip in place with ropes tied to anchor points.

Theoretically, several ladders can be spliced to reach vehicles at the bottom of even longer slopes. Weight will become a problem, however, and a point will be reached where the available manpower will not be able to handle the length and weight of the combined ladders, either to lower them down a hill or to pull them back up. To paraphrase an old saying: Remember, what goes down must come back up!

Ladders can also be used in the ways just described to reach vehicles that have rolled only partway down a hill and come to rest against a tree. The problem is not so much positioning the ladders as it is laying them and working around the wreckage.

A Suggestion: It was suggested that short lengths of 1/2-inch rope can be used for ladder lashing operations. Making 6-foot sections is an excellent way to dispose of lengths of 1/2-inch nylon or kernmantle rope that are no longer fit for rescue operations. Keep a number of short sections of rope on the rescue unit if you are likely to use ladders during off-road rescue operations.

WORKING ON A STEEP SLOPE

While getting to vehicles that are only partway down a hill may not be a problem, working around them may be a real challenge.

Handling a 65-pound hydraulic rescue tool on level ground is one thing; handling the same tool on a 45 degree slope is another thing altogether. Even the most minor tasks can be difficult when a rescuer has to use both hands to accomplish the tasks while attempting to maintain balance with his feet and legs. Once again, ladders and ropes can be used to great advantage.

Using Ladders

If two ladders are rigged for rescuers to descend to a vehicle that is only partway down a slope, one on each side of the vehicle, and the hill is not too steep, roof or wall ladders can be secured at right angles to the descent ladders, one above and one below the wreck. Rescuers should be able to brace their feet against the beams of the ladders and work upright around the vehicle without fear of slipping.

When only one ladder is rigged for descent and the hill is not too steep, roof ladders or wall ladders can be suspended at a right angle to the slope by ropes secured to anchor points at the brow of the hill. If enough ladders are available, an accident vehicle can actually be "boxed" by ladders.

Using Ropes

Rescuers can rig the descent system described earlier in this chapter, put on a prepared harness, or form a diaper seat with webbing and descend to the wreckage by means of a figure-eight device. The rescuers can descend with equipment, and once they are in working positions around the wreckage, they can lock themselves in place by jamming the loose end of the rope between the taut part and the figure-eight descender. Moving up or down to change positions is an easy matter; a rescuer need only unlock, pull himself up the rope or lower himself the required distance, and relock. Moreover, other rescuers can descend on the same lines when it is necessary for one rescuer to work directly above another.

Having sufficient rope but lacking enough harnesses or webbing, figure-eight descenders, and carabiners, rescuers can tie themselves into a bowline on a bight with a chest hitch. They can lower themselves after passing the rope around a smooth object, or they can have rescuers standing at the brow of the hill lower them. Self-lowered rescuers and rescuers who have been lowered by others and then had their lowering lines secured to anchor points will have a problem in adjusting their positions around the wreckage, however.

When it is necessary to have two rescuers work face to face, as when handling a hydraulic rescue tool, one rescuer can be secured in a bowline on a bight/chest hitch with the lowering line attached to the front of his harness. His partner can be in a bowline on a bight/chest harness that has been put on backward by another person so the lowering line extends from his back instead of his chest.

If possible, safety lines should be stretched between trees whenever rescuers must work on a hill that is too steep for a person to maintain his balance. One line should be about a foot off the ground, and another should be about waist level. Thus they will have something to grab for if they lose balance and start to slide down the slope.

PHASE FIVE

Managing Incident Scene Hazards

INTRODUCTION

When asked about the hazards that might be encountered at the locations of motor vehicle accidents, untrained rescuers are likely to list those that are most common: fragments of broken glass and sharp-edged and sharp-pointed pieces of metal and plastic debris. While these things can inflict injury, they are seldom more than nuisances to be dealt with as the rescue effort progresses.

A number of other hazards can severely threaten the safety of victims, rescuers, and spectators. These include downed wires; displaced transformers; damaged utility poles; leaking fuel; fire in, around, or under accident vehicles; instability; and even trains. These hazards must be managed, if not eliminated altogether, before any attempt can be made to reach trapped and injured victims.

RAILROAD GRADE CROSSING COLLISION

Suppose a head-on collision has occurred on a railroad grade crossing. If the grade crossing is used infrequently, as when slow, short freight trains move raw materials into and finished products out of a nearby manufacturing facility once a week, there is no problem. But if the crossing is active, with perhaps as many as a dozen trains passing each day at relatively high speeds, the first hazard management operation must be an attempt to stop the trains. Simply working feverishly in hope of clearing the scene before the next train arrives can lead to disaster.

In the United States, there are more than 250,000 railroad grade crossings, locations where roadways and railroads intersect. In the past 10 years more than 14,000 people have been killed in grade crossing accidents, and more than 53,000 people have been injured.

Collisions occur in a number of ways at grade crossings not protected with gates and/or flashing warning lights. Vehicles collide with trains when visibility is poor, at night, and during bad weather. Speeding vehicles collide with trains when motorists are unable to stop them before reaching occupied crossings, as do cars operated by motorists who think it is smart to race an approaching train to a crossing.

Grade crossing collisions are not limited to unprotected crossings. They also occur at guarded crossings when motorists disregard warning lights and weave around gates even though a 10,000-ton train is approaching the crossing at 60 miles per hour (88 feet per second).

Accidents can also befall emergency service personnel who conduct rescue operations at grade crossings without regard for rail traffic. In areas where rail traffic is light and train schedules are well known, extrication and emergency care operations at a grade crossing can be initiated without delay. When trains are frequent, however, rescuers must take immediate steps to halt rail traffic when that traffic will jeopardize a trackside rescue effort.

Notifying the Railroad Dispatcher of the Situation

Railroad dispatchers control the movements of trains by means of signals and radio communications. However, a dispatcher cannot stop a train until he is made aware of an emergency involving the tracks. Following are steps that you might take if you are a rescue officer.

When you arrive on the scene of a collision that has occurred on an active grade crossing:

- Direct the rescue vehicle driver to park in a safe place adjacent to the tracks, not on the tracks themselves.
- Tell the driver to leave the warning lights on to attract the attention of railroad personnel as well as motorists.

- Quickly assess the situation. Determine whether the vehicle wreckage is on or close to the tracks. Decide whether the hose lines, hydraulic rescue tool hoses, or electric cables must be laid across active tracks and whether any other condition exists wherein a train will threaten emergency service personnel.
- Make your dispatcher aware of the situation.
- Have the dispatcher contact the railroad dispatcher with a request to stop all trains headed for the grade crossing from both directions.
- Be sure that the railroad dispatcher knows the exact location of the crossing. In industrial areas and areas near switching yards, it's possible for a road to be crossed by tracks at several locations.

Locations along railroad rights-of-way are usually identified by mileposts. While marking systems may vary from railroad to railroad, mileposts always indicate the distance from a point of origin. Grade crossings are also provided with markers from which a railroad dispatcher can immediately determine the ownership of the tracks and the exact location of the crossing.

- Have your dispatcher determine from the railroad dispatcher the time that the next train is scheduled to reach the crossing and the direction from which it will approach.

If you learn that there is not much time before a train will reach the intersection:

- Have a rescuer or firefighter attempt to flag the train to a stop.

Stopping Approaching Trains

Unenlightened individuals tend to think that stopping a train is merely a matter of walking a short distance down the tracks, throwing up a hand, and shouting, "Stop!" One has about as much chance of stopping a train in this way as arrogant King Croesus did when he stood at the edge of the ocean and tried to stop the incoming tide with an upraised hand. Here's why:

- For every second it takes the engineer to apply the emergency brakes after he realizes that a collision is imminent, a train that is moving at 60 miles per hour will travel 88 feet.
- A minimum of 15.4 seconds is required for the braking system to begin any significant reduction in the train's speed, in which time the train will travel a distance of 1350 feet.
- Once the braking action starts, the train will travel a total of 1-1/2 miles before it stops.
- Even when moving at only 30 miles per hour, a train will travel for 2/3 mile before stopping after the engineer applies the emergency brake.

Suppose that instead of being the officer who is giving the orders, you are the rescuer who is assigned the task of attempting to stop the approaching train.

- Put on your turnout gear (more for identification than protection) and get two or three flares from the rescue unit. Don't take just one flare; it may not ignite.
- Carry a portable radio with you so you can notify the rescue officer (1) that the train is in sight or (2) that the train has stopped on your signal or (3) that the train has not stopped on your signal and is proceeding to the grade crossing.
- Go down the tracks in the direction from which the train will come to a point 1-1/2 to 2 miles from the grade crossing. Stop when you reach a point where you can be clearly seen by the engineer.
- Place a lighted flare upright between the tracks.

When you see or hear the approaching train:

- Light another flare.
- Swing it slowly back and forth horizontally across your body at a right angle to the track (Figure 5.01).

This is the stop signal used by all railroads. The locomotive engineer should acknowledge the stop signal with two whistle blasts and then stop the train. Do not wave your arms frantically or use any other hand signal. The engineer might misinterpret the signal or disregard it altogether as merely a greeting and not stop the train. Keep in mind that engineers are used to having people wave at them. Don't rely on your turnout gear to give authority to wild arm waving. Engineers claim to have seen some pretty weird sights on their runs.

An important point: A flare should be used to signal both day or night. If a flare is not available, a flag or other brightly colored object should be waved during daylight hours and a bright flashlight or battery-powered hand light should be waved at night.

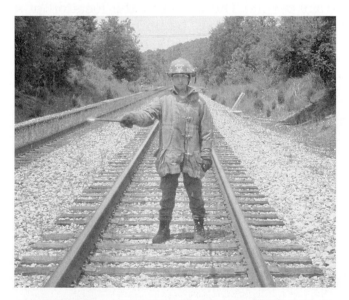

FIGURE 5.01   Stopping Train with Flare

Working On or Near Active Tracks

Let's say that a collision has occurred near to but not directly on the tracks of an active grade crossing. You're the officer in charge of the rescue operation. Circumstances are such that you do not feel it is necessary to stop a train that is likely to reach a crossing before the rescue operation is over, or your dispatcher informs you that a soon-to-arrive train cannot be stopped.

- Provide a rescuer or firefighter with a Freon-powered warning horn or a traffic control whistle and a red flag.
- Instruct the rescuer to go down the tracks in the direction from which the train will come to a point where he can still be seen and heard by rescuers at the crossing.
- Tell the rescuer to sound a warning and wave the flag as soon as he sees the approaching train.

As you proceed with the rescue operation, listen for the rescuer's horn, and also for the train's horn. You may hear the horn being sounded for a distant grade crossing. The grade crossing signal is two long blasts followed by a short blast and one more long blast. The signal is prolonged or repeated until the crossing is occupied by the engine or the lead car. When you hear either the rescuer's signal or the train's horn:

- Have emergency service personnel stand well back from the tracks until the train clears the crossing.

Many emergency service personnel think that railroad torpedoes are used to stop trains, so they carry these explosive devices on rescue vehicles for that purpose. The explosion of one or two torpedoes signals an engineer to proceed at reduced speed, not to stop. Another misconception is that a train can be stopped by laying a metal ladder or pike pole across the rails. While this may have caused a signal to flash in the cab of an engine in the past, it has no effect today.

VEHICULAR TRAFFIC

Accidents invariably produce some sort of traffic problem. If a collision occurs along a two-lane road, the roadway is often completely blocked by wreckage. At the very least, vehicles moving in both directions will be obliged to use one lane or the shoulder of the road in order to move past the accident scene. A collision on a four-lane highway can necessitate the merging of two or three lanes of vehicles into one lane, with the result being a massive traffic jam. Even on a six-lane divided superhighway, a relatively minor accident can cause a tremendous traffic problem. There need be no physical impediment such as wreckage; traffic jams can occur when curious drivers slow their vehicles as they pass an accident scene so they can see what has happened. The slow-moving traffic is often referred to as "gapers' block," or "rubberneckers."

Traffic problems can be minimized in three ways: by controlling lane flow, by establishing a blockade, or by creating a detour.

SPECTATORS

One thing common to all motor vehicle accidents, regardless of severity, is that they attract people. The crowd at the location of a minor incident may be no larger than a few people, while hundreds of onlookers may gather at the scene of a multiple-vehicle, multiple-casualty accident, especially when traffic flow has stopped altogether. It's a quirk of human nature that, instead of being repelled, many people are attracted to the gruesome sights common to motor vehicle accidents. Without close supervision, spectators will often press so close to wrecked vehicles that they interfere with the rescue effort. Onlookers can compromise safety, and they can have a definitely adverse effect on injured persons.

A victim does not need close contact with spectators, whether the contact is physical, verbal, or visual. Onlookers can contribute to a trapped and injured person's fear and apprehension by making comments such as "My God! Doesn't he look awful?" or "Jeez, did you ever see such a mess?" The mere fact that spectators are able to see a victim can cause the person anguish. Men are usually embarrassed when they know that onlookers can see their helplessness, while women are often especially conscious of people watching them if their clothes are torn or disheveled. For these reasons, spectators should be kept at a distance from the wreckage.

UNCONFINED ELECTRICITY

Like many other people, you have probably had an unpleasant experience with electricity. Perhaps you received a mild (but frightening) shock while using a power tool or experienced a fire caused by a frayed cord or a faulty appliance. If you are an experienced medic as well as a rescuer, you may have been required to care for a person who has been electrocuted. You may have seen the severe burns and terrible entrance and exit wounds caused by high-voltage, high-amperage electricity. Fearful as you may be of electricity, however, you cannot simply walk away from a downed wire or expect it to go away. Nor can you always expect someone else to come along and manage the hazard. In a life or death situation, there may not be someone else, especially in rural areas. This is not to say that the officers of your squad should run out and buy lineman's gloves and line-handling equipment. That is a decision that should be made only after careful consideration of the problem of downed wires and consultation with the local power company. Some power companies will do everything they can to discourage the use of lineman's equipment by emergency service personnel; others will offer suggestions for equipment and even conduct training programs.

Broken Utility Pole with Wires Intact; Car Contacting the Pole

If you arrive at the scene and discover that a broken utility pole is suspended or supported by wires:

- Assume the danger zone to be the same as it would be if wires are down, and park the rescue unit at the edge of the zone.
- Advise your dispatcher of the situation and request the immediate response of a power company crew.
- Provide your dispatcher with the number of the nearest standing pole and other pertinent information.
- Ask him to advise you of the estimated time of arrival of the power company crew.
- Then attempt to communicate with the occupants of the endangered vehicle.

If the occupants of the vehicle are conscious and coherent:

- Make them aware of their situation.
- Advise them to remain motionless in the vehicle until power company employees can de-energize the conductors and stabilize the pole.
- Then stand by in a safe place until the power company crew can de-energize the conductors and stabilize the pole.

Broken Utility Pole with Wires Down

Keep these important points in mind whenever you discover that wires are down:

- High voltages are not as uncommon on roadside utility poles as people think. Wood poles sometimes support conductors of as much as 500,000 volts.
- In addition to primary and secondary power conductors, utility poles also support telephone and TV subscriber cables, and conductors for fire alarm, street light, and traffic control circuits.

- Guy wires, the bright, uninsulated wire ropes that lead from utility poles to anchor points in the ground, can become conductors when contacted by a broken wire.
- Voltages of primary and secondary conductors cannot be determined from the size of the wire and the number of standoff insulators.
- The coverings of high-voltage conductors serve more to protect the conductors from the weather than to insulate them, especially when the wires are carrying more than 7000 volts.
- There is no way to tell the direction of current feed.
- Fuses do not always blow and circuit breakers do not always open when power distribution lines go to the ground. The load must be greater than the rating of the safety device.
- When a pole is broken and wires are crossed, every wire supported by the pole may be conducting the highest voltage available, regardless of its purpose or usual load.
- The pole itself or the ground cable attached to the pole may be energized.
- If a wire is not arcing, there is no way to determine whether a downed conductor is energized without a testing device.
- Energized downed wires do not always arc and burn.
- There is no assurance that a dead wire at the scene of an accident will not become energized again unless it is cut or disconnected from the system. When an interruption of current is sensed in most power distribution systems, automatic devices restore the flow two or three times over a period of minutes.
- Ordinary personal protective clothing does not afford protection against electrocution.

Let's say that your rescue unit is safely parked at the edge of the danger zone. The first step is to get specialized assistance on the way and nonessential personnel out of the way.

- Determine the number of the nearest pole you can approach safely.
- Have your dispatcher advise the power company dispatcher of the exact location of the accident, the pole number, and any other pertinent facts.

While you are communicating with your dispatcher:

- Direct other rescuers to clear the danger zone of spectators and non-essential emergency service personnel.

What you do next depends on whether your rescue unit has equipment for moving downed wires: lineman's gloves, and either a clampstick and a hotstick or a weighted throwing line. If your unit does *not* have the proper equipment:

- Do not allow squad members to attempt to move the wire with a wood pole, a wood-handled tool, a tree branch, a natural fiber rope, or anything else that may be moist.

Instead:

- Have them remain outside the danger zone until a power company representative (or specially trained and equipped emergency service personnel) can cut the wire or otherwise disconnect it from the distribution system.
- Prevent spectators and non-essential emergency service personnel from entering the danger zone until the hazard has been eliminated.
- Prohibit traffic flow through the danger zone.

If it appears that they are inclined to do so:

- Discourage occupants from leaving any vehicle contacted by the downed wire.

Uninjured or slightly injured but conscious persons who are still in the vehicles (but not trapped) may not be aware of the electrical hazard. They may not know that a high-voltage conductor is lying on top of the car, or that a wire is lying on the ground directly beneath the door. To open the door and step out may mean instant death.

Many emergency service personnel advocate a procedure whereby victims open a door, crouch in the doorway, and jump clear of the vehicle. It is not likely that an elderly person will be able to do this safely, or an injured person or an obese person or a young child or a person confused as the result of a blow to the head. Any of these people could be fatally electrocuted if he slips and allows one foot to touch the ground while he is crouched in the doorway or if he falls backward after jumping from the wreckage. It is far better for a person to remain in a vehicle until the electrical hazard is controlled.

- Get as close to the vehicle as you can without endangering yourself.
- Quickly gain the occupant's attention and tell him that he must not try to leave the car even though he feels he can do so safely.
- Be forceful in your explanation, but not so forceful that you scare the person.

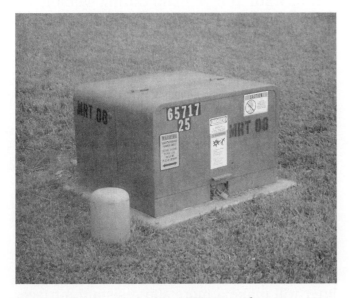

FIGURE 5.02   Pad-Mounted Transformer

When you have gained the occupant's confidence:

- Stay in his sight as long as you can do so safely. If you walk away, the person may think the danger is over and attempt to leave the vehicle.

Pad-Mounted Transformer Damaged by Vehicle

Transformers that are mounted on concrete pads outside a building (Figure 5.02), normally step-down primary voltage in areas where electric power is received and distributed by means of underground cables. These transformers are often found on the front lawns of private dwellings. They're not very pretty, so many homeowners attempt to conceal them by building a falsework of brick, block, or stone or by planting shrubbery around them.

There is very little you can do in a situation when a vehicle has struck a pad-mounted transformer other than call for help and keep people away from the vehicle. You cannot touch the car for any reason (such as gaining access to trapped persons or rigging a tow line) until a power company employee tells you that the transformer has been de-energized.

If you respond to the location and discover that a vehicle has struck a pad-mounted transformer and is resting against or on top of the case:

- Advise your dispatcher of the situation and request the immediate response of a power company representative.
- Request the response of an engine company if one is not already on the scene or on the way.
- Do not touch either the vehicle or the transformer case, even if it appears that service to nearby buildings has been disrupted.

While secondary connections to the transformer may have been broken, the primary connections may still be intact and may be energizing the transformer case and the vehicle with as much as 34,000 volts.

- Instead, stand by in a safe place until a power company representative can assure you that the transformer is no longer energized.

If people inside the vehicle are ambulatory and want to leave the vehicle:

- Persuade them to stay where they are.

If the transformer is burning:

- Approach the transformer from upwind if you can do so safely and attempt to extinguish the fire with a 20-pound A:B:C dry chemical extinguisher.
- Be sure that you do not get so close to the transformer that the extinguisher nozzle contacts the case.

If an engine company is on the scene:

- Have firefighters extinguish the fire from an upwind position with water fog or dry chemical extinguishers.

While you are standing by:

- Keep spectators and other emergency service personnel from the danger zone.
- Have rescuers or firefighters light the scene if it is dark.

VEHICLE ON FIRE

Extinguishing a major vehicle fire is usually the responsibility of people who are trained and equipped for the job: firefighters. It should be routine for an engine company to respond to the location of an incident that has produced injuries and entrapment. Unfortunately, this is not a standard operating practice. In many areas, fire-suppression units remain in quarters until they are called by the rescue officer or the EMS per-

son in charge *after* he arrives at accident locations.

When the fire potential at the scene is high, the delayed response of fire-suppression units can be disastrous. If fire breaks out in a vehicle during the rescue operations and squad members are neither trained nor properly equipped for the emergency, rescue squad members will be able to do nothing more than stand by helplessly and perhaps watch people burn to death until firefighting units respond.

The lack of an automatic response plan is not the only reason for this sad predicament. Normally, first-due firefighting units may be in service at another location. Second-due units may be a considerable distance from the scene. Roads may be blocked during storms. For these and many other reasons, rescue vehicles *must* be equipped with at least several portable fire extinguishers, and EMS personnel *must* be trained in their use.

UNSAFE WORK AREA

What you don't need at the already hazardous scene is anything else that can increase the potential for injury. A slippery road and darkness can do just that. Both you and the people you are trying to help can be injured if you slip during gaining access, disentanglement, or removal activities, and to use tools in darkness near trapped people is to invite disaster.

Making Road Surfaces Slip Resistant

You can be reasonably sure of safe footing if you wear cleats or creepers while working on an icy road. Other emergency service personnel that you may have to rely on during a critical procedure may not have such protection, so steps should be taken to provide a sure footing for them.

Sand can be sprinkled on an icy road, but the sharp, irregular-shaped granules of cat litter will make a more slip-resistant surface. Moreover, cat litter is effective on a larger area than an equivalent amount of sand. Like sand, cat litter can be used to make a fuel- or oil-covered road less slippery. Cat litter can be stored and carried in a gallon plastic milk jug or any other large plastic container that has a handle.

Lighting the Work Area

Emergency vehicle headlights are poor sources of illumination. They cannot be repositioned as needed; they illuminate only one side of an accident vehicle (or two sides if the light strikes them at an angle); they do not provide shadow-free illumination; and they are invariably at the height where they will shine directly into your eyes if you must work facing them.

The initial close-up illumination of a vehicle can be accomplished with a 12-volt trouble light that has a 25- or 50-foot cord terminating in battery clips. When it is possible to connect the light to the damaged vehicle's battery, rescuers who are responsible for gaining access to seriously injured persons have an immediate source of bright light while other rescuers are connecting floodlights to cords and generators.

Good illumination of work areas can be accomplished with floodlights, hand lights, and even personal flashlights. The secret of success is having at least two lights. Use Cyalume Lightsticks for illumination when there are not sufficient hand lights for several work areas or when light is needed near a flammable fuel. Every rescue unit should have these versatile alternative sources of light.

INSTABILITY

Of all the hazard management procedures that might be necessary during vehicle rescue efforts, the least employed is vehicle stabilization. There are many reasons why rescue personnel fail to stabilize vehicles. They may not be trained in stabilization techniques, or they may not be equipped (or so they think). But the principal reason for not stabilizing vehicles is that in many accident situations the involved vehicles *appear* stable, especially in

the eyes of untrained rescuers. Whether they *are* stable depends on factors such as the type of vehicle, the nature and degree of damage to the vehicle, the position in which the vehicle has come to rest, and the character of the terrain under the vehicle.

Following are suggested procedures for stabilizing vehicles in three positions: on all four wheels, on a side, and on the roof. Since stabilization is a team effort, the procedures are written as instructions to a rescue officer, in this case a lieutenant, who is in charge of a team of four squad members. If you are a rescue officer, take note of how each operation is conducted in its entirety. If you are a squad member, pay particular attention to how each task is accomplished to ultimately achieve stabilization.

Stabilizing a Vehicle on Its Wheels

The vehicle that is least likely to be stabilized during a rescue operation is the car that is resting upright on all four inflated wheels, even one that is severely damaged as the result of a front-end or rear-end collision. Why? Because it *looks* stable!

In addition to the usual cuts and bruises associated with an accident, the driver and occupants can also suffer face and skull injuries, knee fractures and dislocations, fractured femurs, dislocated hips, broken ribs, flail chest, and a variety of internal injuries. But the injuries that can be aggravated most by the movements of an unstable vehicle are cervical spine injuries.

Let's say that, instead of colliding at high speed, two vehicles meet at a much lower speed. Collision forces were just enough to crumple the front ends of the vehicles, but more than enough to damage the cervical spine of one of the drivers and two of the passengers in the vehicles. Some of the occupants are sitting upright, while others are slumped in their seats. All the doors of both vehicles are either locked or jammed. If the cars are not rigidly stabilized, the motions that usually result from operations for gaining access may be sufficient to cause damaged cervical vertebrae to shift and sever the underlying spinal cord. Instead of spending a few weeks with a sore neck supported by a cervical collar, some of the occupants may spend the rest of their lives as quadraplegics confined to a wheelchair.

Preventing Forward and Rearward Movements

Preventing the forward and rearward movements of a vehicle that is on its wheels serves two purposes. It keeps the vehicle from rolling down a hill. More importantly, it minimizes dangerous rocking motions that can be transmitted to injured persons during certain rescue operations. Manually widening door openings creates such rocking motions.

USING WHEEL CHOCKS

A well-equipped rescue unit has two pairs of wheel chocks, one to prevent forward movements of the unit after it is parked and one for stabilizing vehicles that have remained on their wheels.

- Position one chock against the front-facing tread of the front wheel and the other chock against the rear-facing tread of the rear wheel on the same side.
- Be sure that both chocks are wedged snugly against both wheels.

USING CRIBBING

If your rescue unit does not have two pairs of wheel chocks, but has cribbing, use 2 by 4's to stabilize a vehicle on its wheels.

- Position one piece of cribbing with the face of the block against the tire tread where the tread contacts the road or ground.
- Hold it in place with one hand while you wedge a second piece of cribbing between the first piece and the road or ground with your other hand.
- Then build a similar chock behind the rear wheel. A finished cribbing chock is shown in Figure 5.03.

USING VEHICLE PARTS OR DEBRIS

There is less chance for a wheel to ride over cribbing placed in this manner if a vehicle is not in gear and a push starts it moving. A wheel can easily ride over a single piece of 2-by 4-inch cribbing laid on the ground.

If you have neither wheel chocks nor cribbing, use whatever you can find on the scene to prevent the forward and rearward movement of a vehicle on its wheels. If they are the deep-dish type, the vehicle's wheel covers will work well.

- Pry two wheel covers from the vehicle.
- Jam one wheel cover under the forward portion of the front wheel and the second cover under the rearward portion of the rear wheel.

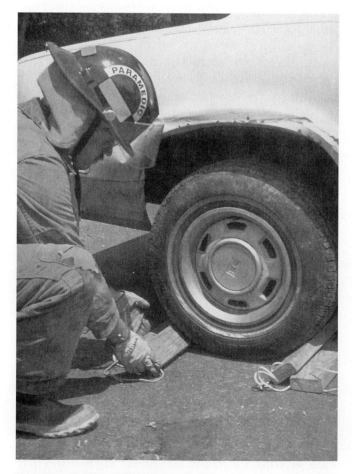

FIGURE 5.03   Cribbing Chock

Deflating the Vehicle's Tires

If you have absolutely nothing else that you can use to prevent the forward and rearward movement of a vehicle, deflate the tires. It is difficult for a vehicle to start rolling when all four tires are flat. Do not waste time by depressing the one-way valve in the valve stems or by removing the valve stems, even if you have the tool designed for the job. Instead:

- Cut the valve stem of each tire close to where it projects from the wheel with a sharp knife or simply pull the valve stem from the wheel with pliers (Figure 5.04).

The valve stem for a tubeless tire has a rubber collar that fits behind the rim; it is held in place by air pressure and can be easily pulled from the wheel.

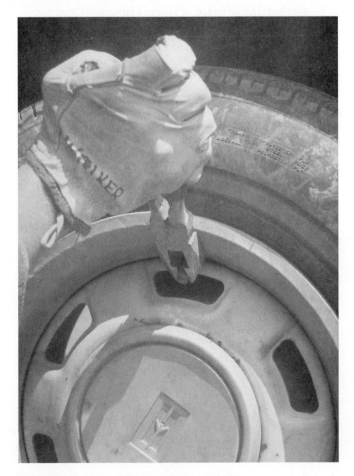

FIGURE 5.04   Pulling Valve Stem

As soon as possible:

- Alert the police officer in charge of the scene that the tires of the vehicle have been purposely deflated.

If the officer is busy with other duties:

- Use chalk or a lumber crayon to mark the tires with a symbol that will tell the officer that the tires are flat as a result of the rescue effort, not the accident. This act of courtesy will assist the accident investigation officers.

An important point: It has been argued that deflating tires is a dangerous procedure, that when the valve stem is removed, the car will suddenly drop and dangerous jolts will be transmitted to injured occupants. This is simply not so. A fully inflated tire will take about 10 seconds to deflate when the valve stem is removed, in which time the vehicle will settle gently onto the steel wheels.

STABILIZING WITH BOX CRIBBING

Cribbing at four points under a passenger car creates an almost rigid structure that defies movement during usual rescue operations. Spring action and tire bounce are virtually eliminated. Following is a procedure that you might lead a team of rescuers through to assure that a vehicle that is on its wheels is truly stable.

When rescuers have placed chocks or other devices against the front and rear wheels:

- Have the rescuers work in pairs, one pair to each side of the car, and build box cribs under the frame rail of the car at four points: one behind the front wheel and another ahead of the rear wheel on each side of the vehicle.
- Instruct the rescuers to build the cribs just to the point where another layer of cribbing cannot be inserted.

A box crib is a simple framework of 2 by 4's. Two pieces of cribbing are laid on the ground parallel to each other about 9 or 10 inches apart. Another layer of two pieces is laid on the first layer, also parallel to each other about 9 inches apart, but at right angles to the first layer. A third layer is added in the same manner, and so on (Figure 5.05).

The last pieces of cribbing that can be installed without lifting the side of the car should be placed at a right angle to the frame rail. If this is not possible, the crib should be rotated 90 degrees. Thus the final layer of cribbing can be positioned at a right angle to the frame. This assures firm contact between the body of the car and the crib.

When the basic cribs are finished:

- Instruct one rescuer from each pair to crouch with his back to the front fender and his hands gripping the fender well.

On your command "lift":

- Have the one rescuer gently lift the side of the car slightly while the other rescuer inserts the last layer of cribbing.

On your command "lower":

- Have the rescuer *gently* lower the front side of the car onto the crib.

- Repeat the procedure to finish the crib ahead of the rear wheels and thus stabilize the car.

Proper stance is important. The position described enables the rescuers to lift with their legs, not the back. Gentle movement is also important. Sudden jerky movements of the fenders, especially movements that are greater than necessary, are transmitted to the vehicle's unprotected occupants.

USING STEP CRIBBING

Step cribbing of the type shown in Figure 5.06 eliminates the need to build cribs in the manner just described.

- Instruct rescuers to work in pairs (a pair to each side of the car) and position the four pieces of step cribbing on the ground at a right angle to the car at locations where they will be inserted: under the frame rail behind the front wheel and ahead of the rear wheel.

When the cribs are in place:

- Have both rescuers move to the front wheel on their side of the vehicle.

On your command "lift":

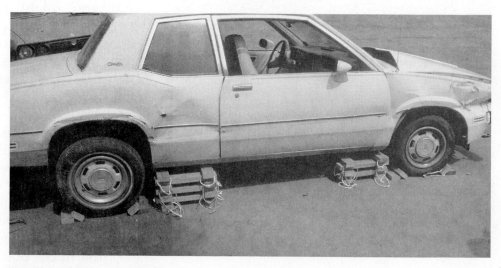

FIGURE 5.05   Box Crib

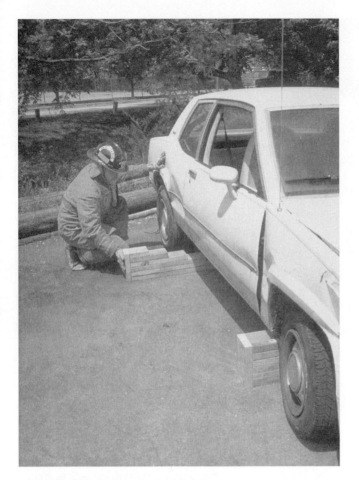

FIGURE 5.06 Step Cribbing

- Have one rescuer of each team crouch and gently lift the fender while the other rescuer moves the pieces of step cribbing into position.

On your command "lower":

- Have the rescuer gently lower the fender to seat the frame rail on the cribbing.
- Repeat the procedure with the rear wheel.

Ideally, a vehicle is stabilized on its wheels at four points in either of the ways just described. However, there may be times when you will not have sufficient cribbing for four-point stabilization, as when it is necessary to use most of the cribbing supply to steady a vehicle on its side. In this case, use the remaining cribbing to stabilize the vehicle at two points, or use other devices for two-point stabilization. Partial stabilization is far better than no stabilization at all.

USING HI-LIFT JACKS

Two of these versatile jacks can be used with cribbing as shown in Figure 5.07, or alone for two-point stabilization if they are not needed for another operation such as raising a crushed roof, displacing a steering column, or lifting the side of a car to reach someone trapped underneath.

- Direct a pair of rescuers on each side of the car to position a Hi-Lift jack so that the lifting toe just engages the edge of the front fender well.

On your command "lift":

- Have the rescuers operate the lifting mechanisms until the front end of the car is supported by the jacks, not the springs.

Just how far the rescuers should lift the car with the jacks will be a judgment call on your part. By means of a few gentle nudges, you should be able to tell when the car is reasonably solid. Notice that the handles are taped vertically to prevent them from being an obstacle and being knocked loose.

USING BUMPER JACKS

Even though they were not designed for the job, notch-style bumper jacks can be pressed into service as stabilizing devices when other tools are either not available or needed for other tasks. Contour-style bumper jacks should *not* be used to stabilize a vehicle on its wheels. By the time the lifting toe of the jack contacts the edge of the fender well, the ratchet mechanisms will be at the top of the jack post. The resulting support itself will be unstable.

If notch-style jacks are not carried on the rescue unit as an emergency lifting and stabilizing device, they can usually be obtained from police cruisers, first responder units,

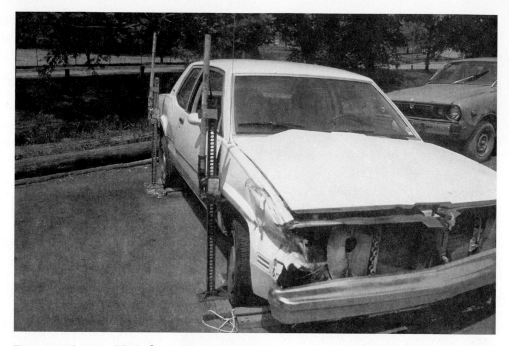

FIGURE 5.07   Hi-Lift Jacks

the cars of volunteers who have responded to the scene, and even spectators' cars.

Do not allow rescuers to attempt to catch the edge of a fender well with this sort of jack; the narrow lifting toe is too short. Instead:

- Have the rescuers work in pairs on each side of the car if there are two jacks and two sets of tools.
- Instruct the rescuers to make an opening in the sheet metal between the fender well and the wraparound portion of the grill, or in the quarter panel, with the pike of a combination forcible entry tool. The hole should be as low as possible in order to keep the ratchet mechanism of the jack close to the base.

Do not allow the rescuers to drive the pike of the forcible entry tool into the sheet metal by swinging the tool like a baseball bat, however. Have the other rescuer of each two-person team strike the anvil portion of the tool with a long- or short-handled sledgehammer. The rescuer holding the tool will have better control.

- Have the rescuers rotate the tool with the pike in the hole until the tool handle is vertical.
- Instruct the rescuers to make a lip in the opening by pulling the handle downward with one hand while holding the head of the tool in place with the other hand, thus corrugating the metal (Figure 5.08).

This is an important step. If the sheet metal is curved or damaged, the rescuer may not be able to insert the lifting toe of the jack into the opening. Moreover, making a lip in the manner just described minimizes the chance that the sheet metal will tear when lifting forces are exerted.

When the openings are made:

- Have a rescuer on each side of the car insert the lifting toe of the jack into the prepared opening and operate the ratchet mechanism until the lifting toe is supporting the vehicle (Figure 5.09).

If sufficient cribbing is available for only two, but not four cribs, they should be built under

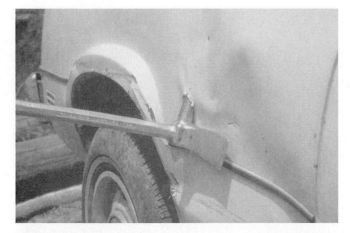

FIGURE 5.08   Making a Hole and Corrugating

the frame rails in front of the rear wheels. Then jacks can be used in either of the ways just described to support the front end of the vehicle and achieve four-point stabilization.

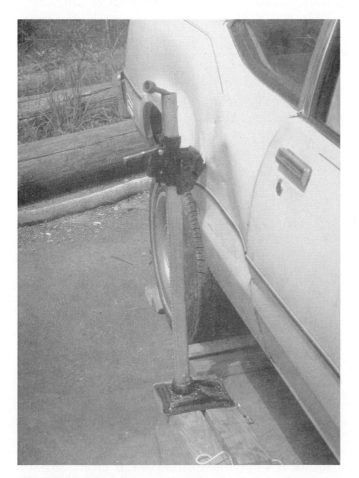

FIGURE 5.09   Bumper Jack

Stabilizing a Vehicle on Its Side

If the vehicle on its side is a truck larger than a pickup truck, the chance is good that once it has rolled onto its side the truck will simply continue to skid in that position until it hits something or stops. And unless the damage is so great that the truck is no longer box shaped or unless the ground under the truck is extremely uneven, the truck is likely to be stable.

This is not usually the case with passenger cars, however. When a more cylindrical than boxlike car rolls onto its side for any of a number of reasons, it is likely to roll several more times and perhaps even tumble end over end before coming to a stop, especially if it was traveling at a high speed before it started to roll. Because of all of the things that can happen to the vehicle and the people in and around it, a passenger car on its side must be rigidly supported in that position.

The Importance of Vertical Stabilization

The correct procedure is to stabilize a vehicle on its side in as near a vertical position as possible. Three benefits will be realized; they are illustrated in Figure 5.10.

First, the vehicle's base of stability will be widened. The base of stability is the distance between the parts of the vehicle that are contacting the ground, in this case the sides and roof edges. The wider the base of stability, the more stable the vehicle.

Second, any downward force exerted on the upper side of the car (a rescuer's weight, for example) will be exerted straight down.

Third, one of several techniques can be used to create an opening through which the injured occupants can be removed safely. Depending on the stabilization method employed and the rescue tools available, a three-sided flap can be cut in the roof and folded down, a section of the roof can be folded back, the entire roof can be folded down, or the roof can be removed altogether.

Stabilizing a Vehicle in the Vertical Position

There are dozens of ways that a passenger car can be stabilized in a vertical position on its side, ranging from simply having people support the car, to supporting the vehicle with pneumatic jacks or hydraulic rams. Several techniques are described and illustrated here to demonstrate that vertical stabilization can be accomplished by rescue personnel regardless of the size of their rescue unit and the nature of its equipment.

Before you read the descriptions of the procedures, consider these two important points.

- Stabilizing a passenger car in the vertical position does require moving the car a bit. This is not as dangerous an activity as it may seem at first glance. You will not be moving the car away from the occupants, but rather moving the car and the occupants as a unit. Even if an injured arm or leg does move a bit during the stabilization procedure, it's far better to risk aggravating such an injury than risk having the unsupported vehicle drop onto its wheels during the rescue effort.
- The procedures described here, while they may appear complicated at first glance, can be accomplished by just a few rescuers when forces are limited.

Now let's consider the procedures. You are the officer assigned to the task of stabilizing a car on its side; you have a team of four rescuers. The car's side and roof edge are contacting the ground, the most common position when a vehicle comes to rest on its side following a rollover.

USING CRIBBING

Approximately 25 lengths of 2- by 4- by 18-inch cribbing are needed for this procedure. It results in excellent four-point stabilization (Figure 5.11).

If occupants are conscious and moving around in the car, perhaps in an effort to escape:

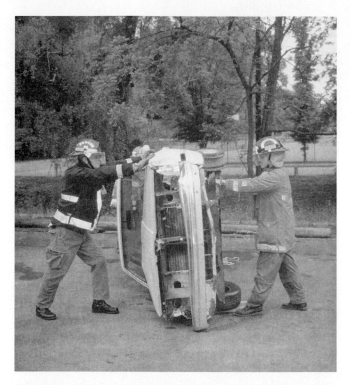

FIGURE 5.10   Car on Its Side with Hi-Lift and Cribbing

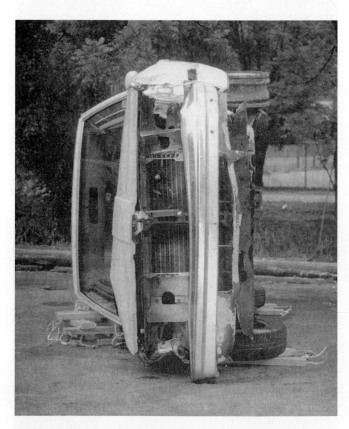

FIGURE 5.11   Stabilization of Car on Its Side with Cribbing on Tire Side

- Stand in front of the windshield where you can be seen.
- Identify yourself and explain what you are going to do.
- Ask the occupants to remain quite still for the next few minutes.

This is an important step. The car is perched precariously as it is, and movements of the occupants may cause the vehicle to topple onto its roof, especially if the roof and roof pillars are damaged.

- Instruct two rescuers to simultaneously build two box cribs, one under the front wheel and one under the rear wheel. Have the rescuers build the cribs just high enough to support the car when it is moved to the vertical position.

Three layers are needed to support most full-sized sedans in the vertical position; only one or two layers will be needed to support a more boxed-shaped small car. While the two rescuers are building the cribs, the other two rescuers can be laying out cribbing on the other side of the car.

Moving the car from the position found to the vertical position is the next step.

- Instruct one rescuer to stand at the rear end of the car.
- Tell the other three rescuers to take positions next to the roof of the vehicle. You stand at the front end of the car where you can clearly see to the left and right.

The rescuers standing at the roof of the car will ease the vehicle into the vertical position and onto the cribbing. You and the rescuer standing at the rear end of the vehicle will be safety persons. Together you will prevent the car from moving so quickly that it settles onto the cribbing with a jolt, which could be harmful to the occupants.

Stance is important. You and the rescuer at the other end of the car must stand where you can either pull the car onto the cribbing

or hold it back if it starts to move too quickly. Do not stand where the car can trap you if it rolls over the cribbing.

When you and the rest of your team are in position:

- Tell the rescuers who are standing next to the roof of the car that, on your command "push," they should gently push on the uppermost portion of the roof.
- Explain that if they push with one hand and crook the fingers of the other hand against the drip molding or the window frame, they will be able to carefully control the speed with which the car moves.
- Tell the rescuer at the rear end of the car either to assist with the movement of the vehicle onto the cribs if it appears to be moving too slowly or not at all or to slow its travel if it appears to be moving too fast.

When everyone is ready:

- Give the command to ease the car onto the cribbing.

If the cribs under the wheels are the right height, the car will be within a few degrees of vertical when it settles onto them. Since most of the weight of the vehicle is being supported by the ground, very little force will be needed to maintain the car vertically during the remainder of the stabilization operation.

- Instruct one of the rescuers to remain in position pushing on the roof.
- Tell him to either angle his body and hold his arms straight against the uppermost portion of the roof or stand sideways with his shoulder against the roof for maximum push and stability.

While that rescuer continues to maintain the car vertically with the wheels against the cribs:

- Have the other two rescuers build two more cribs, one under the A-pillar of the vehicle and one under the C-pillar (Figure 5.12).

The top surface of the last layer of cribbing should be level with the juncture of the A-pillar and the C-pillar with the body of the vehicle, and the layer should be solid instead of open (that is, with the pieces of cribbing touching). Thus it will serve as a base for the piece of cribbing that will be used to "lock" the car in the vertical position.

When both cribs are finished to the level just described:

- Tell the rescuers building them to place one more piece of cribbing on the top of each crib, positioned at a right angle to the roof pillar.
- Tell the rescuers at the cribs that, on your command "push," you and the other rescuer will exert force on the uppermost portion of the roof and push the car against the cribs on the other side.
- Tell them that you will hold the car in this slightly exaggerated position while they push the final pieces of cribbing into the spaces that develop between the top of each crib and the roof pillar.
- Tell them to give the signal "ready" when they have the final piece of cribbing in place and that, on hearing their signals, you will give the command "release," and you and the other rescuer will relax and allow the car to settle onto the cribs.

When everyone is ready:

- Give the series of commands and lock the car in the vertical position.

When pushing forces are relaxed, the car will settle onto the cribs and lock the final pieces of cribbing in place. It will be in as vertical a position as possible, and forces generated by the weight of the vehicle will be exerted straight down into the ground.

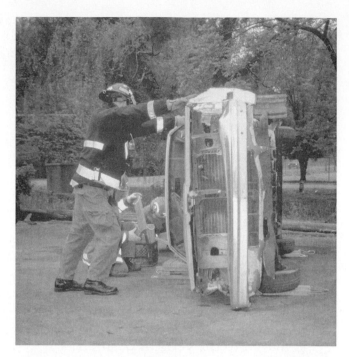

FIGURE 5.12 Stabilization of Car on Its Side with Cribbing at Top Side

As you can imagine, wedges can be used to finish the cribs built under the roof pillars. Experience has shown that this locking procedure is far superior, however; wedges have a tendency to slip.

- Finally, go around the car and check each of the cribs.
- Make adjustments as necessary to assure that all the cribs are tight.

Figure 5.13 shows a car stabilized at four points with cribbing. Note that the car is perfectly vertical and that the base of stability has been increased from 18 inches to almost 5 feet. Moreover, the roof is completely accessible. Depending on the requirements for disentanglement and removal and the tools available:

- A three-sided flap can be cut in the roof and folded down like a door; or
- The roof can be folded down after the A-, B-, and C-pillars are cut; or
- The roof can be folded back after the A- and B-pillars are cut and notches are

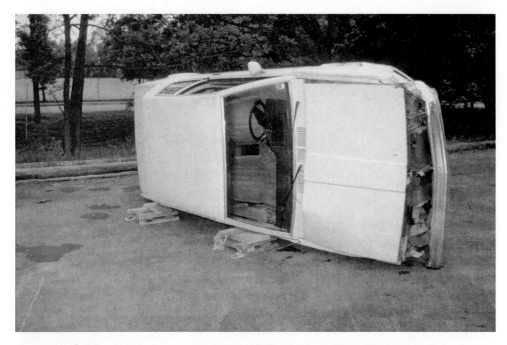

FIGURE 5.13 Stabilization of Car on Its Side with Cribbing Overall

made in the roof edges ahead of the C-pillars; or

- A section of the roof can be removed after cutting the A- and B-pillars, if necessary, and then cutting through the roof from one edge to the other; or
- The roof can be removed altogether after severing all the roof pillars.

If you are reading about this procedure for the first time, you may have formed the opinion by now that stabilizing a car on its side with cribbing is a lengthy and difficult procedure. It is neither. It can be accomplished by four rescuers in exactly the manner described in less than 45 seconds after only a few practice sessions. Rescuers used to working together can usually accomplish the procedure in about 35 seconds.

USING CRIBBING AND A HI-LIFT JACK

Two- or three-point stabilization is possible, depending on the amount of cribbing available. Three-point stabilization can generally be achieved with 12 to 16 pieces of cribbing, while two-point stabilization is possible with half that amount.

If you have sufficient cribbing:

- Have rescuers build a box crib under each wheel.
- Ease the car onto the cribbing.

While two of the team members hold the vehicle in place:

- Have the other two rescuers position and operate the jack.
- Stand at the front end of the car so that you can tell the jack operator to stop when the vehicle is vertical.

The lifting toe of the jack should be positioned under the edge of the roof just behind the A-pillar. It will engage the drip molding and in some cars the window frame.

Figure 5.14 shows a car that has been stabilized on its side with cribbing and a Hi-Lift jack. As you can see, while the vehicle is stable, the jack is in a position where it will prohibit rescuers from folding the roof down or back or removing the roof altogether.

Squad members will still be able to make a three-sided flap in the roof and fold the resulting "door" down, however, and one of the

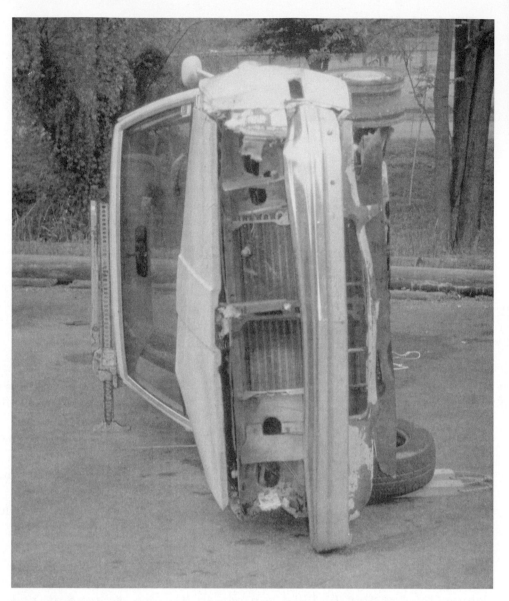

FIGURE 5.14   Stabilization of Car on Its Side with Cribbing and Hi-Lift Jack

vertical cuts can be made as close to the jack as the cutting tool will allow. The jack is supporting the frame of the roof, and cutting the sheet metal will not compromise the frame's integrity in the least. As you examine Figure 5.14, imagine the penalty if the jack were placed farther back along the roof edge away from the A-pillar. It would prevent rescuers from even making a flap in the roof.

If you have only enough cribbing for one crib:

- Have rescuers build that crib under the rear wheel of the car. Then have team members position the jack just behind the A-pillar.

While you watch from a vantage point near the front bumper:

- Instruct the rescuers to operate the jack until the car is vertical.

While this procedure may seem to be a poor substitute for four-point stabilization and perhaps even unsafe, it will result in the vehicle being remarkably rigid. Remember that most of the weight of the vehicle is being supported by the ground, not the cribbing and the jack. In fact, the jack in the illustration is probably not supporting any more than 50 or 60 pounds!

If you have no cribbing available whatsoever, consider using a Hi-Lift jack and a spare wheel to achieve two-point stabilization. Rescuers can acquire an inflated spare wheel from a police car, a responding member's car if yours is a volunteer organization, or even a spectator's car (although a good deal of persuasion may be required!). If the unstable vehicle is a full-sized passenger car or station wagon, the rescuers should try to get a spare wheel from a similar-sized car. If the unstable vehicle is a small one, rescuers should try to get a small wheel.

This is not nit-picking. If rescuers put the wheel from a small car under the wheel of a large vehicle, the vehicle may rotate past vertical when it is pushed by rescuers on the other side. Positioning and operating the jack on the roof side will only rotate the vehicle even farther from vertical. If rescuers put the wheel from a large car under the wheel of a small car, much of the vehicle may actually be lifted from the ground when the jack is operated to move the vehicle to vertical.

When rescuers have a suitable wheel:

* Instruct them to position it under the car's rear wheel so that when the vehicle is moved to the vertical position, the steel wheel of the car will overlap the steel wheel of the spare by several inches.

By positioning the wheel in this manner, you will minimize the possibility that the vehicle will become unstable again if either of the tires deflates during the subsequent rescue effort.

When the wheel is in place:

* Have rescuers ease the car into position against the spare wheel, place the jack so that the lifting toe is just behind the A-pillar, and operate the jack until the vehicle is vertical.

USING A BUMPER JACK AND A SPARE WHEEL

A well-equipped rescue truck, even a small one, carries one or two bumper jacks for times when the Hi-Lift jacks are being used (or are needed) for other tasks. There are two types of bumper jack. The *contour-style* jack has a curved attachment that fits against the bumper. The attachment has a lifting toe that engages the bumper's lower edge. The ratchet mechanism of the *notch-style* bumper jack has a lifting toe that fits into slots provided in the front and rear bumpers.

A contour-style bumper jack is used in the manner of a Hi-Lift jack. A spare wheel is placed under the rear wheel of the car, the car is eased onto the wheel, and the jack is positioned so the lifting toe engages the drip molding of the roof just behind the A-pillar. Care must be taken to assure that the lugs of the detachable lifting portion are fully seated in the corresponding slots of the ratchet mechanism.

Stabilizing a car with a notch-style bumper jack requires some additional steps. The lifting toe is not long enough to engage the drip molding of the roof; therefore, it is necessary to make a receptacle for the lifting toe by punching a hole in the roof.

* Have the team position the spare wheel under the rear wheel and move the vehicle to the vertical position.

While two team members hold the car in position:

* Instruct the third and fourth rescuers to stand by with a combination forcible entry tool (Quik Bar or Halligan Tool) and a drilling hammer while you first mark the location on the roof where the opening will be made, and then decide whether making the opening will endanger a person in the car.

Two points need to be made about creating the opening for the jack. First, the hole in the roof should be made about 4 inches from the drip molding and 4 inches from the windshield edge. This will eliminate driving the pike of the tool into the folded pieces of metal that make up the roof frame. Second, if a rescuer merely stands back and swings the forcible entry tool like a baseball bat, there's a good chance that the pike will sink into the head of a person bunched against the roof.

If you see that an occupant is likely to be struck by the pike of the forcible entry tool:

- Have one of the rescuers make an opening in the windshield large enough for your hand.
- Insert your hand and gently move the occupant's endangered body part 5 or 6 inches from the roof. Remember that the patient may have neck or spinal injuries.

While you hold the person's head in a safe position:

- Instruct the rescuer who has the forcible entry tool to hold it with the pike against the roof surface at the point you marked.
- Instruct the rescuer with the drilling hammer to strike the anvil of the tool sharply with the hammer (Figure 5.15).

When the opening is made:

- Have the rescuer who is holding the forcible entry tool rotate the handle of the tool to the vertical position, and while he holds the pike of the tool in place, pull down on the handle to create a lip at the upper edge of the opening (Figure 5.16).
- Finally, have the rescuers insert the lifting toe into the opening and operate the jack (Figure 5.17) to stabilize the car in the vertical position (Figure 5.18).

People who are unfamiliar with this procedure usually fear that when the jack is operated and the lifting toe is forced against the top of the opening, the narrow toe will

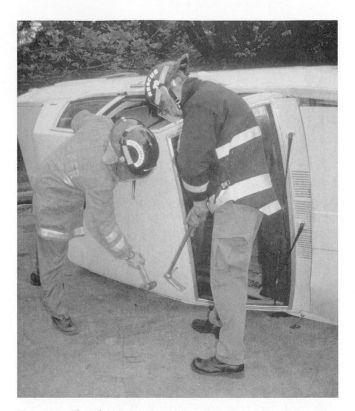

FIGURE 5.15   Striking the Anvil

cut into the sheet metal much like a can opener. Making a lip at the top of the opening with the forcible entry tool eliminates that problem. If any tearing does occur while

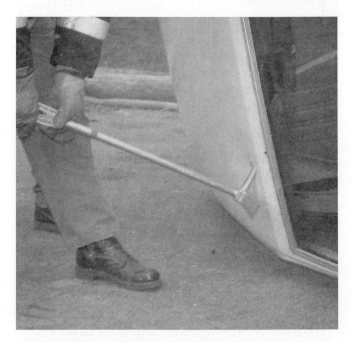

FIGURE 5.16   Rotating the Quik Bar

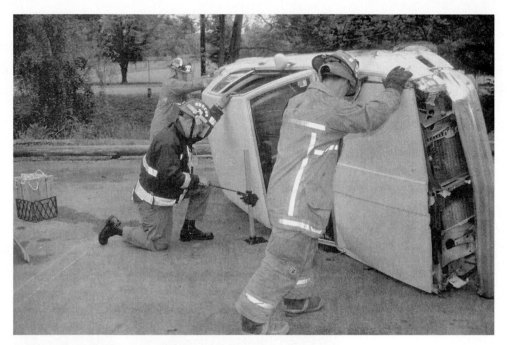

FIGURE 5.17   Inserting the Toe of the Jack

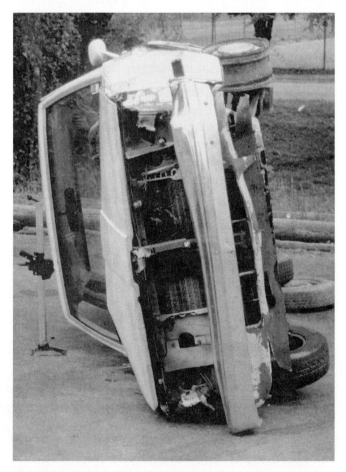

FIGURE 5.18   Stabilized—Jack and Wheel

the jack is being operated, it will be at the side of the opening. The metal will tear for only a fraction of an inch, however. Keep in mind that, as the car moves toward vertical, the weight supported by the jack decreases substantially.

USING TWO SPARE WHEELS

Lacking anything else, a vehicle can be stabilized on its side in about 10 seconds with two spare wheels as shown in Figure 5.19.

- Have one rescuer position the spare wheel under the vehicle's rear wheel so the steel parts will overlap several inches.
- Next, have two members of the rescue team push the car to the vertical position while you and another rescuer act as safety persons.

While one or two rescuers support the car in the vertical position:

- Have another rescuer slide the second spare wheel as far under the A-pillar as possible.

• Next, undertake the locking procedure.

On your command "push":

• Have two or three rescuers push on the uppermost portion of the roof to move the car against the stabilizing wheel on the other side and create additional space between the A-pillar and the wheel.

The A-pillar will rest on the steel rim of the wheel. If it doesn't, as when the wheel is slightly larger than necessary and fully inflated, don't be overly concerned. If the tire deflates while it is supporting the car, the vehicle will rotate a short distance until it settles onto the steel wheel, but not so far that it will become unstable.

Stabilizing a Vehicle with the Jimmi-Jak System™

The Jimmi-Jak System was designed specifically for stabilizing vehicles and other mechanisms of entrapment. Before we consider ways in which this unique tool can be used, let's discuss assembly procedures that are common to all operations.

As with any mechanical device, a few simple safety precautions must be observed while using the Jimmi-Jaks.

• Do not attempt to defeat the pressure relief safety feature of the controller. The internal mechanisms are sealed. If you discover at any time during maintenance activities that the seals are broken, return the controller to the dealer for inspection, testing, and resealing.
• Never drag a jack by its air supply hose; damage to the nipple and/or failure of the hose can result.
• Use only Jimmi-Jak attachments and accessories with the jacks. They have been specially designed for the system.
• Operate the Jimmi-Jak System only if you are trained to do so.

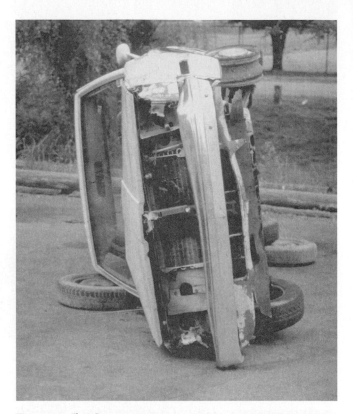

FIGURE 5.19   Stabilized—Wheel and Wheel

ASSEMBLING THE COMPONENTS

All of the base plates and attachments are readily interchangeable with all of the jacks. Simply align the keyway of the jack to the pin of the base plate or attachment and push the components together; then turn each part so the pin locks into the slot of the keyway.

The jacks of the Jimmi-Jak System can be extended manually, with carbon dioxide or nitrogen from a cylinder, or with compressed air from a cylinder, compressor, or truck air brake system. A pressure regulator is recommended when the air supply exceeds 150 psi and required when the jacks are pressurized by a compressed gas cylinder.

To operate the System from a compressed air cylinder:

• Check to see that the regulator exit valve is closed and that the T-handle of the regulator is turned out to the point of no resistance.
• Connect the pressure regulator to the compressed air cylinder. Turn the hand

wheel only finger-tight; do not use a wrench.

- Open the cylinder valve. Pressure in the supply cylinder will be indicated by the high pressure gauge on the regulator.
- Turn the T-handle of the regulator until the low-pressure gauge indicates approximately 150 psi.
- Connect the hose that leads from the regulator to the inlet on the side of the dual dead-man controller. Push the coupling onto the nipple until you feel it lock in place. Gently pull and twist the coupling to assure that the connection is secure.
- Connect the green and yellow air supply hoses to the discharge ports of the controller. The hoses have double safety couplings. They must be pushed firmly onto the nipples while the collets are held retracted. When disconnecting the hoses from the controller and the jacks, it is necessary to pull back on the collet while at the same time pulling the coupling free from the nipple.

To pressurize the jacks (and to either lift a load or improve stabilization):

- Pull the spring-loaded handles of the controller air flow valves toward you. Feather the controls until the load is lifted the desired distance or stabilization is assured.

You may hear the sound of air being released during lifting or stabilization operations. Air being released from the controller is a sign that the system has reached its maximum operating pressure and that the relief valves have opened. Air being released from a jack indicates that the piston is fully extended.

To release air from the jacks to lower a load or destabilize a vehicle:

- Push the controller air flow valves forward. The load will cause the pistons to retract.

MAKING THE JACKS INTO RIGID STRUTS

Pressurizing the jacks is not necessary for most stabilization operations. The piston of each jack can be extended manually, and the jack can be made into a rigid strut in the following manner:

- Fit the base plate and the desired attachment to the jack. Be sure that the attachments are securely locked in place.
- Position the base plate under or near the object that must be stabilized. Then pull the piston out from the barrel of the jack until the attachment contacts the load.
- Be sure that the rotating collar is seated firmly against the barrel of the jack.
- Insert the locking pin into the opening in the piston that is closest to the collar. Be sure that the fixed washer of the pin is not resting on the outer surface of the collar.
- Rotate the collar until the inclined planes of the collar are lodged firmly against the shaft of the pin.
- Turn the rotating T-handle of the collar to lock the setscrew against the barrel of the jack. Do not overtighten the screw; finger-tight is all that is necessary to lock the collar in place.

You can be sure that a jack is firmly supporting a load by gripping both T-handles of the collar and rotating it with two hands after the locking pin is in place. Be careful, however; forcefully sliding the rather shallow inclined planes of the collar against the locking pin adds considerable mechanical advantage to your efforts. You can actually lift a heavy load a short distance just by forcefully rotating the collar.

Stabilizing a Vehicle on Its Side When the Roof Edge Is Contacting the Ground

An advantage of the Jimmi-Jaks over other stabilizing devices is that they can be used to stabilize a vehicle on its side either in the position found or fully vertical. In either case:

- Station rescuers at both ends of the vehicles so they can manually stabilize it while you are assembling and positioning the equipment.
- Assemble both A-jacks with a base plate and a pointed attachment.
- Position the assembled jacks against the upper surface of the car, one at the hood and the other at the trunk lid.

The next step is to make an opening in the hood and trunk lid that will serve as a receptacle for the points of the jacks. The holes should be from 8 to 12 inches above the level of the points of the fully retracted jacks.

While rescuers continue to support the vehicle:

- Strike the sheet metal with the point of a combination forcible entry tool or the pike of a fire ax. If you are concerned about the stability of the car, or if there is not sufficient room to swing the tool, have another rescuer strike the head of the tool with a hammer while you hold it in place. The resulting hole should be 3/4 inch to 1 inch in diameter.
- Reinsert the point or pike of the tool in the opening, and while you hold the head of the tool with one hand, rotate the handle with your other hand until the tool is vertical.
- While you continue to hold the head of the tool so that the point or pike is in the opening, with your other hand, pull the handle of the tool downward.

This will create a lip at the upper edge of the opening—a lip that will make insertion of the tool easier and prevent the sheet metal from tearing when the jack is supporting a load.

While other rescuers continue to support the vehicle:

- Manually extend the piston of the jack until the point of the attachment is well seated in the opening. If necessary, manipulate the body of the jack to assure that the base plate is flat on the

roadway. The swivel will compensate for the angle of the jack.

While you hold the attachment in place with the point in the opening:

- Push the locking pin through the openings in the piston that are closest to the inclined planes of the rotating collar.
- Rotate the collar until the jack becomes a rigid strut; then turn the T-handle finger-tight to lock the collar to the barrel of the jack.
- Repeat the procedure for the other jack (Figure 5.20).

With the two jacks in place, there is no opportunity for the car to roll onto its roof. The stabilization task is not finished, however, until another jack is positioned against the underside of the vehicle, regardless of whether the vehicle is being stabilized vertically or in the position found.

While rescuers continue to support the vehicle:

- Move to the underside of the car and assemble a B-jack with a base plate and a suitable attachment.

You will have to look at the underside of the car to determine which attachment will be best suited for the task. You may be able to catch the drive shaft or the edge of a frame member with the V-block attachment. Or you may be able to force a wedge into the junction of frame members. Or it may be necessary to capture a frame member or an opening in the frame with a J-hook, in which case you will have to rig a slotted wedge with a chain.

When the attachment is in place and the jack is properly positioned:

- Insert the locking pin into the piston and turn the collar against the pin until the jack becomes a rigid strut. Turn the collar forcefully to move the car against the jacks on the other side (Figure 5.21).

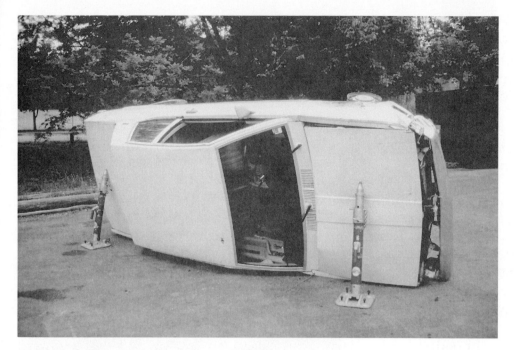

FIGURE 5.20 Stabilized—Jimmi-Jaks

If you feel that hand-adjusted jacks will not provide sufficient rigidity (as when there is considerable damage to the vehicle), assemble the air supply components, connect supply hoses to the jacks that are supporting the hood and trunk lid, pressurize the jacks, and adjust the pins and collars. When the collars are tight, bleed air from the system and remove the supply hoses from the jacks so they are not tripping hazards.

Stabilizing a Vehicle on Its Side on Soft Ground

Operations can become complicated when jacks are used to stabilize a vehicle on soft ground. Instead of the lifting toe moving up when the jack handle is operated, the base of the jack can sink into the ground and continue to sink until it reaches a firm base. This problem can be eliminated by placing a 24-inch jack plate under the jack. Thus the base will be expanded from about 35 square inches to 576 square inches. If the jack is supporting 60 pounds when the car is vertical, a jack plate will reduce forces exerted on the ground from a little more than 1-1/2 pounds per square inch to 1/10 pound per square inch.

No jack plates? No problem! Simply position the base of the jack in the well created by the steel wheel of an inflated spare tire (Figure 5.22).

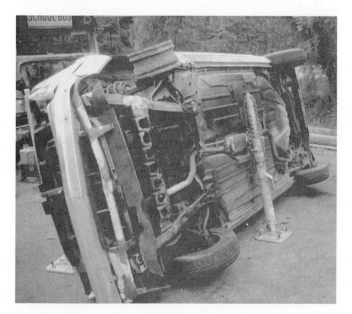

FIGURE 5.21 Stabilized—Jimmi-Jaks

Stabilizing a Vehicle with the Wheel Edges on the Ground with Jimmi-Jaks

The principal advantage of using Jimmi-Jaks to stabilize a car that has come to rest on its side and wheel edges is that the vehicle does not have to be moved to vertical prior to stabilization.

While several rescuers at each end of the vehicle are supporting it in place:

- Make an opening in the hood and trunk lid with the point of a forcible entry tool or the pike of a fire ax, about 12 inches from the road surface. Use the tool to form a lip in each opening.
- Assemble the A-jacks, each with a base plate and the slotted wedge attachment.
- Position the jacks next to the openings made in the trunk lid and hood.
- Manually extend the piston of each jack a few inches and insert the locking pin.
- Capture the ring of a J-hook with the slip hook of one of the chains supplied with the Jimmi-Jak System. Insert the point of the J-hook into the opening made in the hood or trunk lid, and while you hold the J-hook in place, pull the chain tight and drop the nearest link into the slot of the wedge.
- Repeat the chaining procedure with the other jack (Figure 5.23).

While rescuers continue to support the vehicle:

- Move to the underside of the car with a B-jack that has been fitted with a base plate and an appropriate attachment.

Again, the choice of an attachment will depend on where you can find a suitable jack point. You may be able to catch the drive shaft or the edge of a frame member with a V-block, or you may be able to insert the point of an attachment into an opening in the frame.

- Make the jack into a rigid structure by pinning the piston and rotating the collar (Figure 5.24).

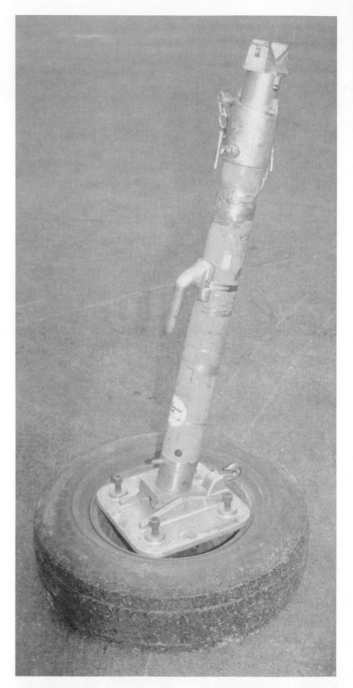

FIGURE 5.22   Stabilized—Jimmi-Jaks on Wheel

If there is slack in the chains, or if you feel that the stabilization should be more rigid:

- Connect the air supply to the jacks at the trunk lid and hood.
- Direct a rescuer to stand by each of these jacks, pull the pin, and rotate the

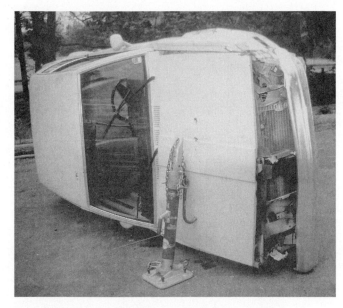

FIGURE 5.23   Stabilized—Jimmi-Jaks

collar so that the T-handles are parallel to the vehicle. Thus they will not snag in the chain when the jack is pressurized.

When the rescuers have prepared the jacks:

- Pressurize the jacks and lengthen the pistons until the chains are tight.

While you maintain air pressure in the jacks:

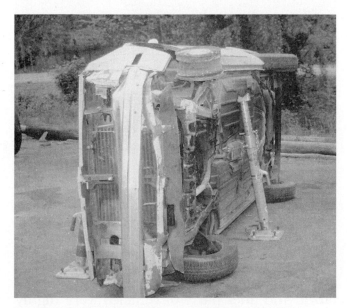

FIGURE 5.24   Stabilized—Jimmi-Jaks

- Direct rescuers to insert the locking pin in each jack.

When the pins are in place:

- Gently bleed air from the jacks and allow the locking pins to settle onto the collars. Since the chains will be under tension, it will not be necessary for rescuers to adjust the collars.
- Bleed the rest of the air from the system and uncouple the supply hoses from the jacks so they are not tripping hazards during subsequent rescue operations.

Stabilizing a Vehicle on Its Roof

Depending on the forces exerted on the vehicle during a rollover, a passenger car is likely to come to rest upside-down in one of these positions:

- Horizontal, with the roof crushed flat against the body of the vehicle, and both the trunk lid and hood contacting the ground
- Essentially horizontal, resting entirely on the roof, with space between the hood and the ground, and space between the trunk lid and the ground
- Front end down, with the front of the hood contacting the ground and much of the weight of the vehicle supported by the A-pillars.

When the roof of a car is crushed flat against the body of the vehicle, as when all the roof pillars have collapsed, the car is essentially a steel box resting on the ground with the occupants completely encapsulated in the wreckage. This is one time, and the only time, when stabilization is unnecessary. Since the structure is rigid and no part is suspended, there is nothing to stabilize. Getting to the occupants will be extremely difficult, however.

In the situation illustrated in Figure 5.25, a major portion of the body of the vehicle is supported by roof pillars. As long as the pillars

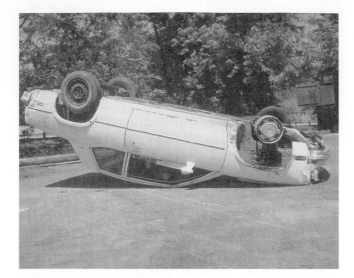

FIGURE 5.25   Vehicle on Roof

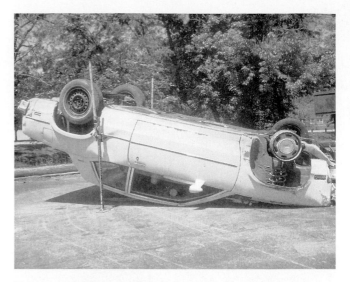

FIGURE 5.26   Stabilized—Hi-Lift Jacks

remain intact, there will be openings through which it may be possible to reach at least some of the occupants. But if the pillars collapse, as may be the case when the pillars are weakened during the rollover, the elevated portion of the vehicle will come crashing down.

Stabilization of an upside-down car involves supporting the elevated portions of the vehicle (Figure 5.26). There is no real secret to success. Use cribbing and jacks, if you have them, or cribbing, jacks, and spare wheels (Figure 5.27). If you have neither cribbing nor jacks and it is not likely that another rescue unit or rescue-equipped fire apparatus can reach the scene for some time, stabilize the vehicle with spare wheels.

Regardless of the procedure you use while you accomplish the stabilization, be sure to stay outside the danger zones; that is, anywhere under the vehicle where you might get trapped if the roof pillars collapse and the vehicle drops.

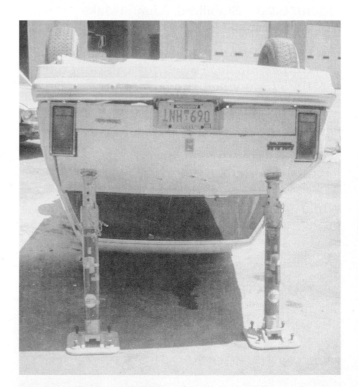

FIGURE 5.27   Stabilized—Jimmi-Jaks

HAZARDS PECULIAR TO VEHICLES

Following are components of a vehicle that may be hazardous to rescuers other than the sharp metal parts, sharp-pointed objects, and broken glass produced by a collision.

The Vehicle's Electrical System

It is standard operating procedure for many rescue units to permanently disable the electrical system of *every* accident vehicle by cutting a battery cable. This was a reasonable practice when wiring insulation and the fabric and fiber parts of vehicles were highly combustible. Today, however, permanently disabling a vehicle's electrical system may actually hinder a rescue operation.

Consider the value of leaving electrically operated accessories operable.

- Being able to reach through window openings and operate door lock switches eliminates the need for time-consuming forcible entry operations.
- If you can lower windows by operating a switch, you eliminate the likelihood of patients being injured during window removal efforts.
- Being able to move the seat backward by pressing on a switch will create 6 inches or more of working space between the driver and the steering wheel.
- Pushing a button in the glove box to open the trunk lid sure beats having to expose the lock mechanism with a cutting tool and operate the lock with a screwdriver.

You can't carry out any of these time-saving procedures if you don't have power, however. If you deem it necessary to disable a vehicle's electrical system, do it temporar-ily by unbolting the ground cable (black) from the battery. Take care as you work around the battery. Remember that in some cars, the cooling fan will come on even though the engine is not running.

Catalytic Converters

Car manufacturers started installing emission control systems in 1975 in an effort to reduce the concentrations of undesirable exhaust gases and thus improve the quality of the air we breathe. One of the components of a car's emission control system is the catalytic converter located on the underside of the vehicle between the engine exhaust pipe and the muffler (Figure 5.28).

The converter has a stainless steel shell, a diffuser, and catalyst-coated ceramic cores. The catalyst changes the carbon monoxide in exhaust gas to carbon dioxide and changes hydrocarbons to carbon dioxide and water. The catalytic action does not alter all the exhaust gas, however.

When a catalytic converter is operating properly, the internal temperature ranges from 1300° to 1500° F, while the outer shell reaches a temperature of about 1000° F. But when the engine is not properly tuned, the

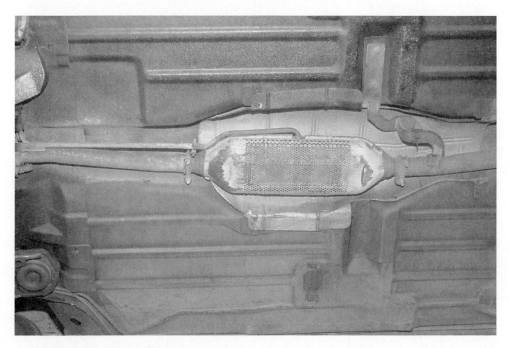

FIGURE 5.28 Catalytic Converter

internal temperature can be as high as 3000° F and the shell can become red-hot. Shielding prevents the transfer of heat to the floor of the vehicle and other vehicle components, but there is no shielding under a converter. Thus you must be extremely careful when working around the underside of a car that is on its side, especially during stabilization operations. Even the momentary contact of a turnout coat–protected arm could result in a nasty burn.

Hydrogen sulfide and sulfur dioxide (which have the odor of rotten eggs) can be emitted through the broken shell of a converter. Both are toxic, but for the emission to be sufficient to pose a threat to rescuers working nearby, the car's engine would have to be operating.

Drive Shafts

The drive shaft that transfers power from a vehicle's transmission to the differential is not solid steel, but rather a length of steel pipe with a cap welded to each end (Figure 5.29).

Since it is sealed at both ends, a steel drive shaft becomes a pressure vessel when it is heated as by flames from burning fuel. If it is not cooled, pressure within the shaft can quickly reach the point of violent rupture with fragmentation. Flying pieces are not a great problem when a vehicle is on its wheels, but when a vehicle is on its side, fragments from an exploding drive shaft can travel with great force for a considerable distance. A rupture from one end of a drive shaft to the other is not uncommon.

If you are called on to extinguish fuel burning under a vehicle that is on its side, be sure to cool the drive shaft initially, and then from time to time while you extinguish the fire. Operate the hose line from a position that is not directly in line with the drive shaft.

Struts

A variety of spring-loaded, gas- and liquid-filled struts can be found on passenger cars. MacPherson struts provide the normal dampening action of shock absorbers while at the same time serving as a structural link of the front suspension. Other struts assist with the movement and hold hatches and hoods in place (Figure 5.30).

Since they are essentially closed containers, gas- and liquid-filled struts can rupture

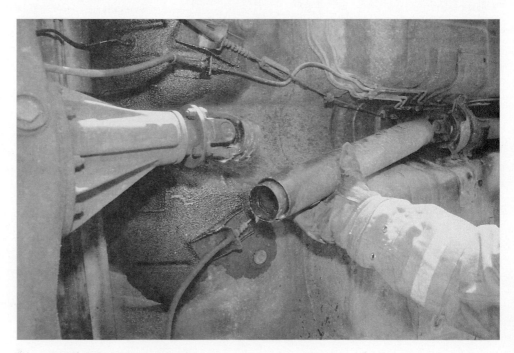

FIGURE 5.29   Drive Shaft

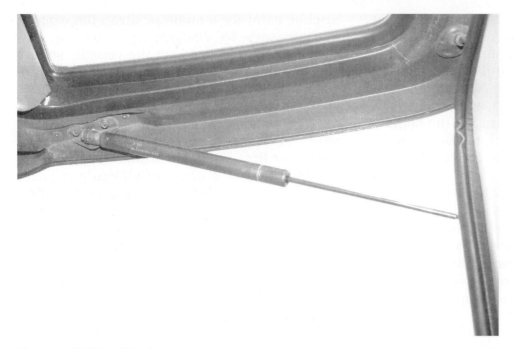

FIGURE 5.30 Struts

when heated. Nearby rescuers can be contacted by burning fluid and/or flying bits of debris. When you are fighting a fire in a vehicle that has struts, maintain a respectable distance until you are reasonably sure that the struts have been cooled.

When it is necessary to remove the roof of a hatchback vehicle, do not sever the assist struts along with the roof pillars. To do so may cause the violent release of parts.

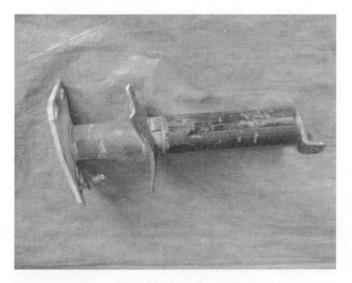

FIGURE 5.31 Shock-Absorbing Bumper

Energy-Absorbing Bumpers

In 1973, car manufacturers started installing energy-absorbing mechanisms on front and rear bumpers in an effort to reduce car repair costs. Where steel brackets simply transmitted collision forces to fenders and other body components, the energy absorbers, like shock absorbers, dampen the potentially damaging forces. The first mechanisms were designed to absorb impacts of up to 5 miles an hour; today's bumper mechanisms are required to absorb the forces created by only a 2-1/2 mile an hour crash (Figure 5.31).

There are two types of energy-absorbing mechanisms. The most commonly used one operates on the principle of the shock absorber. The unit consists of a piston tube that has a bumper bracket at the end and a cylinder with a stud that secures it to the frame of the vehicle. The piston tube is filled with an inert gas under pressure, while the cylinder is filled with a hydraulic fluid. The gas pressure in the piston keeps the energy absorber in the fully extended position at all times.

Upon impact, the piston tube is pushed into the cylinder, and hydraulic fluid is forced into the piston tube through a metering orifice. It is the controlled flow of fluid that provides the energy-absorbing action. The hydraulic fluid does not simply squirt into the piston tube, however; it displaces a floating piston within the tube, which, in turn, compresses the gas behind it. After impact, the pressure of the gas acting on the floating piston forces the hydraulic fluid back into the cylinder and thus extends the energy absorber to its original length.

Another type of energy absorber, the isolator, is a rubber and metal sandwich. When the bumper impacts with something, the rubber portion of the isolator stretches. After impact, the rubber returns the bumper to its original position unless the blow was so severe that the rubber was ripped from its metal base.

Much has been said about the dangers of energy-absorbing bumpers to emergency service personnel during rescue operations. Some authorities recommend chaining bumpers or even drilling shock-type energy absorbers and releasing pressure when they are found to be compressed as the result of an accident.

While it's true that an impact-compressed shock-type energy absorber *might* suddenly return to its normal extended position during a rescue operation, it's highly unlikely that it *will* return. Only a few instances of sudden extension have been reported in the 20 years that energy-absorbing bumpers have been used. In dozens of cars that have been frontal-impact and side-impact crash tested and dozens more that have been damaged in actual accidents, the energy-absorbing bumper mechanisms were found to be either destroyed (and thus rendered harmless) or so buried in the wreckage that they would pose no threat whatsoever. Therefore, we feel that chaining bumpers and drilling shock-type energy absorbers are totally unnecessary steps that consume time better spent on other hazard management and extrication procedures.

If you see that the shock-type energy absorbers are compressed, simply stay out of the area in front of them and warn other rescuers to do the same. If you must create an anchor point for a chain or strap (as when it is necessary to displace the steering column), kneel at the side of the vehicle, secure the chain or strap around the wheel housing, and carry the end to the hood either over the bumper or behind it.

A far more hazardous condition exists when shock-type energy absorbers are exposed to fire. They are miniature pressure vessels and, as such, can violently rupture when heated. When fighting a car fire, quickly cool the energy absorbers, and then combat the fire from a position where you are not likely to be hit by flying debris if the absorbers do rupture.

VEHICLE SAFETY SYSTEMS

Much has been done by automobile manufacturers to make their products safer. Door locks prevent motorists from being thrown from their vehicles upon impact with another vehicle or object. Steel girders protect a car's occupants during broadside crashes. Passenger restraint systems have evolved from simple lap belts. Fuel tanks are in places where they are less likely to be damaged during rear-end collisions. Antilacerative windshields lessen the possibility of terrible facial injuries resulting from forceful contact with the windshield during a frontal collision, and so on.

Some of these features posed problems for emergency service personnel until training programs could be modified. Today, well-trained rescuers can enter automobiles and disentangle trapped persons quickly regardless of the safety systems present. However, one safety feature of automobiles remains an enigma and, in the minds of many rescuers, a threat to their personal safety.

Air Bags

Up to now, emergency service personnel never thought much about air bags since so few cars were equipped with them. A member of an active rescue squad could respond to hundreds of motor vehicle accidents in a year and never see a car equipped with air bags. Such is not the case today. Air bag systems are available in a large number of vehicles, and now every new car sold in the United Sates is required to have some form of automatic crash protection, with air bags being the preferred system (Figure 5.32).

Much has been written and said about the dangers of air bags to emergency service personnel and accident victims alike. So much has been said, in fact, that rescuers throughout the country are expressing fears and even hesitating to perform two procedures that have been used successfully for years to create working space in front of injured drivers: displacing and severing steering columns.

"Dangerous," "flammable," "explosive," "toxic," "carcinogenic," "mutagenic," "lethal," and "deafening" are some of the terms that have been used singly or in combination to describe the components and operation of air bag systems. These fears and descriptions have resulted from word-of-mouth scuttlebutt, magazine articles, misinterpreted technical reports, product information sheets, EPA reports and product descriptions in hazardous material action guides, and, most unfortunately, warnings from vehicle rescue instructors. Oh yes, the authors of this book included! Like many other people, we fell into the trap of passing on bits of information from seemingly reliable sources without first determining whether those bits of information were fact or fiction. We humbly apologize to people that we have mislead in past training programs.

In an effort to set the record straight, we discussed air bag systems with personnel at the General Motors Proving Ground and Mercedes-Benz and finally with sales and engineering personnel of Morton Inc., at Ogden, Utah, the principal supplier of air bag components to U.S. and foreign car manufacturers.

The chemical compound that burns and releases the gas that inflates air bags is sodium azide. It's true that sodium azide is a dangerous commodity. In the book *Emergency Handling of Hazardous Materials*, prepared by the Bureau of Explosives and published and distributed by the Association of American Railroads, Washington, DC, sodium azide is included in the poison B category and described as a colorless, crystalline, water-soluble solid that will burn and may explode if large quantities are involved in fire or subject to shock. The book also states that toxic oxides of nitrogen are produced in fires involving sodium azide.

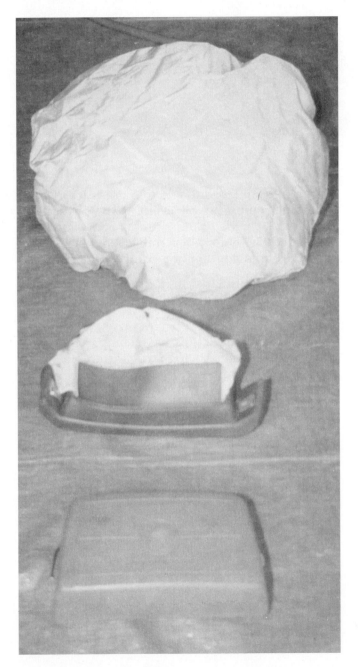

FIGURE 5.32 Air Bags

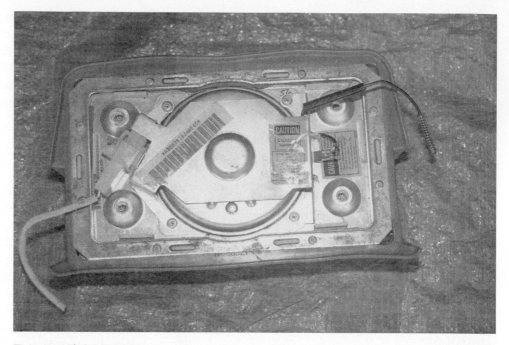

FIGURE 5.33   Air Bag

The key words in that particular product description are "large quantities." This means anything from barrels, trucks, and warehouses full of sodium azide, not 90 grams of the chemical stored in a 4.3-inch-diameter container that is mounted in the hub of a car's steering wheel (Figure 5.33).

Myths and Facts About Air Bags

Let's look at some of the other myths that have caused emergency service personnel to be fearful of air bag systems and pertinent facts provided by the people who know. Shown in Figure 5.34 is a cutaway of a typical air bag.

MYTH: The actions of rescuers during certain disentanglement operations can cause the inflation of air bags.

FACT: If a vehicle has not been involved in a front-end collision, nothing that a rescuer does while displacing or severing a steering column can accidentally cause the inflation of an air bag.

MYTH: An air bag inflates with up to 12,000 pounds of pressure. If an accidental inflation occurs while a rescuer is in the space between the driver and the steering wheel, the rescuer is likely to be crushed.

FACT: An air bag inflates to a pressure of 4 psi. In the improbable event of an accidental inflation, the bag would simply conform to the rescuer's body for a few milliseconds with no more than a gentle nudge and then deflate.

MYTH: In a similar vein, a driver's slamming into an inflated air bag is like slamming into a brick wall.

FACT: Accident victims have compared contact with an air bag to being struck in the face with a soft pillow.

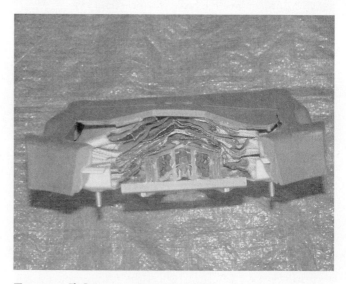

FIGURE 5.34   Air Bag Cutaway

MYTH: The gas that is produced when sodium azide burns is toxic *and* flammable. A closed passenger compartment filled with the gas generated by the sodium azide will pose a potentially lethal threat to victims and rescuers alike.

FACT: The 60 liters of gas produced by the burning sodium azide (a little more than 2 cubic feet) is 99% nitrogen. The remaining gases are nontoxic, nonflammable byproducts of combustion.

MYTH: Hydrogen gas is used to inflate the air bags of some cars.

FACT: Hydrogen gas never was, is not now, and never will be used to inflate air bags for reasons that should be obvious.

MYTH: If an air bag does not deflate immediately, the driver may be suffocated much in the way that a person can be suffocated when his face is covered with a soft thin plastic bag (a garment bag, for example).

FACT: Deflation occurs as soon as a forward-moving individual contacts an inflated air bag; gas is forced through several unrestricted openings in the bag. The time that a person's face may be in contact with a fully inflated bag is measured in milliseconds, not minutes.

MYTH: The canister of sodium azide (the gas generator) is mounted within the steering column of a car at a point where, if the column is displaced by rescuers in the usual manner, it will detonate with fearsome consequences.

FACT: The gas generator is mounted in a module that forms the hub of the steering wheel, not in the body of the steering column. As for "detonating with fearsome consequences," see the next myth/fact combination.

MYTH: Sodium azide is so explosive that, when a canister detonated during a car crushing operation, the force of the resulting explosion blew out the sides of the crusher.

FACT: Sodium azide in a gas generator does not explode; it burns. The gas generator is designed to provide controlled and contained combustion when electrically activated. Each gas generator design has been required to pass a rigorous qualification test monitored by the federal government prior to going into production.

MYTH: Air bags inflate with a deafening roar.

FACT: The inflation of an air bag has been compared to the bursting of an inflated paper bag at fairly close range.

MYTH: The sodium azide container will explode if subjected to fire.

FACT: The gas generator of an air bag system has a safety feature that prevents explosion in a fire situation. At approximately 350° F, the ignition of a small charge of smokeless powder causes the gas generator to operate as in a frontal crash situation. The sodium azide burns, nitrogen inflates the bag, and the bag deflates.

MYTH: Electromagnetic radiation (radio waves) will cause sodium azide containers to detonate.

FACT: A device built into the gas generator prevents radio waves from causing an accidental inflation under any circumstances. Mercedes-Benz personnel drove air bag–equipped vehicles in close proximity to the antennas of one of the most powerful radio stations in Europe without a single accidental deployment.

MYTH: Air bag systems are adversely affected by climatic changes.

FACT: Cold has no affect on the gas generator of an air bag system, nor do high ambient temperatures or moisture.

MYTH: The residue that is deposited on the surface of a deflated air bag is harmful.

FACT: Approximately 1 gram of an ashlike residue is produced when the sodium azide in a gas generator burns. Some of it is deposited on the surface of the air bag as the bag deflates. However, only 20 milligrams of the residue, an amount that will cover the head of a pin, can be considered problematic. If you would happen to get the entire amount on ungloved fingers and then wipe your eyes with those fingers, your eyes would probably smart as if contacted by a drop of lemon juice.

And so it goes. For every myth listed here, there is probably another one in circulation causing concern if not actual fear in rescuers about the safety of working near undeployed air bags. These concerns and fears are unfounded. It is the consensus of the people queried during the preparation of this section that air bags pose no threat to emergency service personnel during rescue operations. One respondent to our questions replied, not in an effort to be flip, but as a way of reinforcing the safety of air bags, that just about the only way for a rescuer to be harmed by the components of an air bag system is to remove the gas generator from its housing, pry the canister apart, and eat the sodium azide pellets!

How Air Bags Work

Even though air bag systems are essentially the same, rather than talk in general terms, we will discuss how one particular system works: the Mercedes-Benz Supplemental Restraint System. (Remember that while we are referring to one particular vehicle restraint system, many of the different functions and components discussed may be found on a number of other vehicles.) A representative of the U.S. headquarters of Mercedes-Benz provided a great deal of the information that served as a base for this section.

The Supplemental Restraint System is so firmly integrated into the design of the passenger compartment of Mercedes cars that it is virtually invisible. You can tell that a Mercedes car has air bags by the SRS embossed on the padded hub of the steering wheel (which is actually the air bag and gas generator package), by the SRS labels that are attached to the radiator cowl and the inside of the glove compartment door, and by a distinctive ETR/DRIVER-AIRBAG tag that is attached to the VIN plate located on the A-pillar of the driver's side of 1986 and later cars.

Some other makes and models of cars have distinctive markings on the cover of the air bag and gas generator module and some do not. All cars that are equipped with air bags have an identifier at the location of the VIN number, however.

The Mercedes-Benz Supplemental Restraint System has three key elements built into the forward part of the car's interior.

- The air bag itself, which, along with the gas generator, is contained in a module that is an integral part of the steering wheel assembly.
- A padded knee bolster integrated with the lower edge of the instrument panel on the driver's side. The bolster helps prevent the driver's body from being forced down and forward as a result of a frontal impact.
- A unique emergency seat belt tensioning retractor concealed within the car's B-pillar.

The functional brain of the Mercedes Supplemental Restraint System is the electronic crash sensor located at the forward end of the transmission tunnel. When the vehicle is involved in an accident, the sensor gauges the direction and magnitude of impact, and if it is a frontal impact equal to or greater in force than a 12-mile-an-hour crash into a solid barrier, the Supplemental Restraint System goes to work.

The sensor causes a chain reaction that ultimately results in the generation of gas and the inflation of the air bag. An electric current causes a filament similar to that in a flash bulb to glow. The glowing filament ignites a squib, which ignites a small amount of ignition booster material, which in turn ignites the sodium azide gas generant, thus producing the nitrogen necessary to inflate the bag. While this sounds incredibly complex, the sequence of events is completed in 5 milliseconds, or five one-thousandths of a second!

Nitrogen gas from the burning sodium azide passes around baffles and through screens to the air bag, which is secured to the top of the gas generator. The pressure of the inflating bag causes "doors" in the air bag/gas generator module to open, and the bag pops out and forms a cushion between the driver's head and upper body and the steering wheel. In a total of 25 milliseconds, less time than it takes to blink an eye, the air cushion is ready and waiting even before the driver's body can begin to move forward.

A controlled deflation through four apertures in the bag's underside begins with the impact of the driver's body against the air bag. The bag is deflated within 1 second.

In Mercedes cars, the front passenger's emergency tensioning retractor operates simultaneously with inflation of the air bag. The retractor consists of a piston within a cylinder and a gas generator. The piston is connected by a cable to the seat belt retractor or reel. Triggered by the crash sensor, the generator instantaneously produces gas pressure that drives the piston up the cylinder. The cable that is attached to the piston turns back the seat belt reel and tightens the belt loop. Before the passenger's body can even begin to move forward in reaction to the impact, his three-point seat belt is tightened and he is firmly restrained. The tightening is gentle; there is no jolting sensation, and the passenger will not be flung back against the seat. He is simply held in place. The seat belt can be released after the collision by depressing the quick release button in the usual manner. It is anticipated that other cars will have similar devices within the next few years.

In addition to built-in safeguards against inadvertent or inappropriate deployment, the Mercedes-Benz Supplemental Restraint System is designed to help assure that when it *should* deploy, it *can* deploy. The system incorporates an energy accumulator; its purpose is to store sufficient energy to deploy the air bag and activate the emergency tensioning retractor even if the car battery is disconnected or destroyed during an impact and normal power is lost. Also incorporated in the system is a step-up transformer that will deliver sufficient voltage to operate the system even if the battery is not fully charged.

Considerations During Rescue Operations

The question most often asked by rescue personnel is, "How should the chain or strap be rigged for a displacement operation if a steering column has an undeployed air bag?" There is considerable (but unnecessary) concern about exerting any force or pressure on the air bag/gas generator module.

Since the gas generator is an integral part of the air bag module, and since the air bag module is an integral part of the steering wheel assembly, and since it is just about impossible to cause an accidental deployment of an air bag, a pulling chain or strap can be positioned in any manner. It can be wrapped around the hub of a nonarticulated column for maximum leverage or lower on a column that has a tilting and telescoping steering wheel.

Severing the steering column should not be a problem in any car that is equipped with air bags. It's not likely that a steel saw blade passing through the wiring harness in the column will create a condition similar to the one that exists when the crash sensor is sending a signal to the gas generator. Nonetheless, a good practice is to disconnect the battery from the electrical system before severing the column of a car that has air bags.

If you elect not to displace or sever the steering column of a car that is equipped with air bags, but rather to remove a part or all of the rim of the steering wheel, take care to make the cuts close to the rim. Thus you will not be cutting into the bag storage area. There is no danger in doing so, just the inconvenience of having to deal with the loose floppy bag.

If you use hydraulic shears to separate the rim from the steering wheel, you could conceivably cut into the bag storage compartment or even into the gas generator. To avoid problems, be careful to keep the blades close to the rim.

Be aware that if you respond and discover that an air bag has deployed, heat could be a problem. The aluminum body of the gas generator becomes very hot, as hot as a hand-held steam iron, as the sodium azide burns. A gas generator starts to cool as soon as the chemical is burned away, but if you reach the scene quickly and working around the steering wheel is a priority operation, keep your fingers away from the generator. Normally, the gas generator is well concealed by a plastic housing, but forces created by the crash may have broken the housing and left the gas generator somewhat exposed.

SUMMARY

The fifth phase of a vehicle rescue operation begins as soon as the officer-in-charge has completed the assessment and developed a plan of action. Hazard management activities may not end until the rescue operation is complete and emergency service personnel are ready to leave the scene.

Motor vehicle accidents can cause a number of hazards to be spread over a wide area. Efforts must be undertaken to control these hazards, if not eliminate them altogether, so that rescuers can work in relative safety.

PHASE SIX

Gaining Access to Trapped Persons

INTRODUCTION

In the days of "you crash—we dash" rescue operations, gaining access was not a very complicated operation. Rescuers would simply make an opening in the wreckage large enough for EMS personnel to crawl through and reach the victims. While the idea was good, the practice was flawed; EMS and rescue personnel were stomping on people like grapes in a vat. The problem became more acute as cars became smaller after the gas crunch of the 1970s. With the acceptance of the smaller, fuel-efficient vehicle, compacts are quite common on today's roadways. Getting a 200-pound (or heavier) rescuer through a window opening of a subcompact car containing four adults is like trying to squeeze 15 pounds of something-or-other in a 5-pound bag!

With time came changes. With improved tools and better training, rescuers discovered that they were able to gain access to trapped persons quicker, so instead of making a single opening in wrecked vehicles, they made multiple openings. As a result,

EMS personnel were able to carry out assessment procedures and initiate emergency care measures without being hindered by doors, windows, B-pillars, and the bodies of other victims. The standard operating procedure became: Open doors. If doors cannot be opened quickly, remove windows. If nothing else is possible, make openings in the body of the vehicle.

With time has come the need for even more changes. Training programs such as the Basic Trauma Life Support course and the Pre-Hospital Trauma Life Support course have made EMS personnel aware of the need to reach injured persons in the shortest possible time and, when necessary, to care for the occupants as if everyone has a spinal injury. To help EMS personnel meet those goals, rescuers must have a new plan for gaining access—a plan that assures quick access to all occupants while at the same time creating good working space. The first thing that must be done is to stabilize the vehicle to ensure that it will not move through spring action while the following steps are taken.

When responding to a crash involving two vehicles in a head-on collision, the initial opening is made so that medical personnel or rescuers can reach into the passenger compartment (or climb into the compartment, if possible) and protect the occupants with a covering.

How and where an opening will be made will be a matter for your judgment; there is no one formula to follow. The easiest way to enter a closed vehicle that has collided head-on with another vehicle or an object is to break or remove the rear window. If there is no one in the rear of the passenger compartment, you might consider breaking the rear side windows. If your team members are quite proficient in the use of a hydraulic rescue tool and the tool is ready for immediate use, you might have them force open a door. Removing the windshield will create the largest opening, but a conventional removal may be difficult because of the extent of damage to the glass caused by the impact, and a destructive removal may be dangerous because of the proximity of the front seat occupants. Whatever you decide, have team members make the opening quickly.

When there is an opening in the vehicle:

- Have rescuers cover the occupants as much as possible with a lightweight tarp, or an aluminized rescue blanket if there is any danger of fire.

If there is room in the vehicle, and entry can be made without fear of aggravating injuries or causing new ones:

- Have a medic climb into the vehicle to continue patient protection measures.

When the occupants are properly protected:

- Have rescuers remove or cut through the windshield.
- Have rescuers expose the entire interior of the vehicle by folding back a section of the roof, removing a section of the roof, or removing the roof altogether.

Again, the choice of a technique will be a matter for your judgment. Consider the space needed, the tools available, and the team members' abilities to use those tools.

With the roof out of the way, EMS personnel can properly assess the injured persons and initiate lifesaving efforts, and rescuers can make additional openings in the vehicle and undertake disentanglement operations that will create even more working space.

Is this a technique that should be adopted as a standard operating procedure? Not at all. Certainly you would not elect to remove the roof when a vehicle has only one minimally injured occupant. Nor would you remove the roof when the occupants are conscious and able to discuss any injuries with you. But when the occupants are unconscious and probably seriously injured, there is no reason not to remove the roof right away.

Remember: Quick access and the creation of working space will help EMS personnel achieve their goals of reaching injured persons quickly and caring for patients as if everyone has a spinal injury.

On the pages that follow, you will find many ways for gaining access through the doors, windows, and body of a vehicle. The fact that they are presented in a certain order does not mean that they should necessarily be accomplished in that order.

Before we discuss any procedures for gaining access, however, let's see what a car is made of, and let's look at the terms that will be used throughout the rest of the book.

THE ANATOMY OF A CAR

A car is comprised of many systems. There is a fuel system, an electrical system, an exhaust system, an emissions control system, a cooling system, a steering system, a suspension system, a brake system, and more. Components of some of these systems have been mentioned in earlier sections, and other components will be discussed later in the text. What we are concerned with here is the body system, for it is the body components that rescuers have to disassemble, distort, displace or sever during gaining access and disentanglement operations.

Like beauty, the body of a car is more than skin deep. True, the body's surface metal gives a car its distinctive sweep, the particular look that sets it apart from other vehicles. However, there is much below the body surface that is vital to the basic outer structure. In other words, a car body consists of more than just a few doors and fenders hung on to a shell.

The body shell is a rather complex assortment of large sections of steel that have been stamped into a definite shape. At the bottom of the assembly is the floor pan. This is the foundation, stamped with bulges and curves to conform to the space requirements of the engine, transmission, and rear axle. The stamping must also reflect the ultimate size and shape of the passenger compartment.

If the car has a separate frame, the floor pan is bolted to the side rails, but kept from actual contact by large rubber cushions. If the car is of unitized construction without a frame, the floor pan is attached to various metal pieces that make up the center section of the chassis. Most cars have two floor pans. One is for the passenger compartment; the other extends rearward and makes up the floor of the trunk.

The cowl assembly is often called the firewall because it separates the passenger and engine compartments. The cowl is a stamped piece of steel; it has a number of openings for wires, tubes, and other components essential to the vehicle's operation. The cowl assembly does not stop at the height of the instrument panel but continues up both sides of the dashboard in formed pillars and stops when it meets the roof panel. These pillars, which also provide the frame for the windshield, are called A-pillars.

On the opposite end of the cowl assembly is the rear quarter panel. This assembly runs from the rearmost part of the rear door edge, around the back, and to the rear door on the other side. On a number of cars, the rear quarter panel is integral with the rear fenders. A major difference between this and other panels is its inner construction. Unlike the floor pan and the cowl assembly, the rear quarter panel is made up of an outer skin and inner panels that serve as reinforcements for the rear passenger compartment, the trunk, and the wheel housings. Most of the inner panels are not readily visible, but without them, the construction would be weak and vibrations in the rear section of the car would be severe.

The center body pillar is called the B-pillar. All cars have a center body pillar, regardless of whether they are two- or four-door vehicles. Made of heavy stock and formed for strength, the B-pillars extend from the floor pan straight upward. On a four-door sedan, the B-pillar reaches to the roof assembly and is welded to it. On a four-door hardtop, the B-pillar rises only as high as the door level. On a two-door hardtop, the B-pillar is incorporated into the rear quarter panel. In addition to providing strength to the body of the vehicle, B-pillars serve as foundations for locks and hinges of the front and rear doors.

While we generally think of C-pillars as parts of the roof assembly that join the roof to the rear quarter panel on each side, some four-door sedans have C-pillars that, like B-pillars, extend from the floor pan to the roof assembly. In these cars, the portions that join the roof assembly to the rear quarter panel are properly called D-pillars. Since the C- and D-pillars of sedans come together at the edge of the roof, and for the sake of simplicity, we will refer only to C-pillars when discussing sedans and to D-pillars when discussing station wagons.

Doors and deck lids complete the basic car body system. The front deck lid that covers the engine compartment is more commonly called the hood, and the rear deck lid is usually called the trunk lid for obvious reasons.

Doors are comprised of an inner and outer panel. The inner panel provides strength and the outer panel is merely a metal shell. The inner panel has a variety of openings and offsets for the attachment of window mechanisms and door locks. The upper section of each door serves as a window frame. Cars built after the mid-1970s have an internal side rail between the inner and outer panels. The rail resembles the steel guardrail that can be found along roadways and is installed to absorb much of the impact of a broadside collision. The deck lids are similar to doors in that they have an inner panel with crossbars for strength, and an outer panel or "skin."

While you need not know the location and purpose of every nut, bolt, and other component in a car, you should know where you can find weak and strong points. Knowing the weak points, like single thicknesses of sheet metal, will help you make decisions about gaining access. Knowing strong points, as where roof pillars join the floor pan, will help when you must decide where to place powerful tools during displacement operations.

Just as EMS personnel should have a working knowledge of medical terminology, so, too, should rescuers have a working knowledge of terms commonly used in connection with car components. To that end we have included a diagram and commonly used terms in Figure 6.01.

GAINING ACCESS THROUGH DOOR OPENINGS

Today's cars are made with safety in mind. Improved locking and latching mechanisms prevent doors from flying open on impact, and doors themselves have been substantially strengthened. Nonetheless, most doors can be opened without great difficulty. There are two distinct advantages to quickly opening doors:

- Opening a door exposes more of an injured person's body than does merely opening a window. A more complete assessment can be made, and severe lower body injuries can be cared for quicker.
- Opening a door also creates an opening through which occupants can be removed.

A number of tools can be used in a variety of ways to open both damaged and undamaged vehicle doors. However, the quickest and

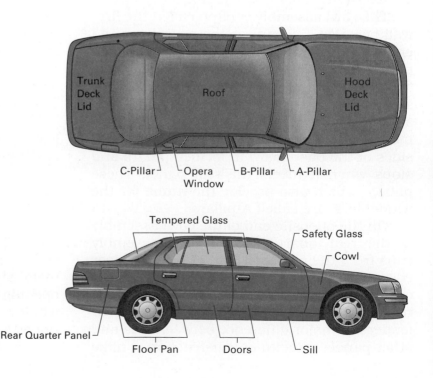

FIGURE 6.01   Anatomy of a Car

easiest way to open a door is to walk up to the door, operate the latch mechanism, and pull the door open in the manner intended by the manufacturer. This works even when damage to the vehicle is severe. Remember: Try before you pry!

Unlocking and Unlatching Undamaged Doors That Have an Accessible Lock Knob

Obviously you can gain access to injured persons trapped inside a crashed vehicle by simply smashing a window, reaching in, and unlocking the door. But how about gaining access to sick persons in vehicles in non-accident situations? What if you are called to the parking lot of a supermarket to open a locked car so EMS personnel can care for an elderly person who may be suffering the effects of a hot day. A sick, elderly man does not need (1) to have to worry about his unlocked car remaining in a public parking lot, (2) to remove hundreds of pieces of broken glass from the interior of the vehicle, and (3) to replace an expensive tempered glass window that is not covered by insurance while trying to exist on a modest fixed income. There are several alternatives to breaking a window to reach a sick or injured person in a vehicle.

Asking an Uninjured Occupant to Unlock the Door

The following technique is usually successful when the uninjured occupant of a locked vehicle is conscious and able to move his arms:

- Rap on the window to gain the person's attention.
- Call out instructions for the person to operate the lock mechanism. Shout if you must; the person may be hard of hearing.

At the same time:

- Wiggle a finger outside the window as if you were operating the lock knob.

The pantomime action is important. A person who is confused or has an altered level of consciousness may not be able to understand your verbal instructions, nor may a non-English-speaking individual, a small child, or a person who is hard of hearing. Most will be able to comprehend the lock-operating movements of your finger, however. If a person is unconscious or otherwise unable to operate the lock mechanism, you will have no alternative to unlocking a door from outside the car.

An important point: The word "uninjured" in the paragraph that precedes the instruction is emphasized for a reason. The technique just described should be used only to gain the attention of an uninjured person. If a person who has a cervical spine injury as the result of an accident suddenly turns his head almost 90 degrees in response to a rap on the window, the chance is good that he will aggravate the injury.

While manufacturers are moving away from them in favor of more secure devices, the majority of the more than 170 million motor vehicles registered in the United States have door locks operated by exposed-to-view (and therefore accessible) knobs.

Some cars and trucks in this category have doors with mushroom-head lock knobs; that is, knobs with expanded heads that can be easily gripped with the fingers. Others have doors with so-called "anti-theft" lock knobs—straight-shanked pieces of plastic that defy pulling with a hooked tool. It's hard to believe that people will install devices that cost less than a dollar apiece and expect them to make their $25,000 cars theft-proof. But people do just that and in great numbers!

Using a Noose Tool to Unlock Doors

A door that has either type of lock knob can be opened easily and quickly with a noose tool. In addition to the noose tool, you will need two short flat pry bars and a wood or hard rubber wedge.

- Lay the tools on the roof directly in front of the door you want to open.

With one hand:

- Insert the prying edge of one tool into the space between the window frame and the roof.
- Move the window frame away from the roof.

With your other hand:

- Insert the prying edge of the second tool into the slightly enlarged opening.
- Alternately pry and reposition the tools until you have an opening of an inch or two between the window frame and the roof edge.

While you hold the window frame away from the roof edge with one tool:

- Insert the wedge into the space to maintain the opening (Figure 6.02).
- Then insert the noose tool into the opening, and capture the lock knob with the noose (Figure 6.03).

While you hold the body of the tool with one hand and pull on the T-handle with your other hand:

- Lift the lock knob to unlock the door (Figure 6.04).

Don't unlatch the door just yet. With the window frame under tension because of the wedge, the door may spring open with considerable force as soon as you operate the latch mechanism. Instead:

- Insert the end of one of the prying tools into the space between the window frame and the roof edge.
- Exert force on the prying tool and enlarge the space just enough to remove the wedge.
- Release your hold on the tool and remove it.
- Finally, unlatch the door and open it.

A variety of tools can be used to operate mushroom-head lock knobs, including lengths of wire, coat hangers, and wire flare stands. If the doors have frameless windows, a screwdriver, another long, thin tool, or a saw blade can be used to move lock knobs to their unlocked position.

A straight-shank anti-theft lock knob can be operated with a wire-and-washer tool. A wire flare stand can be used to move an anti-theft knob that has flats (as opposed to being round its entire length). If the car has frameless windows, a saw blade or a sharp-edged tool will usually bite into the knob enough for it to be lifted.

The procedure for unlocking a door that has a frameless window is essentially the same. You just have to be a little more careful than when working with a framed win-

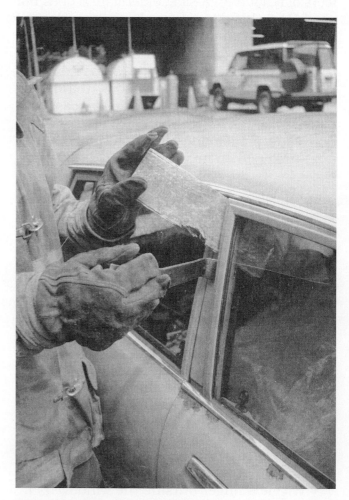

FIGURE 6.02   Inserting Wedge

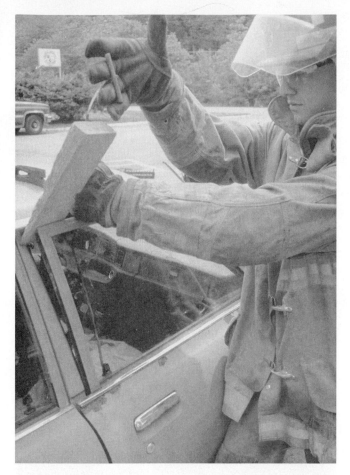

FIGURE 6.03 Noose Tool, Unlocking Door

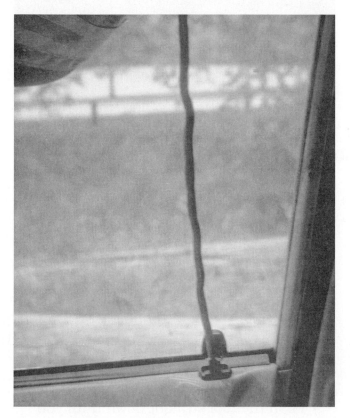

FIGURE 6.04 Lifting Lock Knob

dow. When you pry an unframed window away from the roof, the steel tool will be close to the most vulnerable part of a tempered glass window—the unprotected edge. Be careful not to strike the glass edge with the tool during the prying operation; the glass may shatter even when only lightly struck.

STRAIGHTENING THE WINDOW FRAME IN A NON-EMERGENCY SITUATION

A problem with the procedure just described is that it sometimes distorts the window frame to the point where a gap will remain between the window frame and roof edge after the door is closed. You can correct the problem easily.

- Lower the window.

With the door fully open:

- Stand on the inner side of the door with your knee firmly against the door panel just below the window.
- Grip the upper corner of the window frame.
- Give the frame a couple of sharp pulls toward you (Figure 6.05).

This should return the frame to its proper position. If it does not, repeat the procedure with another rescuer either at your side or at the other side of the door facing you. Exert pushing and pulling forces together on your command.

This may seem like an insignificant and unnecessary operation, but it's not. If you have taken the trouble to unlock a door instead of smashing a window to reach a sick person, take just a few more seconds to straighten the window frame, especially in a non-emergency situation. Returning the window frame to its normal position may prevent the owner from having to pay a costly and unnecessary repair bill. This "extra effort" is what separates good rescuers from those that are not so good.

Unlocking and Unlatching Doors That Do Not Have an Accessible Lock Knob

Car manufacturers have made door locks more complicated in an attempt to reduce the number of auto thefts. The doors of some late-model cars are locked by sliding a knob horizontally, others by depressing a rocking knob. Needless to say, different tools and techniques must be used to open these doors.

Using a Locksmith's Tool to Unlock Doors

One way of unlocking doors equipped with other than exposed lock knobs is to use a tool specially designed for the task; there are several models. A flexible flat metal blade is inserted between the window glass and the weatherstripping, and the tool is manipulated until the end of the tool or a groove or hook engages the lock mechanism.

These tools are used by locksmiths, lockout specialists, parking garage personnel, repossessors, and, undoubtedly, car thieves—all people who can use the tools successfully because they use them frequently. These tools are often recommended for emergency service units, but unless rescuers are familiar with the procedure required for a particular make and model car, using one of these tools can be time-consuming and frustrating. More often than not, a rescuer's being able to unlock a door with a locksmith's tool is a matter of luck.

Using the Slide Lock Tool to Unlock Doors

A special tool used effectively to unlock car doors with sliding bar locks is the Slide Lock Tool, manufactured by the Sliding Lock Tool Company of Louisville, Tennessee. Unfortunately, use of the tool is limited to General Motors vehicles manufactured from 1980 to date. Nonetheless, it is an inexpensive, easy-to-use tool worth carrying.

To make an opening for the tool:

- Use a short pry bar tool or a long thin tool such as a screwdriver to move a

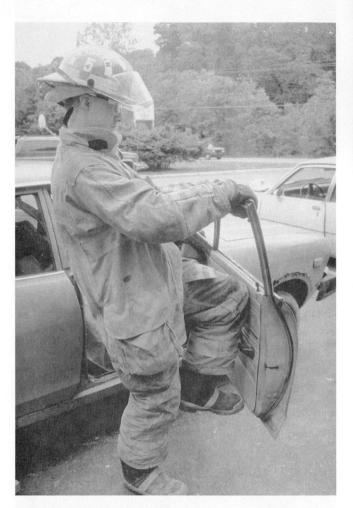

FIGURE 6.05 Straightening Door Frame

small portion of the weatherstripping away from the window glass directly above the lock cylinder.

While you maintain the opening with the prying tool:

- Insert either end of the Slide Lock Tool into the space and push it down about 4 or 5 inches.

While you hold the end of the tool in one hand:

- Rotate the tool 1/4 turn clockwise (until the part of the tool in your hand is at a right angle to the glass).
- Push the tool straight down until you sense a "spongy" feeling that indicates

the hook of the tool has engaged the lock rod.
- Inch the working end of the tool along the lock rod until it is as close to the lock cylinder as possible.

While you continue to hold the end of the tool in one hand:

- Disconnect the wire from that end with your other hand and rotate the tool slightly in a counterclockwise direction. This will cause the hook to capture the rod snugly.
- Finally, pull the wire with your free hand toward the hinged side of the door to move the sliding rod and thus unlock the door.

Opening Front Doors with a Steel Awl

A steel shanked awl can be used to unlock a front door when nondestructive means fail. This rather simple procedure works most of the time.

Hold the awl in one hand while striking it with the drilling hammer. Make a small hole next to or just below the key insert on the door (Figure 6.06). Rotate the tool to open the hole just large enough to insert the awl fully. Then back it out and reinsert it while "aiming" it toward the rear of the key lock. There is a small horizontal tab on the rear of the key lock which controls the rods leading to the manual mushroom/slide lock and the lock box. On some cars, moving the awl up will unlock the door, while on others, moving it down will manipulate the tab (Figure 6.07).

Opening Doors That Cannot Be Unlocked and Unlatched by Conventional Means

Prior to 1967, vehicle doors were not very secure. People were often thrown from cars when a head-on or rear-end crash caused doors to fly open after the mating parts of door latches separated.

The doors of most of the cars on the road today are prevented from opening as

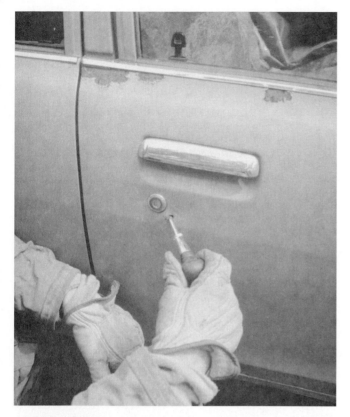

FIGURE 6.06 Using Steel Awl

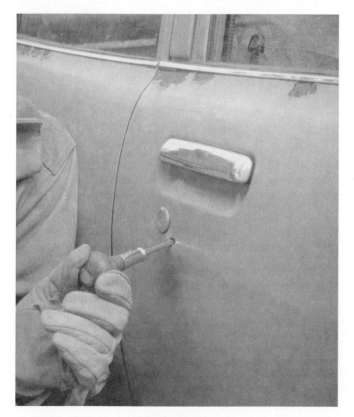

FIGURE 6.07 Using Steel Awl

the result of a collision by the combination of a safety bolt set in the door frame and a receptacle set in the door body. A fork in the receptacle prevents the door from swinging open, and a flange on the safety bolt prevents the bolt from pulling out of the receptacle in the door. Latch mechanisms must be able to withstand at least 2750 pounds of pull or shearing force, but in reality, most door locks can withstand pulling and shearing forces in excess of 4000 pounds.

If you have a hydraulic rescue tool, opening a badly damaged door that has a safety bolt is seldom a problem. These powerful tools generate prying forces far in excess of 4000 pounds. However, hand-powered hydraulic jack and spreader assemblies that were often used successfully to pry open the doors of older cars will not develop forces sufficient to open doors that have safety bolts. These tools are rated according to the force exerted on the face of the piston of the jack, not the force available at the tips of the spreader. Only 600 pounds of force is available at the tips of a 6-inch spreader powered by a 4-ton hydraulic jack.

It seems reasonable to assume that the forces available at the end of a long-handled prying tool are not sufficient to pry open a door that is held closed by a safety bolt, even when the tool is manned by two or three strong rescuers. It can be done, however.

The secret to easily opening the jammed doors of wrecked vehicles is unlocking and unlatching doors before you attempt to force them open. If you can disengage the latch receptacle from the safety bolt, then opening a jammed door will involve no more than moving the door away from its frame. This can often be done with a tool as small as a 15-inch pry bar.

There are four steps to opening a badly damaged door that is secured with a safety bolt: (1) making an opening in the door panel, (2) unlocking the door, (3) disabling or destroying the latch mechanism, and (4) prying the door open.

Making an Opening in the Door Panel

A number of tools can be used to make a three-sided flap in the sheet-metal panel of a vehicle door, including a panel cutter, a flat-blade screwdriver, a can-opener type tool, and an air-operated chisel.

USING A HAMMER AND PANEL CUTTER

The Schild Tool shown in Figure 6.08 is specifically designed for making openings in sheet metal. This sturdy tool has a handle, a striking surface or anvil, a point for making a starting hole, and a two-part curved blade. The crescent-shaped part of the blade farthest from the handle is for cutting light sheet metal, while the crescent-shaped part closest to the handle is for cutting heavier sheet metal.

When you first see a Schild Tool, you may wonder how the blade cuts; it is about 1/8-inch thick and not at all sharp. Do not attempt to put an edge on the blade with a grinder as some people have done. The blade will become firmly wedged in the work as

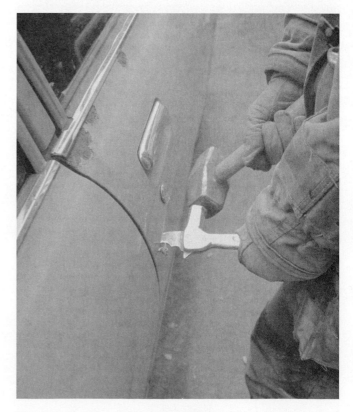

FIGURE 6.08   Using Schild Tool

soon as you start to cut. Sheet metal is cut with a blunt tool, not one with a sharp edge.

To make a starting hole in a door panel:

- Hold the tool in one hand with the starting point against the door panel about 2 inches above and 3 or 4 inches to the hinge side of the door handle.
- Sharply strike the anvil of the tool with a drilling hammer or other heavy short-handled striking tool.
- Drive the starting point completely into the door panel (Figure 6.09).

Making a starting hole in this manner is important. From a hole in this location you will be able to drive the tool both to the side and downward. If you attempt to make a starting hole in the lip of the door, the piece of metal that forms the latch side of the door will prevent sideward movement of the tool. Next:

- Insert the tip of the cutting blade into the starting hole, with the cutting edge facing the latch side of the door.

While you hold the tool at a right angle to the door:

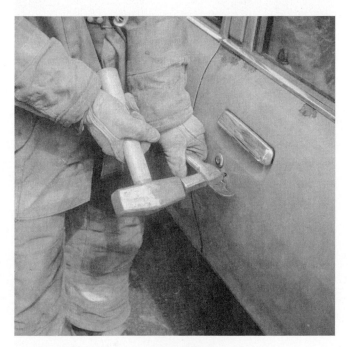

FIGURE 6.09   Using Schild Tool

- Repeatedly strike the anvil sharply with the hammer.
- Continue to drive the tool in this manner until it is prevented from moving farther by the metal that forms the latch side of the door (about one inch from the door edge) (Figure 6.10).

There may be a tendency for the blade to wander as you drive it from the starting hole to the door edge. If this happens, simply tap the side of the anvil projection to make the necessary course correction.

When you cannot drive the tool any farther to the side:

- Remove the blade from the cut and reinsert the tip into the starting hole, this time with the cutting edge facing down.
- Drive the tool downward with the hammer to a level several inches below the bottom edge of the lock cylinder.

To turn the tool to make a horizontal cut:

- Either alternately strike the anvil and the side of the tool to turn the blade without removing the blade from the cut; or
- Remove the tool and reinsert the tip of the blade in the vertical cut with the cutting edge facing the latch side of the door.
- Drive the tool as far as possible toward the latch side of the door.

Finally:

- Insert the point of the tool into the very end of the first horizontal cut and drive the tool down until it joins the very end of the second horizontal cut. This will free a section of the outer door panel.

A procedure that was used by rescuers for many years to expose a door's lock and latch mechanisms was to make a three-sided flap in the panel. The problem with that technique was that the rods attached to the latch operator and lock cylinder of some cars prevented the flap from opening far enough. Moreover, many rescuers experienced difficulty in detaching the rods because of the lack of working space.

By freeing a section of the door panel, you can usually create an opening large enough for your hand to pass through to reach the lock and latch mechanisms. If connecting rods are in the way, you will have working space to either remove or cut them.

Before we go on to the step of unlocking the door, let's consider the use of other tools for making an opening in the door panel.

USING A HAMMER AND SCREWDRIVER

A large flat-blade screwdriver makes an excellent sheet-metal cutting tool. Do not hold the tool in the manner of a chisel, however, as many rescuers are prone to do. You will drive the tip of the screwdriver into the sheet metal, and the metal will grip so tightly that you may have a problem pulling it free.

To make a starting hole in the door panel:

- Hold a corner of the screwdriver blade against the metal and strike the side of the blade with a hammer.

To make the cut:

- Hold the screwdriver at an angle so 1/4 inch to 3/8 inch of one side of the blade is in the starting hole.
- Strike the side of the screwdriver blade with the hammer to drive it through the metal.
- Stop periodically and withdraw the screwdriver slightly so that only 1/4 or 3/8 inch of the blade is in the door. The wider the cutting edge, the more difficult it is to cut the metal (Figure 6.11).

USING A CAN-OPENER TYPE TOOL

The can-opener portion of the Pry-Axe and similarly constructed combination forcible

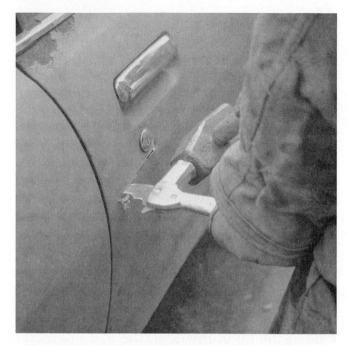

FIGURE 6.10   Using Schild Tool

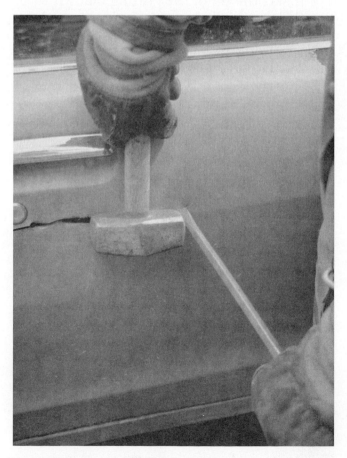

FIGURE 6.11   Using Screwdriver

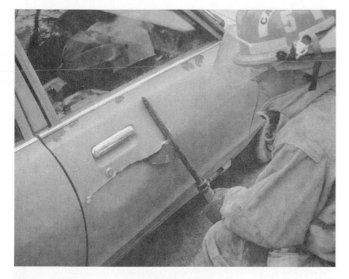

FIGURE 6.12   Using Can Opener

entry tools will easily cut door panels. Make a starting hole with the pike of the tool and make cuts in the manner suggested for the panel cutter (Figure 6.12).

Openings made with can-opener tools usually have sharp jagged edges. Be careful when you put your hand into the opening made by pulling the flap aside, even if you have gloves on.

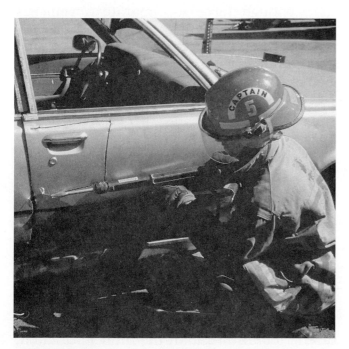

FIGURE 6.13   Using Air-Operated Chisel

USING AN AIR-OPERATED CHISEL

An air-operated chisel will make an opening in a door panel in less time than it takes to tell about it. A benefit of using an air chisel for this task is that once the tool is set up, it can be used for other procedures, like removing or folding back the roof, displacing B-pillars, and so on. Conserve air for other more difficult tasks by keeping the pressure down to 70 or 80 pounds while making openings in door panels (Figure 6.13).

Unlocking the Door

Once you have made an opening in the door panel, unlocking a door is usually a simple matter. Seldom is a door's lock and latch mechanism damaged to the point where it cannot be operated.

With the help of your flashlight:

- Locate the part of the lock mechanism that is operated by the lock cylinder, or in a car so-equipped, the rod that leads from the tailpiece of the lock cylinder to the lock mechanism.
- Operate the part with your finger, or pull or push on the rod to unlock the door.

Disabling the Latch Mechanism

Unlocking a door does not unlatch it. After making a flap in the door panel and unlocking the door, you must operate the latch mechanism. If the door is jammed, you must take steps to keep the latch in the open position while you pry the door from its frame.

With the help of your flashlight:

- Examine the latch mechanism.

By tracing the path from the hinged door handle or the push button (depending on the make and model of the car) to the latch and lock mechanisms, you should be able to clearly see how the latch operates.

- Attempt to unlatch the door by finger pressure on the mechanism.

To keep the latch in the open position while you pry the door from its frame:

- Jam a flat-blade screwdriver between the moving latch parts.

If you cannot operate the latch mechanism by hand:

- Drive the face plate of the lock off with a 2-inch ripping chisel or an air-operated chisel (Figure 6.14).
- Then pry the latch parts from the case.

There is no plan to follow since lock and latch mechanisms are different. When the face plate is off, you can pull the lock fork and other moving parts away from the case with a small prying tool and thus disable the latch. Once the safety bolt is free of the latch, opening the door involves no more than moving it away from the body of the vehicle.

Using Hand Tools to Force Open a Jammed Door

A door that cannot be pulled open after it has been unlocked and unlatched can usually be forced open with a combination forcible entry tool.

To gain maximum leverage:

- Have another rescuer hold a piece of cribbing in place against the car body while you wield the tool.

When the rescuer is in position:

- Insert the wedge end of the tool into the space between the door and the door frame.
- Then exert force on the tool as you use the piece of cribbing as a fulcrum. The door should pop open.

A rescuer who can exert 100 pounds of force on a 42-inch forcible entry tool can develop more than 300 pounds of prying force on the edge of a door when a piece of cribbing serves as a fulcrum. This should be more

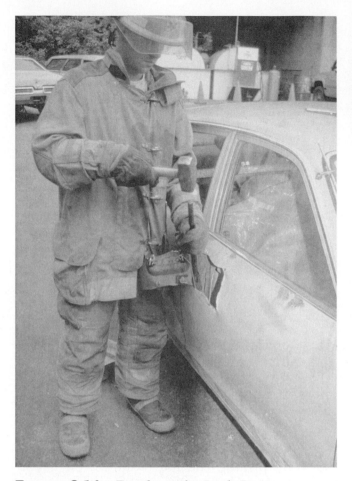

FIGURE 6.14   Breaking the Lock Box

than enough force to separate a vehicle's door from its frame (Figure 6.15).
Remember: The secret to success in forcing open jammed doors with hand tools is unlock, unlatch, then pry.

Using Powered Tools to Open Vehicle Doors

At this point, you may be inclined to ask why a rescuer would bother to use a powered tool when simple hand tools can be used to gain access in so many situations. There are two good reasons.

First, powered tools lend greater force and speed to rescue operations. Needless to say, hydraulic rescue tools develop more force than a rescuer wielding a pry bar, and time can be saved when a rescuer can open a severely damaged door with a hydraulic rescue tool rather than the unlock, unlatch, and pry technique described earlier.

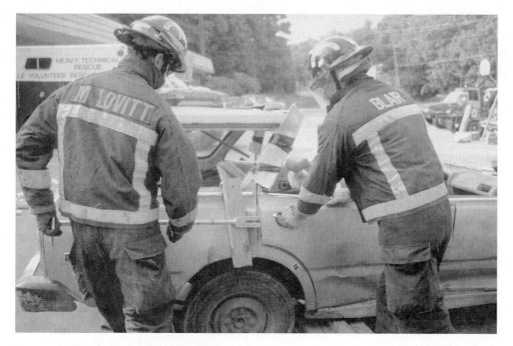

FIGURE 6.15   Prying the Door

Second, in many cases, powered tools enable rescuers to carry out gaining access and disentanglement operations in a single nonstop effort. A rescuer using a hydraulic rescue tool can remove a door immediately after opening it, and thus eliminate a major impediment to subsequent emergency care, packaging, and removal procedures.

Hydraulic tools are not the only powered tools that can be used for gaining access. An air-operated chisel or a reciprocating saw can be used to sever door bolts and an impact wrench can be used to unhinge doors. At no time is the argument that rescue is a science of alternatives more true than during the gaining access phase of a vehicle rescue operation.

OPENING VEHICLE DOORS WITH A HYDRAULIC RESCUE TOOL

Vehicle doors can be forced open in two ways: by prying the latch away from the safety bolt and swinging the door open on its hinges or by breaking the hinges and pivoting the door on the safety bolt. The decision as to which technique to use is usually influenced by the nature and degree of damage to the door. Following are procedures that you and another rescuer can use to force open doors with a hydraulic rescue tool.

Let's say that you have stabilized the vehicle, and the occupants are properly protected. Don't just attack the door with the tool. Carry out some preliminary steps that will make the job safer and easier.

Removing Windows. Forcefully opening a door that has a window in place can result in victims and rescuers being sprayed with glass particles. This will not be any problem since patients are protected and you and the other rescuers are wearing protective gear. However, glass fragments all over the car and the ground outside will be a nuisance and could become hazardous during subsequent operations.

If the window of the door you are going to open is rolled up:

* Remove it before you force the door. (The techniques for window removal are discussed later in this phase.)

If the window is rolled down and you can see that it is not broken:

- Run a strip of duct tape over the glass opening the length of the door. If the glass shatters, it will not come out; or
- Tap the edge of the glass with a steel tool. The window will shatter and the fragments will drop down into the body of the door.

If the door you are going to force open is a rear door with a window that will not roll down completely into the body of the door:

- Lay a lightweight tarp over the window, then shatter the glass. The tarp will keep the fragments from flying.

Creating Working Space for the Tips of the Tool. The gap between the latch side of a door and the adjacent pillar of an undamaged vehicle seldom exceeds a quarter of an inch. When the door is damaged as the result of a side impact collision, the gap can be quite large. But if the vehicle has been involved in a head-on or rear-end collision, there may be no gap at all between the edge of the door and the adjacent pillar.

When the door gap is narrow, rescuers will often try to simply wedge the tips of a hydraulic rescue tool into the existing opening. Or they will use the tool like a battering ram in hopes that the tips will find their way into the gap. Both efforts waste valuable time. There are better ways to create working space for the tips.

Using a Forcible Entry Tool. Use this procedure while your partner is preparing the tool for service:

- Insert the duckbill of a combination forcible entry tool as deeply as possible into the doorgap several inches above the safety bolt.
- Use a short sledgehammer to drive the duckbill in if the gap is extremely narrow.

While you support the head of the tool with one hand:

- Force the claw end of the tool downward with your other hand to distort the door lip and thus widen the gap.

- Then reposition the duckbill farther down into the gap and repeat the procedure. You should not have to remove the tool from the door gap to reposition it.
- Continue the prying/repositioning/prying procedure until you have widened the gap from several inches above to several inches below the safety bolt.

By the time your partner finishes assembling the tool, you will have created ample working space for the tips (Figure 6.16).

Using the Spreading Tool to Create Space for the Tips. When the rescue tool is ready for immediate service, you can use either of the following two procedures to move the edge of the door away from the adjacent pillar.

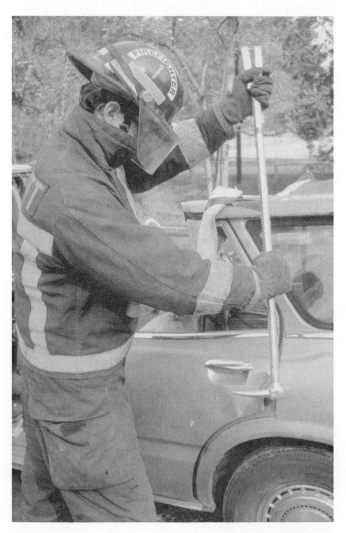

FIGURE 6.16   Making an Opening with Quik Bar

- Position the tool so the arms will spread vertically in the window opening.

While you hold the tool in position:

- Spread the arms slowly until the upper tip is seated against the upper window frame and the adjacent roof edge, and the lower tip is resting against the inner door panel.

Proper positioning of the lower tip is important. If the side of the tip pushes against only the outer panel of the door, it will simply peel the panel away, not push the door body outward as desired.

When the tips are properly positioned:

- Spread the arms of the tool to the maximum opening (Figure 6.17).

The window frame and roof edge will move up slightly until a rigid base of metal is created. Then the pushing effort of the arms will be concentrated on the more resilient door body, and as the lower arm moves, the door body will roll down and out. As it does, the latch edge of the door will be pulled away from the adjacent door panel and working space will be created for the tips (Figure 6.18). You can use this method for pulling a pushed-in door away from a patient.

Be aware that as the upper portion of the door body moves down and out, the latch form may separate from the striker bolt. If it does, the door will open.

Squeezing the door body will also create working space for the tips.

- Open the spreading tool just enough to capture the upper portion of the door body between the arms.
- Close the arms to squeeze the inner and outer door panels together.

The latch edge of the door should move away from the adjacent pillar just enough that a gap will be created sufficient for the tips (Figure 6.19).

Forcing the Latch Away from the Safety Bolt. This relatively simple procedure can be diffi-

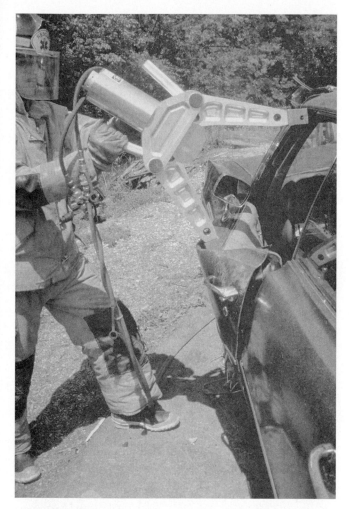

FIGURE 6.17   Making an Opening with Spreader

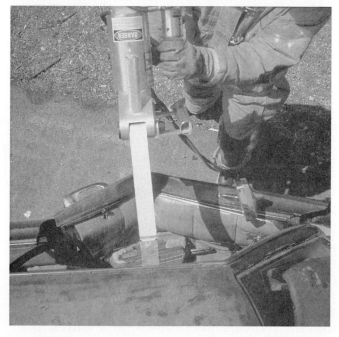

FIGURE 6.18   Pulling Door Away from Patient

cult and time-consuming when the tips of the hydraulic rescue tool are not deeply seated into the door gap. The following procedure will reduce the time it takes to open doors.

- Insert the tips as far as you can into the gap.
- Spread the arms just a bit to widen the gap.
- Close the arms and push the tips in deeper.
- Repeat the procedure until the tips are seated deep in the door gap.
- Then spread the arms to move the latch away from the safety bolt.

When the latch separates from the safety bolt:

- Swing the door open.

An important point: Do not allow your partner or another person to lean backward against the door in an attempt to keep it from flying open. Rescuers have been injured when doors that were under a great deal of tension "exploded" outward. If you are concerned about the sudden, violent movement of a door after the latch separates from the safety bolt, secure the window frame of the door to the B-pillar with a web strap or rescue chain before you pry it open. The loop should be large enough to allow the door to move a little after the latch separates from the safety bolt.

OPENING A FRONT DOOR BY BREAKING THE HINGES

When a car is struck broadside with sufficient force to displace the B-pillar inward, a large gap usually forms between the door edge and the front fender. Often this gap is wide enough to expose the underlying hinges. At the same time, the gap between the door edge and the B-pillar may be narrowed as the sheet metal of the door is distorted by the collision. In such cases, you should consider opening the door by breaking the hinges and pivoting the door on its safety bolt.

Before doing anything else:

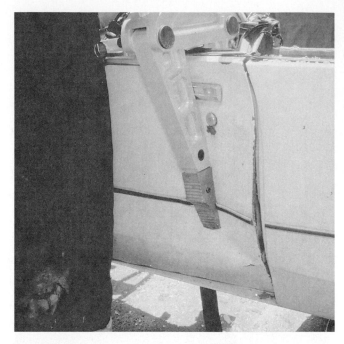

FIGURE 6.19   Creating a Gap with Spreader

- Check the gap between the door and the fender.

If the opening is not large enough for you to reach the hinge plates with the tips of the rescue tool:

- Squeeze the door as previously shown, only this time at the front of the door (Figure 6.20).
- Displace metal as necessary with either a forcible entry tool or the rescue tool itself.

Doors that contain a lot of plastic or light metal flex so much as to make it a frustrating task trying to pop the hinges. When using the hydraulic spreader, hold it vertically rather than horizontally. Work the tips into the top of the door frame at the A-pillar. By continually opening and closing the tips, you will allow the spreader to run down the A-pillar to the top hinge. This gives you much more bearing surface to work the spreader arms. Once the top hinge is broken, continue to push the arms straight down and break the bottom hinge. Two different vehicles are shown in Figures 6.21

and 6.22, and Figures 6.23 and 6.24. Both are worked from the top down.

This can be a dangerous operation for you, your partner, and the person in the car next to the door. If you and your partner are standing too close when the bottom hinge breaks and the latch separates from the safety bolt, the door can drop onto your feet. If the door twists while forces are being exerted by the rescue tool, the person next to the door could be injured. Avoid accidents while you are breaking hinges by:

- Standing well behind any point the door is likely to drop onto if it breaks free;
- Positioning a spine board between the occupant and the door as soon as a suitable opening is made; and
- Having your partner maintain a constant pull on the door with a web strap wrapped around a portion of the window frame.

When the door is completely off the hinges, it can be pivoted on the safety bolt. Be careful! Keep your feet from under the door.

Depending on the damage resulting from the collision and the prying effort, the latch may or may not separate from the safety bolt. If it does not, force the latch and the safety bolt apart with the rescue tool. Thus, you will have accomplished a gaining access and a disentanglement step in one operation.

OPENING REAR DOORS

The rear doors of a four-door sedan can also be opened in two ways. If you need to open a rear door but not the front door of the same side, pry the latch away from the safety bolt and swing the door open on its hinges. But if you have to open both doors of the same side, save time by breaking the hinges of the rear door and pivoting the door open on its safety lock after you open the front door. The rear door hinges of most cars are completely accessible when the front door is open (or off). Take the same safety precautions as you would when breaking the hinges of the front door: taking the proper stance, protecting

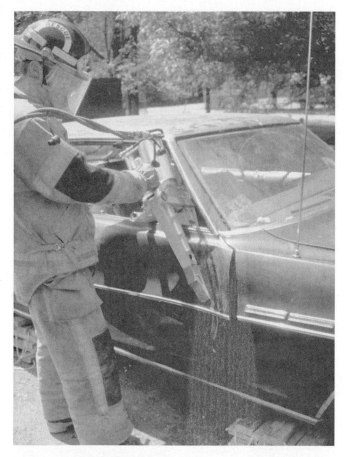

FIGURE 6.20   Creating a Gap with Spreader

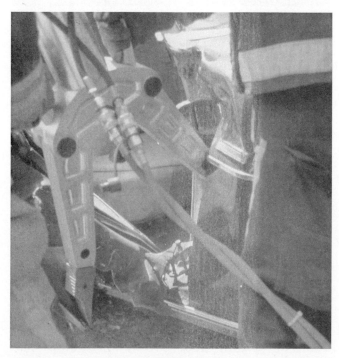

FIGURE 6.21   Working with Spreader from Top Down

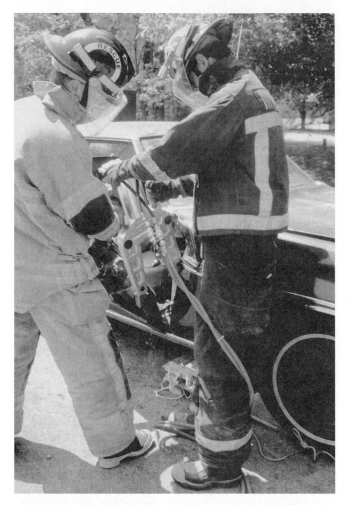

FIGURE 6.22   Working with Spreader from Top Down

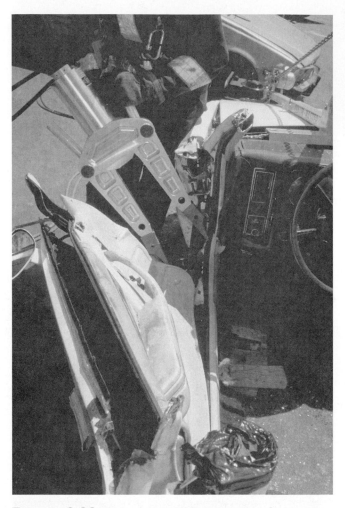

FIGURE 6.23   Working with Spreader from Top Down

the person next to the door, and having your partner pull the door away from the car with a web strap.

OPENING REAR DOORS BY SEVERING THE HINGES

You can open the rear doors of most four-door sedans by severing either the safety bolt or the hinges. Cutting the hinges is in order if the construction of the rear door or the extent of damage is such that reaching the safety bolt will be difficult, or if the open door will be an impediment to emergency care and removal activities.

While another rescuer supports the door:

- Cut the hinges with the saw—first the top hinge, then the bottom.

When both hinges are cut:

- Pivot the door on its safety bolt. The door may or may not pull free from its safety bolt.

If the door does not pull free from the safety bolt when you pull it open:

- Either cut the bolt while your partner supports the door; or
- Secure it in the widest open position with a chain or strap that is anchored to the bumper or frame member.

Unhinging Rear Doors. Unhinging the rear doors of a four-door sedan is a snap. Remember that the rear door hinges of almost every car are exposed after the front door has been either opened or removed.

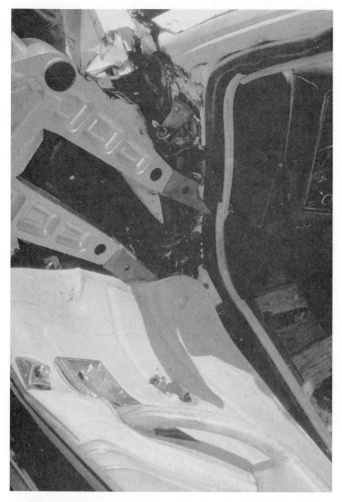

FIGURE 6.24 Working with Spreader from Top Down

While your partner holds his weight against the door:

- Remove the hinge bolts (Figure 6.25).

When all of the hinge bolts have been removed:

- Pivot the door on the safety bolt.

If the latch does not pull free from the safety bolt:

- Sever the bolt with the air chisel or the reciprocating saw.

As the saying goes, there's good news and there's bad news. The good news is that unhinging doors is a quick and easy technique.

The bad news is that it cannot be done with every car. Some cars have hinges secured to the body of the vehicle with threaded studs installed from inside. These hinges cannot be disassembled in the ways just described. Before you start an unhinging procedure that may not work, widen the gap between the fender and the hinge side of the front door and look inside to see how the hinges are secured. If you see hex-head or round head Phillips machine bolts, the door can be unhinged.

OPENING DOORS BY SEVERING THE SAFETY BOLT

The blade of a reciprocating saw can usually cut through hardened safety bolts in less than a minute.

"Bottoming out" is a problem in this procedure, so be sure to use high-speed shatterproof blades, not the ordinary metal-cutting blades that come with the saw. Bottoming out is when the point of the blade strikes a solid object during the cutting effort, in this case the lip of the B-pillar against which the door closes.

An ordinary blade is likely to break when the point contacts a solid surface. If it does, you will have to stop and change the blade—a sometimes difficult and time-consuming task in stress, low light, and bad-weather situations. A shatterproof blade will merely bend, and you have to stop only long enough to straighten the blade by hand while it is still in the holder.

Severing Door Bolts with a Reciprocating Saw. As is the case when using a hydraulic rescue tool, creating working space is an important step when using a reciprocating saw to sever a safety bolt (Nadar Bolt). You must have unrestricted access to the bolt.

While your partner is assembling the equipment:

- Widen the gap between the door lip and the B-pillar with a forcible entry tool (Figure 6.26). Follow the procedure suggested for creating working space for the tips of a hydraulic rescue tool.

Before you get into position to cut:

- Quickly depress and release the saw's operating trigger as many times as necessary to fully extend the blade.

While it may seem inconsequential, this last step is important. If you start the cut when the blade is in the fully retracted position, the point of the blade may bottom out on the first stroke. If this happens, you'll have to stop and straighten the blade.

While your partner stands at your side or behind you and illuminates the work area with a flashlight:

- Hold the handle of the saw with one hand, and cradle the body of the saw in your other hand, which is resting firmly against the side of the vehicle.
- Adjust the position of the saw in your hand so the point of the fully extended blade is not contacting the inner lip of the B-pillar.

When you are ready:

- Depress the trigger and start the cut.

   If the saw is a variable speed model:

- Keep the speed very low until you are sure the point of the blade is not striking the inner lip of the B-pillar.

When you are sure that the blade will move freely:

- Bring the saw speed up to maximum.
- Exert downward force with both hands to facilitate the cut.
- Have your partner continually lubricate the saw blade during the cutting process (Figure 6.27).

When the blade passes through the bolt:

- Withdraw the saw and pull the door open. Use a pry bar if the door remains jammed after the bolt is cut.

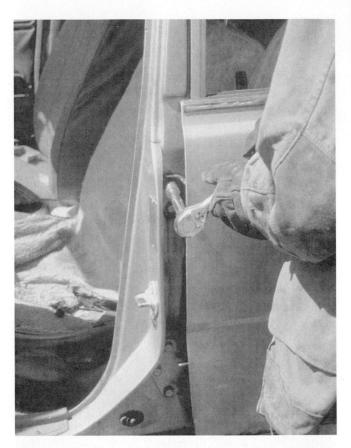

FIGURE 6.25   Unbolting Rear Door with Hand Socket

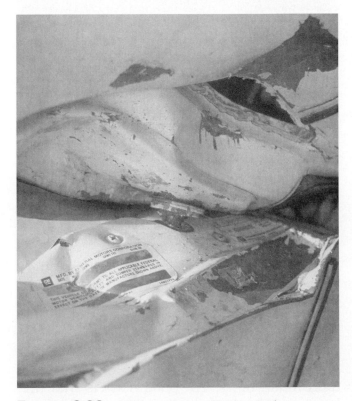

FIGURE 6.26   Widen Gap to Nadar Bolt

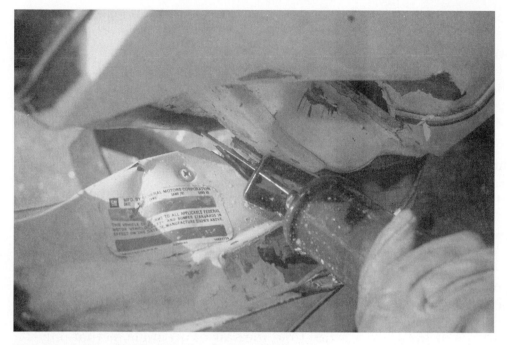

FIGURE 6.27   Cutting Nadar Bolt

Removing the door altogether can be accomplished by cutting the hinges while the door is fully open. Cutting hinges with a reciprocating saw takes time, however. If the injured person next to the door needs immediate attention, let EMS personnel carry out lifesaving measures and remove the doors during the disentanglement phase of the rescue operation.

OPENING VEHICLE DOORS WITH AN AIR-OPERATED CHISEL

Attempting to cut a door bolt of any diameter with a low-pressure air-operated chisel is seldom, if ever, successful. Cutting heavy door bolts may be impossible even with a high-pressure air gun (200 to 300 psi) that has a new chisel.

If you have a high-pressure air gun and a sharp chisel and you think you can sever a particular door bolt, try it. Check your progress after a minute or so. If the chisel is making its way through the bolt, then by all means, continue. If you've made little or no progress, abandon the procedure rather than waste time. Instead of trying to cut the bolt, make several cuts into the B-pillar and free the bolt and its attachments. You'll have

to improvise the procedure as you go, and it will be a "nibbling" operation, but will probably work.

Cutting hinges can be equally difficult. Stamped hinges can be cut with a high-pressure air-operated chisel, while cast hinges cannot. Stamped hinges have smooth, irregular-shaped parts with rounded edges. Cast hinges have square edges and a grainy appearance. A cross section of a cast hinge would appear rectangular.

OPENING VEHICLE DOORS BY REMOVING HINGE BOLTS

Pairing a reciprocating saw or an air-operated chisel with an impact wrench enables a rescuer to disassemble a vehicle's components as well as sever them. Impact wrenches are available with either an electric or air-operated motor. Thus the impact wrench can be operated from the same power source as the cutting tool.

Having both electric tools connected to a "Y" or junction box at the end of an extension cord eliminates the need for changing plugs in the middle of a rescue operation. Likewise, having both air-operated tools connected to a "Y" or manifold eliminates the need to uncouple and couple supply lines during a critical procedure.

Remember: Heavy-duty impact sockets must be used with either an air-operated or an electric impact wrench. The high torque and constant hammering will ruin an ordinary socket in just a few seconds.

Unhinging Front Doors. The bolts that secure the front door hinges to the body of a vehicle are concealed behind a portion of each fender. In most cars a metal fender stiffener lies directly over the hinge bolts.

If you are going to use an air-operated chisel:

• Install a wide cutting chisel instead of the panel cutter. While a panel cutter will cut through the sheet metal of the fender without difficulty, it will either ride over or cut only a part of the stiffener.

If you are going to use a reciprocating saw:

• Install a short shatterproof blade.

To expose the hinges:

• Make a starting hole in the fender with the pike of a forcible entry tool just below the break in the fender (the point where the vertical portion of the fender meets the horizontal part), and about 8 inches from the door edge.
• Insert the air-operated chisel or the blade of the reciprocating saw into the opening.
• Make a horizontal cut from the starting hole to the door edge.
• Cut through the fender and the underlying stiffener at the same time.

Making this cut with a reciprocating saw takes a little care. Instead of holding the tool so the sole plate is flat against the metal (as it would normally be held), hold the saw at an angle so that only the rear edge of the sole plate rides on the metal. This will prevent the point of the blade from bottoming out on underlying components.

After making the horizontal cut:

• Replace the wide chisel with a panel cutter if you are using an air gun; there is no other underlying stiffener to be concerned with. The blade of the wide chisel will be difficult to keep in the cut, while the T portion of the panel cutter will ride on the surface of the metal.
• Then reinsert the chisel or the blade of the reciprocating saw in the starting hole and make a vertical cut downward to a point just below the level of the bottom door hinge.

If you are using a reciprocating saw:

• Hold the saw at an angle so that only the rear edge of the sole plate contacts the fender and only the forward portion of the blade cuts through the metal. This prevents bottoming out.

When you finish the vertical cut:

• Pull the resulting flap down to expose the hinges (Figure 6.28).

While your partner holds his weight against the door:

• Remove the hinge bolts from bottom to top with the impact wrench. You may have to use either a straight or universal extension in close quarters (Figure 6.29).

When all of the bolts have been removed:

• Pivot the door on the safety bolt (Figures 6.30, 6.31, 6.32).

If the latch does not pull free from the bolt as you pivot the door:

• Sever the bolt with either the air chisel or the reciprocating saw while your partner supports the door.

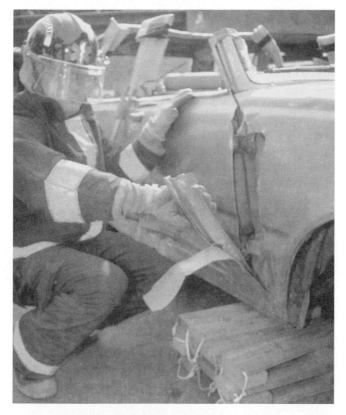

FIGURE 6.28   Exposing Hinges

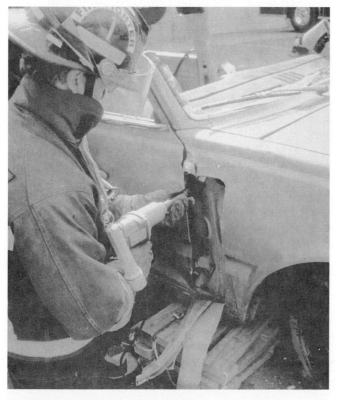

FIGURE 6.29   Unbolting Door with Impact Wrench

GAINING ACCESS THROUGH WINDOW OPENINGS

There was a time in the history of vehicle rescue when breaking windows was just about the only known way of entering a vehicle when doors were either locked or jammed. The technique was simple. A "rescuer" simply bashed in the windows with whatever tool was available! Firefighters used axes, rescue personnel used sledgehammers, ambulance attendants used jack handles, and police officers used riot sticks and probably even gun butts. Today, rescue operations are a little more "patient friendly," if we can paraphrase a computer term. When possible, windshields and rear windows are removed rather than broken, and when breaking glass is absolutely necessary, it's done in such a manner that danger to occupants is minimal. There's a reason.

The Dangers of Indiscriminately Breaking Glass

Bashing in windows sprays occupants with pieces of glass ranging in size from powder particles to small shards and 1/4-inch chunks. Glass debris finds its way into unprotected eyes, ears, nostrils, mouths, and, of course, open wounds. Large chunks of glass can be picked from an open wound, but very finely divided particles may remain unnoticed deep in the wound. If they are not removed (as by debridement), they will continue to damage tissues even after the wound is closed.

Before we discuss procedures for safely disposing of vehicle windows, let's consider what the windows are, how they contribute to safety, and how they are mounted.

Types of Automotive Glass

Automotive glass has an interesting history. The idea of windows on automobiles wasn't even considered until 1908. Even then, the only piece of glass was a flat windshield sold at extra cost. The 1910 Owen was the first automobile to have a windshield provided as

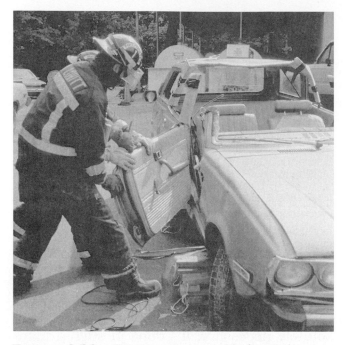

FIGURE 6.30   Pivoting Door on Nadar Bolt

standard equipment, and side windows did not appear on cars until 1917.

The first "safety" glass appeared in 1926. That year's Stutz had a windshield with lengths of wire running horizontally every seven inches to keep glass shards together if the windshield were broken. The 1926 Rickenbacker had the first laminated windshield—a sandwich of two clear panes of glass with an inner layer of clear celluloid. Today, safety glass is installed in passenger cars in two forms: laminated windshields and tempered glass side and rear windows.

Windshields

While they appear to be single panes of glass, windshields are actually two pieces of plate glass bonded by high temperature to a thin sheet of opaque plastic. The resulting lamination, or "sandwich," is a strong, clear window. When something strikes a laminated windshield with sufficient force to break it—like a stone from outside or a head from inside—the glass fractures, and cracks radiate away from the point of impact like a spider's web. Small bits of glass fall away from the point of impact, but unlike the

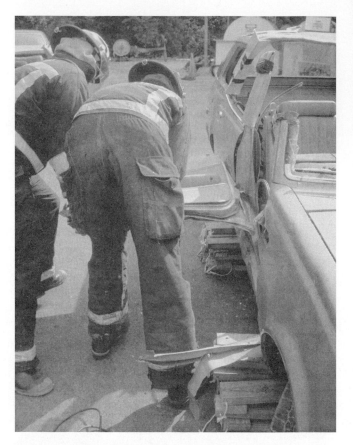

FIGURE 6.31   Pivoting Door on Nadar Bolt

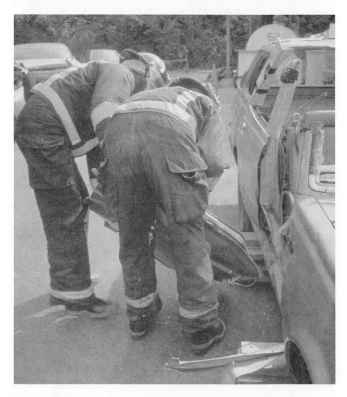

FIGURE 6.32   Pivoting Door on Nadar Bolt

shards produced when a plate glass window breaks, most of the broken pieces of a laminated windshield remain adhered to the plastic inner layer.

A laminated windshield will usually keep unrestrained occupants inside a vehicle during a low-speed front-end collision. If injuries do result from striking the glass, they are usually limited to a concussion and/or minor lacerations of the forehead and scalp. However, in some instances, cervical spine injuries can also be a result of a low-speed collision.

ANTI-LACERATIVE WINDSHIELDS

A few automobile companies both foreign and domestic have been using a windshield which has an extra layer of butzite (plastic) on the interior. This is to prevent the occupants from encountering glass in the event of a collision. You must be very careful when handling this type of windshield, as the exterior glass shards break away very thin and extremely long.

Though the idea was good, the windshields were extremely expensive and subject to damage on the interior. Most have been discontinued, however, be aware there are many on the road.

Side and Rear Windows

The side and rear windows of passenger cars are most likely a single sheet of glass—but glass that is tempered much like steel. Tempered glass windows are tough—approximately five times stronger than laminated windows—and because they are tough, tempered glass windows can often withstand crash forces severe enough to virtually destroy a vehicle. Nonetheless, tempered glass windows can be easily broken with a simple hand-held tool. When tempered glass windows do break either by accident or design, they shatter into 3/16- to 1/4-inch chunks rather than shards. These chunks can cut flesh, to be sure, but the resulting wounds are usually shallow, one-drop-of-blood punctures, rather than the deep, profusely bleeding lacerations and incisions common to long, sharp shards of plate glass.

Removing Windshields and Rear Windows

For years, windshields and rear windows were installed in a rubber gasket that had a slot for the glass and a slot for the lip of the pinch weld—the frame in which the window is set. In 1964, car manufacturers started installing windshields and rear windows against a strip of polysulfide adhesive laid in the pinch weld, and in 1974 the manufacturers changed from polysulfide to urethane for a much stronger bond. Windshields and rear windows are still mounted with a urethane adhesive, although some manufacturers are also producing cars with gasket mounted windows.

Because you are likely to encounter both installations during vehicle rescue operations, and since a different removal procedure is required for each, you must be able to recognize whether a windshield or rear window is gasket-mounted or adhesive mounted.

Look at the side of the window. If you see glass, then what appears to be about a quarter-inch of a black plastic or rubber material, then chrome trim, you will know that the glass is mounted in a U-shaped gasket. If you see glass, then chrome trim, you will know that the window is mounted with an adhesive material.

Removing a Gasket-Mounted Windshield of an Older Car

The gasket-mounted windshield or rear window of an older car can be quickly removed by simply cutting away the exposed lip of the gasket. The linoleum knife included on the suggested equipment list in Phase One is especially well suited for the task because of its hooked blade. However, any knife can be used if a linoleum knife is not available.

- Use a short pry bar or other prying tool to remove any chrome trim from the sides and top of the windshield. Don't bother with the trim at the bottom of the windshield. The glass will pivot on that edge (Figure 6.33).

Starting at about the midpoint of the windshield:

- Slide the point of the knife under the retaining lip of the gasket and drive the point into the body of the gasket while holding the knife blade as flat as possible against the glass.

In one continuous movement from the starting point:

- Draw the knife toward you along the top of the windshield and down one side (Figure 6.34).
- Twist the knife handle slightly to assure that the blade slides on the glass. Otherwise it will cut through the retaining lip of the gasket.
- Don't try to sever the retaining lip completely in one pass of the knife; instead
- Make several progressively deeper cuts.

When you have severed all of the retaining lip of the gasket on that side:

- Go to the other side of the car and repeat the procedure.

When all of the retaining lip of the gasket has been removed:

- Carefully work the end of your pry bar behind the upper edge of the windshield close to the midpoint and attempt to pry the glass away from the frame.

If you meet resistance to the point where the glass is likely to break if you continue to exert force on the prying tool:

- Check to see that all of the gasket's retaining lip has been removed. Just a

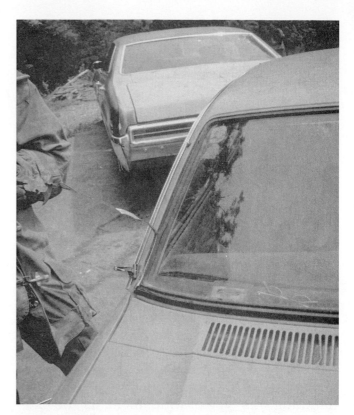

FIGURE 6.33 Removing Gasket-Mounted Windshield

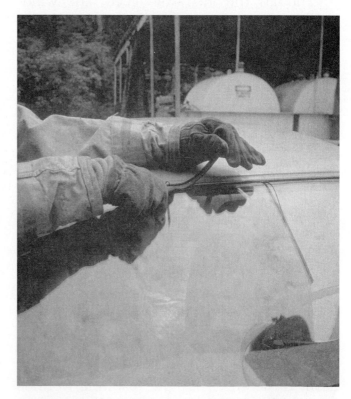

FIGURE 6.34 Removing Gasket-Mounted Windshield

few small projections of gasket can prevent the quick and clean removal of a windshield.

When you have a large enough opening between the edge of the glass and the frame:

- Grip the upper edge of the glass with your hands.
- Pivot the glass on its lower edge.
- Pull the glass from its frame and carry it to a safe place (Figure 6.35).

Needless to say, considerable time will be saved if two rescuers work together to remove a windshield, one on each side of the car.

An important point: If you lubricate the knife blade with the soap solution you use to lubricate hacksaw blades, you'll find that cutting the gasket is much easier.

Removing a Gasket-Mounted Rear Window Intact

A gasket-mounted rear window is removed in the same manner as a gasket-mounted windshield. However, a little more care is neces-

sary in prying the window from the frame. The weakest part of a tempered glass window is its edge. A slight tap with a steel tool can cause a tempered glass window to shatter.

When you have stripped away all of the retaining lip of the gasket:

- Gently work the end of a flat pry bar behind the edge of the glass at about the midpoint of the window.
- Do not drive the bar in with your hand or another tool; to do so may cause the window to break.

When there is an opening between the glass and the frame:

- Insert the tip of the pry bar so that 3 or 4 inches of the tool are behind the glass.

With the body of the bar pivoting on the window frame and the prying edge pushing against the glass:

- Move the window away from the frame just far enough for you to get your fingers behind the glass.

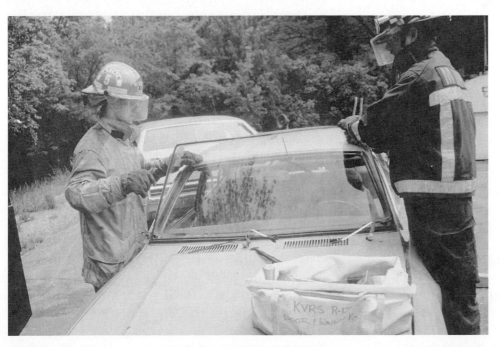

FIGURE 6.35 Removing Gasket-Mounted Windshield

While you support the window with one hand:

- Remove the prying tool.
- Then pivot the glass on the lower edge, remove it from the frame, and carry it to a safe place.

Removing the Gasket-Mounted Windows of Newer Cars

In older cars the windshield and rear window are simply set in the channel of the gasket. In new cars that have gasket-mounted windshields and rear windows, the glass is held in the channel with an adhesive. To remove these windows it will be necessary to cut the leg of the gasket away in the conventional manner, then separate the glass from the remainder of the channel with a windshield knife. The procedure for using a windshield knife is outlined in the following section.

REMOVING AN ADHESIVE-MOUNTED WINDSHIELD OR REAR WINDOW INTACT

An adhesive-mounted windshield is removed with a knife that has been designed specially for the task. The knife is used in such a way that the glass is separated from the adhesive.

With a short flat pry bar or other prying tool:

- Remove the chrome from the two sides and the upper edge of the window.

It is not necessary to remove the piece of chrome that covers the bottom edge of the windshield or rear window. The window will pivot on the lower edge of the glass.

- Next remove any trim clips that will interfere with movement of the windshield knife. Most can be pulled away with the edge of a prying tool or the blade of a screwdriver.

To insert the blade of the windshield knife behind the glass:

- Hold the tool so the knife blade is parallel to the edge of the glass in the space between the window and the window frame.
- Exert downward force on the tool handle to press the knife blade into the adhesive material.

As you exert downward pressure:

- Turn the handle of the tool to work the knife point blade behind the glass.
- Continue to rotate the handle until the knife blade is behind the window and at a right angle to the edge of the glass.

Untrained rescuers invariably try to insert the knife blade by holding the tool so the blade is at a right angle to the window, then jamming the point under the glass. This usually causes the blade to break.

While you hold the handle of the tool with one hand:

- Pull on the T-handle to draw the tool across the top of the window and down the near side. This action will separate the glass from the adhesive (Figure 6.36).

It's important to hold the tool handle perpendicular to the glass. If you hold the tool so the handle angles slightly toward you, the sharp edge of the knife will bite into the window frame and stop. If you hold the tool so the handle is angled away from you, the knife edge may break through the edge of the glass, especially if the window has fracture lines that extend to the edge of the glass.

When you have half the top edge and one side of the glass separated from the adhesive:

- Move to the other side of the vehicle and repeat the procedure.
- Insert the short pry bar behind the glass at about the midpoint of the window and pry the upper edge of the window away from the frame. The glass will pivot on the bottom edge.

You may encounter resistance as the glass moves away from the top and sides of the window frame and pulls strings of adhesive away from the window frame, especially during a hot-weather rescue operation. If this happens, use a linoleum knife or other knife to sever the "strings" while you hold the upper edge of the window away from the frame with your hand or the prying tool.

Finally, depending on your needs:

- Either fold the windshield down; or
- Remove it from the vehicle altogether.

If you elect to remove the windshield altogether and have trouble separating the glass from the bottom edge of adhesive by rocking the window from side to side, cut the adhesive with a knife.

PROBLEMS IN REMOVING WINDSHIELDS AND REAR WINDOWS INTACT

While removing adhesive-mounted windshields and rear windows in the manner just described can usually be done quickly and easily, this will not be the case all of the time. Fractures that extend to the edge of a windshield, the age of the vehicle, weather, a do-it-yourself sealing job, and the width of

the adhesive strip may make removing a window with a windshield knife impossible. Following are some suggestions for dealing with these problems.

Broken Glass. Removing a windshield that has fracture lines extending from the point all the way to the edges of the glass will be difficult, if not impossible. There will be a tendency for the knife blade to pop out from behind the glass when it reaches a fracture, regardless of how careful you are to keep the tool handle vertical, or how gently and steadily you pull on the T-handle. If a windshield has many fractures, you will save time by either making an opening in the glass, or cutting the windshield from the frame, depending on your needs.

Older Glass. The adhesive of an older car may be so hard that even if you can get the point of the windshield knife behind the glass, you may not be able to pull the tool with the T-handle. Don't waste time if you find this to be the case. If you must remove a windshield, cut it out. If you must remove a rear window, break it.

Cold Glass. It is extremely difficult to separate a windshield or rear window from its

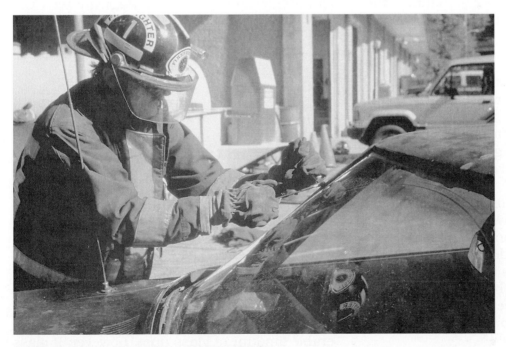

FIGURE 6.36   Using Windshield Knife

adhesive in cold weather, even in a new car. The heat from an incandescent floodlight kept in motion a few inches from the edge of the windshield can be used to soften the adhesive.

If cold prevents you from removing an adhesive-mounted window quickly and no incandescent floodlight is immediately available, abandon the procedure and cut or break the glass.

Home-Sealed Windows. Saturday mechanics attempt to seal leaking windshields and rear windows with a silicone preparation available in auto supply stores. The sealant does more than keep rain out of a car, however; it also keeps rescuers out!

A home-sealed windshield can usually be easily identified by the beads (or globs) of a nearly clear substance adhered to the chrome trim, the window frame, and the glass. Seldom will a motorist go to the trouble of removing the chrome trim, squirting the sealant into the space between the edge of the glass and the window frame, and then replacing the trim.

If you see that a windshield or rear window has been sealed in this manner, don't bother trying to remove the glass with a windshield knife. You probably will not be able to insert the knife edge behind the glass, let alone separate the glass from the original adhesive. Either cut or break the window.

Wide Adhesive Strips. While the strip of adhesive in the pinch weld of most cars is about 5/8-inch wide when the glass is against it, some new cars have adhesive strips up to 1-1/4-inch wide. The long blade windshield knife must be used to remove these windows.

Incidentally, don't be alarmed if you look at a windshield or rear window installation of a new car and see a black strip around the window that is much wider than your knife blade is long. The black is ceramic paint that is applied to the glass to hide welds, the adhesive strip, and imperfections in the pinch weld. The adhesive strip itself will not be more than 1-1/4-inch wide.

CUTTING OUT WINDSHIELDS WITH UNCONVENTIONAL TOOLS

Using an Ax. Since there is no equipment to assemble and set up, the fastest way to forcefully remove a windshield is with an ax. Cutting can be accomplished while kneeling on the hood of the vehicle or standing at the side.

Starting at the midpoint of the windshield:

- Cut across the top and down one side with short strokes.
- Use just enough force to drive the cutting edge of the ax through the glass, and keep the blade as close to the window frame as possible. This will minimize the problem of jagged edges remaining after the windshield has been removed.

When you have cut through half the top and one side of the windshield:

- Have your partner stand at that side and support the cut portion with his hands. Then move to the other side of the vehicle and repeat the procedure.

When both sides and the top have been cut through:

- Make a fourth cut along the bottom edge and remove the windshield altogether.

Oh yes . . . be sure to keep your mouth shut when you are removing a section of windshield with any cutting tool. Glass fragments may find their way into the opening and lacerate your gums and tongue and the roof of your mouth. If you swallow some of the glass debris, you could be in for some serious gastrointestinal trouble.

Using a Reciprocating Saw. Because of the high-speed back-and-forth action of the blade, fragmentation is not as severe as when a windshield is cut with an ax or an air-operated chisel. The operation does produce a considerable amount of glass dust, however. If glass dust spreading away from the vehicle will be a problem, as when another accident vehicle is close, use strips of duct tape to mask the part of the windshield that will be cut.

Your best position for this procedure may be on the hood of the car. It might be difficult to reach the midpoint of the windshield with the saw from a position at the side of the vehicle.

After protecting the occupants (and masking the glass, if necessary):

- Climb onto the hood and punch a starting hole in an upper corner of the windshield with the pike of a forcible entry tool.
- Insert the saw blade into the opening and guide the tool across the top of the windshield and down until the blade is near the dash.
- Reinsert the blade into the starting hole.

In one continuous movement:

- Guide the saw across the top of the windshield and down the other side. Be sure to keep the shoe of the tool pressed firmly against the glass (Figure 6.37).

Depending on your needs:

- Either break the glass from side to side along the bottom edge of the windshield and fold the window down; or
- Make a fourth cut with the saw and remove the windshield altogether.

If you elect to remove the windshield rather than fold it down, be sure to keep the saw blade at a level where it will not contact the dash.

Using an Air-Operated Chisel. Reduce the problem of fragmentation and conserve your air supply by operating the gun at a pressure of 30 to 40 psi. The widest curved chisel available should be installed in the safety retainer.

If you feel that glass dust outside the vehicle will pose a threat to rescuers or emergency service personnel, use strips of duct tape to mask the path that the chisel will take.

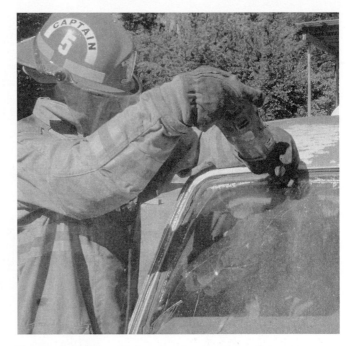

FIGURE 6.37   Using Reciprocating Saw on Windshield

After protecting the occupants (and masking the glass, if necessary):

- Make a starting hole in a lower corner of the windshield with the chisel. One or two quick bursts of air should be sufficient.

While you hold the gun with one hand and support the shank of the chisel with your other hand:

- In one continuous movement, guide the chisel up one side of the windshield, across the top, down the other side, and across the bottom to the starting point (Figure 6.38).

If you allow your gloved hand to glide on the surface of the windshield while you firmly support the shank of the chisel, you can prevent the end of the chisel from punching through the glass.

Using a Glas-Master Glass Removal Tool. All of the above mentioned methods of removing or breaking out windshields are discussed in length simply to give you an arsenal from which to draw, for any event or circumstance you may happen upon. Keeping this in mind,

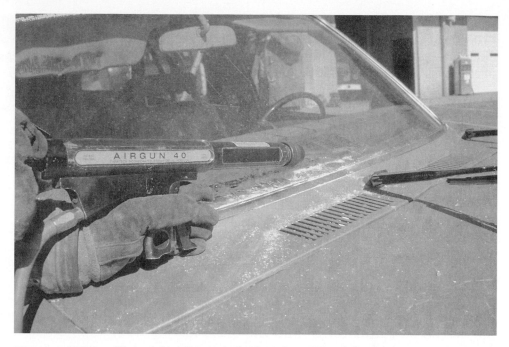

FIGURE 6.38   Using Air-Operated Chisel on Windshield

a tool to bridge all or most of these problem areas is the Glas-Master saw. This tool does not rely on any power source, is light in weight, and is easy to train with for best results. It therefore becomes the tool of choice for most situations.

The Glas-Master saw is equipped with a hook for making a starter hole in safety glass (Figure 6.39) and a spring-loaded center punch for taking out tempered glass without scattering glass to the inside of the vehicle. Cutting action is accomplished on the backstroke, the same as the reciprocating saw, thus pulling the saw into the work and depositing glass chips to the outside (Figure 6.40). The saw has other uses with different blades, such as cutting soft plastics found on many new model autos.

Disposing of Side and Rear Windows

In some rescue situations you will be able to simply break a tempered glass window to make an opening in a vehicle. In other situations you will have to take rather elaborate steps to protect the occupants from glass fragments.

Breaking Tempered Glass Side and Rear Windows

A tempered glass window in its fully closed position is tough. If you strike the center of the window with the flat face of a short sledgehammer, you will have to exert consid-

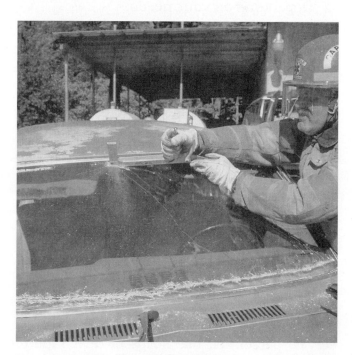

FIGURE 6.39   Using Glas-Master on Windshield

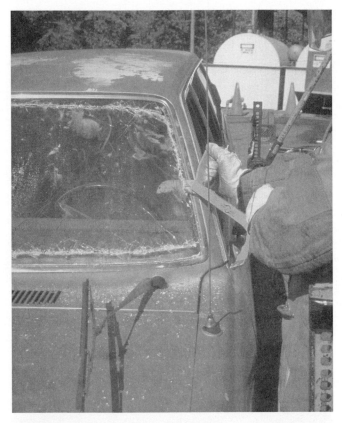

FIGURE 6.40   Using Glas-Master on Windshield

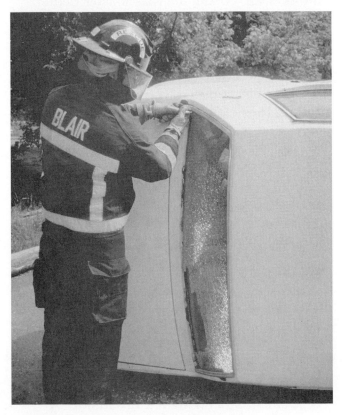

FIGURE 6.41   Using a Center Punch

erable force to break the glass. When a blow is sufficient to stress the glass to the breaking point, fragments will explode into the vehicle (along with the hammer, if you do not have a tight grip on the handle). Glass fragments propelled into a vehicle in this manner can penetrate unprotected eyes and flesh.

Rolled-up tempered glass side windows can be broken in such a way that the fragments will remain in the window frame until they are removed by hand. The secret of success is to use a sharp-pointed tool. The pike of a forcible entry tool can seldom be used successfully, however. While the pike may be sharp enough to break the glass, the quickly widening shank of the pike stresses the fragments and causes them to separate. The best tools for the job are spring-loaded center punches and ordinary steel prick punches. Both have sharp points and very narrow shanks.

USING A SPRING-LOADED CENTER PUNCH

Using a spring-loaded center punch to break tempered glass windows eliminates the need for a hammer. Set the spring for maximum impact if you have an adjustable model.

- Position the point of the tool against the glass in a corner of the window; this is the least resilient part of the window.
- Then position your hand around the tool in such a way that when the point passes through the glass, the frame will prevent your hand from following.

When your hand is in position:

- Push the sliding part of the tool toward the window until the spring mechanism "fires" and drives the point of the punch through the glass (Figure 6.41).

Proper positioning of your hand and the punch is important. If you simply operate the punch without resting your hand on a part of the door, it's likely that when the glass breaks, your hand will drive fragments into the interior of the vehicle. This is exactly what you are trying to avoid by using the center punch!

- After the glass shatters, use the blunt end of the tool to make two or three finger holes in the upper edge of the window.
- Strike the glass gently to assure that fragments drop straight down instead of being propelled into the passenger compartment.
- Insert your gloved finger into the holes and pull glass fragments out until you have a slot large enough for your hand.
- Then insert your gloved hand into the slot and push fragments out with your palm and fingers until all of the window has been removed.

As when using a spring-loaded center punch, don't just place the point of the prick punch against the glass and whack the punch with a hammer. Your hand may hit the glass and push fragments inward.

- Cradle the punch between your palm and curved fingers.
- Position the heel of your hand against the door so the point of the punch is contacting a lower corner of the window.
- Tap the end of the punch with the hammer to break the glass.
- Remove the fragments in the manner suggested after using a spring-loaded punch.

When using the Glas-Master for breaking tempered glass, place the top of the T-handle against the door panel and the front guard against the window post. Place the punch in the corner of the side glass (Figure 6.42). Push the punch into the window approximately 3/4 inch. The glass will shatter without a follow-through (Figure 6.43).

Facilitating Entry into a Vehicle Through Window Openings

Reaching all the occupants of a small car from positions outside the vehicle is usually not a problem, nor is reaching the occupants adjacent to the doors of a large car. On the other hand, getting to passengers seated on the middle of the front and rear seats may be extremely difficult.

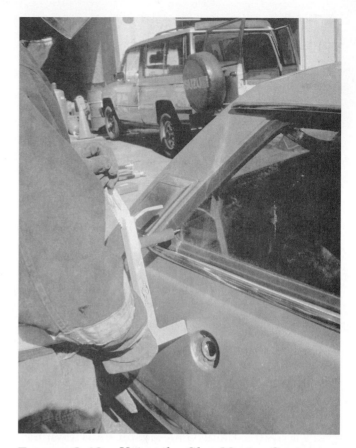

FIGURE 6.42   Using the Glas-Master Center Punch

There is an alternative to climbing through window openings and walking on, kneeling on, or crawling over other injured occupants to reach these folks, however. Use a long spine board as a work platform. In Figure 6.44, the EMT is working from a spine board placed by other emergency service personnel or helpers recruited from the onlookers. Note how the EMT can reach everyone in the vehicle.

ENTERING THROUGH THE BODY OF A VEHICLE

In several situations you may not be able to enter a vehicle through window or door openings, as when:

- One vehicle is sandwiched between two other vehicles.
- A car has been struck broadside by another vehicle and pushed against a building.

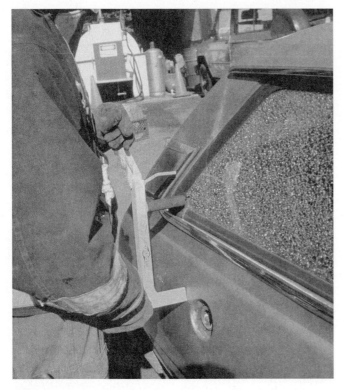

FIGURE 6.43 Using the Glas-Master Center Punch

- A number of vehicles damaged in a freeway accident are so close together that the doors cannot be opened and rescuers cannot enter through window openings.
- A vehicle that has come to rest on its side has doors so severely damaged that opening them will be a difficult and lengthy procedure.

In any of these situations, you might be able to enter the vehicle through the windshield or rear window opening. To do so may necessitate your crawling over some of the patients in order to reach others—a procedure that may aggravate existing injuries and even cause new ones. A better idea is to enter the vehicle from the top.

ENTERING THROUGH THE ROOF OF A VEHICLE

A number of techniques can be used to enter a vehicle on its wheels when doors and side windows are inaccessible. You can:

- Make an opening in the roof;
- Fold back a section of the roof;
- Remove a section of the roof; or
- Remove the roof altogether.

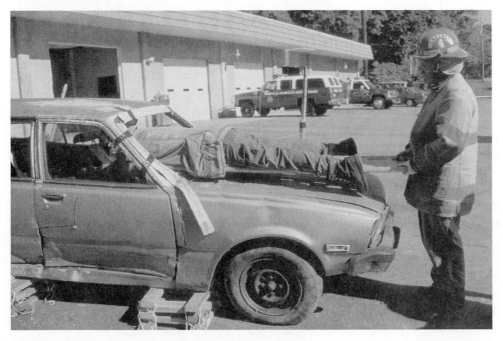

FIGURE 6.44 Working Off of a Spine Board

All four procedures are discussed in detail in Phase Eight. Your choice of a technique will depend on the nature and extent of damage, and the accessibility of door roof pillars. Whatever you do, strive to make the largest opening possible so you can reach all of the trapped persons.

ENTERING AN OVERTURNED VEHICLE

A rollover often occurs when a passenger car is struck forcefully from the side or when the driver loses control of his vehicle and the side wheels drop off the roadway onto a depressed shoulder.

You may arrive and find that an overturned car is simply resting on its top with the roof pillars intact. In this case, you may be able to enter the car through a door or window opening after you have stabilized the vehicle. Or, you may discover that the roof is crushed flat against the body of the vehicle and that the occupants are totally encapsulated in the wreckage. This is a terribly frustrating situation that taxes the abilities of even experienced rescue personnel and is likely to be more common now that convertibles are available once more. Or, you may find the car is in a drainage ditch tightly pinning the doors shut.

Making an Opening in the Floor

Making an opening in the floor is usually no problem; it is the weakest part of a car, especially in areas where salt is used on icy roadways.

If most of the roof is crushed flat against the body of the vehicle, you will be able to assess only the situation in the rear of the passenger compartment. The front seat will effectively seal the front of the compartment from view or touch. Therefore, you will have to make openings in the front foot wells.

One way to free accident victims from this form of encapsulation is to remove the entire floor and the attached seats. This procedure involves removing the drive shaft if it is a rear drive, the exhaust system, and the

emergency brake cable, and then cutting the floor. The task is doubly difficult if only hand tools are available. However, if a reciprocating saw or a good air chisel is on hand, the time needed to remove the floor is dramatically reduced.

As mentioned, the first step is to clean off the bottom of the vehicle. Using the power saw, cut the drive shaft at the universal joint and pull it toward the rear to slide it out of the spline in the transmission. Next cut the brake cables and cut off the exhaust system. Be careful that the catalytic converter does not burn you. Cut the fuel lines at the rear where they enter the fuel tank. Plug them with golf tees (Figure 6.45).

The foot well in the rear seat is very obvious when viewed from the bottom. Punch out the drain hole cover to give yourself an opening for the reciprocating saw. Use the short saw blade to prevent "bottoming out." Push the handle of the large screwdriver through the hole first to make sure no body parts are near the intended saw path (Figure 6.46). Remember you are under the rug so

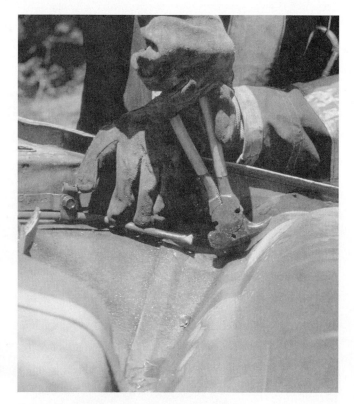

FIGURE 6.45   Plugging a Gas Line

there shouldn't be a problem. Make a three-sided cut the full size of the raised portion of the floor pan (Figure 6.47). Bend back the flap and push the rug in and out of the way. At this time you should be able to determine if any of the victims are in the way. Have a rescuer crawl through the opening to stabilize the victim(s) (Figure 6.48). Make sure you run duct tape around the sharp edges of the opening before entering.

When removing the entire floor, the reciprocating saw or a good air chisel is run around the perimeter of the passenger compartment (Figure 6.49). The only problems normally encountered are around the transmission supports; it may be necessary to cut the brackets.

Next, cut the seat belts to the front seat and with long pinch bars or Halligan Tools (Figure 6.50), pry the entire floor up. You may have to cut the rug (Figure 6.51). Continue lifting (Figure 6.52) until the entire

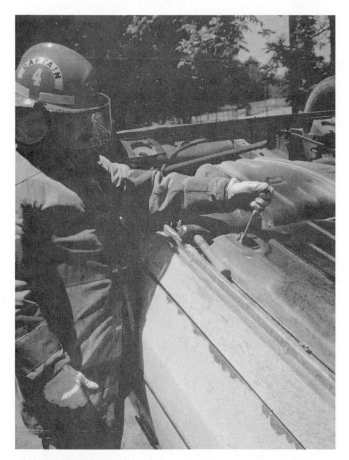

FIGURE 6.46   Pushing Screwdriver Through Drain Hole

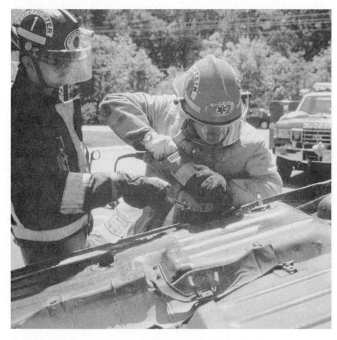

FIGURE 6.47   Making Three-Sided Cut

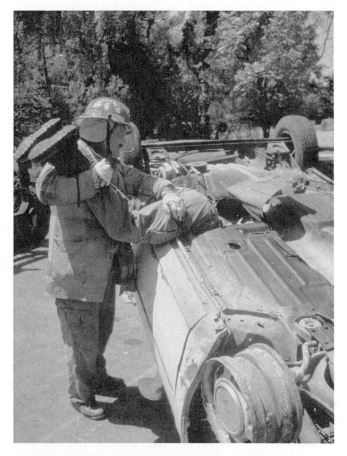

FIGURE 6.48   Medic into the Opening

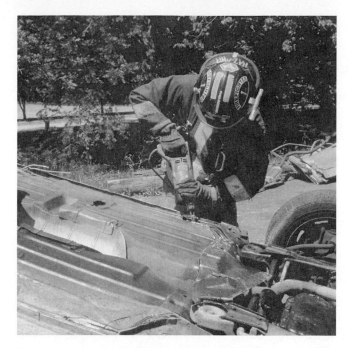

FIGURE 6.49   Cutting Out the Floor

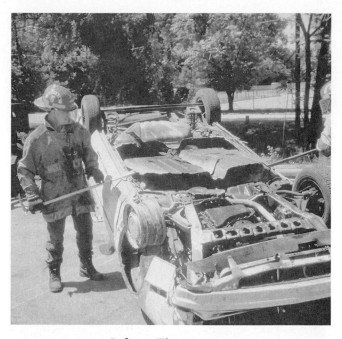

FIGURE 6.50   Lifting Floor

floor is out of the vehicle with front seats attached (Figure 6.53). You will be surprised at how easily this entire operation is accomplished in 15 to 20 minutes.

Lifting One End of the Vehicle to Make the Roof Accessible

A procedure that is used successfully by rescue units confronted with this situation is to lift one end of the vehicle, then cut the roof pillars and move the victims away from the vehicle on the roof. While rescuers have air bags to lift the car, pneumatic shoring devices to support it, and powered tools to remove the roof, you can use a wrecker and the tools carried on the ambulance to accomplish those tasks.

Incidentally, the A-pillars of cars manufactured after 1979 are supposed to be able to support the weight of an overturned car without collapsing. This was mandated to minimize the problem of accident victims being totally encapsulated in the wreckage.

A wrecker needs to be positioned so that a vertical lift can be made. Thus there is little chance that the car could skid backward on the edge of the trunk lid as the front of the car is raised. With the wrecker

in position and the winch cable attached to chains secured to two dependable anchor points, the winch operator should lift the front end of the car just enough to take the weight off the A-pillars, a distance of about an inch.

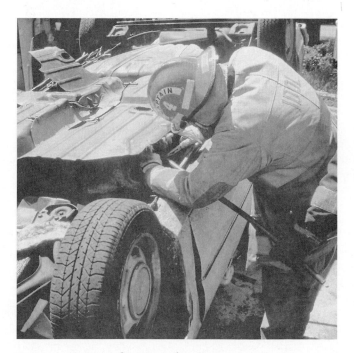

FIGURE 6.51   Cutting the Rug

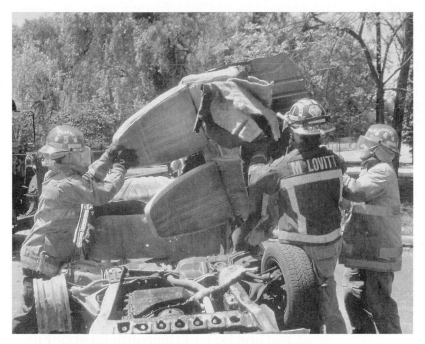

FIGURE 6.52 Pulling Out
Entire Floor with Seats

As the rescuers sever first the A-pillars and then the B-pillars, the weight of the victims will cause the roof to slowly drop to the ground. The wrecker operator should then lift the front end of the car just enough for the rescuers to sever the C-pillars. As the front end goes up, the roof will remain on the ground.

When the C-pillars are cut, the winch operator should lift the car again, but just enough that the roof section with its passengers can be moved from underneath the vehicle. The rescuers can then pull the roof section away from the wreckage to a point where the injured persons can be properly cared for. As you may have determined, this

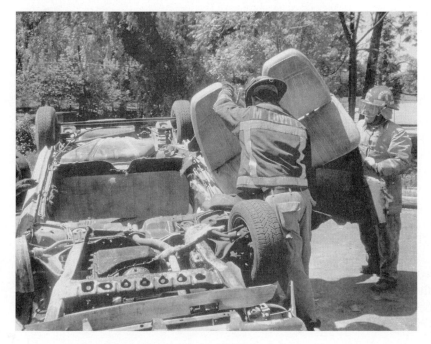

FIGURE 6.53 Pulling Out
Entire Floor with Seats

technique allows the removal of seriously injured people without the twisting or bending of body parts.

Variations in the procedure may be necessary because of the nature and extent of damage to the vehicle. That's why there has been no attempt made here to list the steps of the procedure one-by-one as has been done in the rest of the book. However, two things must remain constant in all operations of this nature. The wrecker operator must be proficient in the use of his equipment, and the winch cable must be secured to at least two anchor points that will not fail during the rescue effort.

You may be wondering how quickly this task can be performed. On the average, allow about 15 minutes from the time the wrecker is in place until the roof is pulled away from the vehicle. A similar procedure will be discussed and illustrated in Phase Eight, with rescuers using air bags and pneumatic jacks.

OPENING THE TRUNK OF A PASSENGER CAR

Trunk compartments are not usually thought of as passenger spaces; therefore emergency service personnel are seldom inclined to search trunks during vehicle rescue activities. Unfortunately, bodies have been discovered in trunk compartments long after the conclusion of rescue operations, and long after any lifesaving efforts might have been effective. In addition to those of fraternity pledges, the bodies of crime victims have been discovered in car trunks, as have the bodies of teenagers who were on their way to a drive-in movie when the accident occurred.

Include a trunk check as a part of routine forcible entry procedures. Look not only for hazardous materials that might pose a threat to you, the victims, and the bystanders, but also for human cargo.

The easiest way to open a car trunk is to use the key. But if the key is not available, or if the lock is damaged, entry can be made with hand tools. Don't waste time trying to pry the lid up with a forcible entry tool, however. Although they do not appear to be very sturdy, most trunk latch mechanisms resist prying. And don't punch the lock cylinder in with the pike of a forcible entry tool. While the procedure works sometimes, more often than not you will jam the tailpiece of the lock in the latch mechanism. Instead, use a technique that is successful almost all of the time.

Using Hand Tools

You will need a drilling hammer, a short sledgehammer, a Schild panel cutter or other tool suitable for cutting sheet metal, and a screwdriver with a fairly narrow blade.

To remove the lock cylinder:

- Use the point of the panel cutter to make a starting hole in the trunk lid about an inch to one side and an inch above the lock.
- Drive the cutting edge of the tool downward to a point slightly below the lock.
- Make a horizontal cut from the starting hole to a point about an inch beyond and an inch above the other side of the lock.
- Make a third cut from that point down to a point slightly below the lock (Figure 6.54).

With the screwdriver:

- Pry the flap containing the lock cylinder out and down. This action will pull the rectangular-shaped tailpiece of the lock out of the slot in the latch mechanism.
- Look into the opening and locate the rectangular slot in the latch mechanism.
- Then insert the tip of the screwdriver into the slot and twist the tool to unlatch the trunk lid.

Using Powered Tools

Unlocking and unlatching a trunk lid is hardly a job for which you would go to the

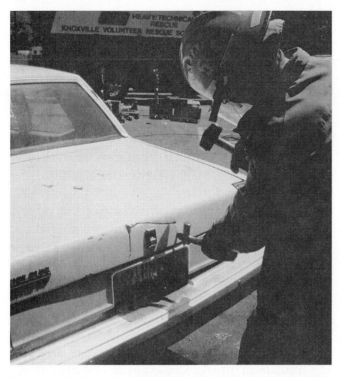

FIGURE 6.54 Opening Trunk with Schild Tool

trouble of setting up a powered tool. However, if you have assembled an air-operated chisel or a hydraulic rescue tool for other tasks, use it to open the trunk lid as well.

If you have an air-operated chisel, use it in the manner just suggested. Keep the pressure low to conserve air for disentanglement operations. If you have a hydraulic rescue tool, first use a forcible entry tool to widen the gap between the trunk lid and the body of the vehicle. Then alternately pry and reposition the tool for a better bite until the lid pops open.

REACHING A PERSON WHO IS TRAPPED UNDER A VEHICLE

Thus far we have discussed procedures that might be used to reach persons trapped *within* accident vehicles. Now let's consider techniques you might use to gain access to a person trapped *under* a vehicle.

A number of accidents can result in this predicament. A pedestrian can become trapped under a vehicle after being struck, knocked down, and run over by the front wheels. An unbelted driver can be trapped under his own car when collision forces eject him from the vehicle. A weekend mechanic can become trapped under his car when a makeshift jack stand fails. Regardless of the cause of entrapment, extricating an individual from this predicament involves more than simply pulling him from under the vehicle by his hands or feet.

Lifting One Side of the Vehicle

Obviously the car is both a mechanism of entrapment and injury. But there may also be other mechanisms of injury that you cannot see yet.

If the person trapped under a car is small, you might be able to pull him from under the car by his shoulders or arms. But what if his chest or abdomen is in intimate contact with a sharp metal edge? Worse yet, what if a sharp-pointed object has penetrated the person's abdomen when the car dropped onto him? If you simply pull the person from under the car, you might rip his abdomen from diaphragm to genitalia, thus gutting him! When you consider the reduced distances between the ground and the bottoms of modern cars, especially compact ones, it should be clear that the same fate would be likely should you attempt to pull *anyone* from under a car.

How can you avoid such a disaster? First stabilize the vehicle, then lift either one side or an end, then remove the person. Lifting a vehicle to reach a person who is trapped underneath is a team effort. Let's say that you are the officer-in-charge of a four-rescuer team.

Selecting the Side to Be Lifted

The ideal way to remove a person from under a vehicle is to move him onto a long spine board with a rope sling. Thus the side of the vehicle closest to the person's head is the side that should be lifted after the other side is cribbed.

Chocking the Wheels

Using wheel chocks makes additional pieces of cribbing available for other stabilizing operations. While the other team members are preparing the equipment:

- Have one rescuer position one wheel chock ahead of the front wheel and the other chock behind the rear wheel of the side opposite the one to be lifted.

Preventing Side Drop

Preventing side drop is an important step. When one side of a vehicle is lifted, there is a tendency for the other side to drop slightly as the springs on that side take on more weight. Even a slight drop might cause a sharp-pointed object to penetrate the patient's body or a sharp-edged object to lacerate the person's chest or abdomen.

As soon as the wheel chocks are in position:

- Direct rescuers to build cribs under the frame rail of the side opposite the one that will be lifted, one crib just behind the front wheel well and the other crib just ahead of the rear wheel well.

- Have the rescuers build the cribs to the level where they can't insert another layer of cribbing without lifting that side of the vehicle (Figure 6.55).

If necessary:

- Have the rescuers rotate the cribs so the last layer of cribbing can be laid at a right angle to the side of the vehicle.

This will assure that the other side of the vehicle will rest on solid cribs, and that pivot points at the top of the cribs will be as wide as possible.

When both cribs are built to the level where another layer of cribbing cannot be inserted:

- Have two of the rescuers each crouch with his back to the front fender and his hands gripping the edge of the fender well.

On your command "lift":

- Have these rescuers gently lift the side of the car just a few inches while the other rescuers insert the final layer of cribbing at a right angle to the side of the car.

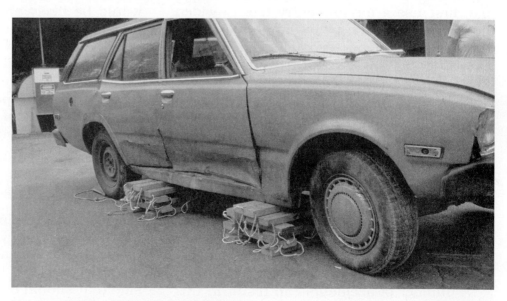

FIGURE 6.55   Preventing Side Drop

The two cribs will serve as pivot points and will prevent that side of the vehicle from dropping when the other side is lifted.

Making the Lift

Rescue units have a number of devices that can be used to lift the side of a car, including jacks, a hydraulic rescue tool, and air bags.

USING A HI-LIFT JACK

The Hi-Lift jack is well suited for this task for several reasons. The jack is capable of lifting 7000 pounds. The positive locking action of the sliding steel pin all but eliminates the possibility that the jack will slip when supporting a load. Moreover, setup time is minimal when compared to other tools.

As soon as the wheel chocks and cribs are in place on the other side of the vehicle:

- Direct one rescuer to lie on his belly close to the patient's legs in a position where he can see the person's chest.
- Have two rescuers prepare to build cribs under the frame rail behind the front wheel well and ahead of the rear wheel well.

Exactly where cribs are built under the side of the vehicle to be lifted will depend on the patient's position. If he is situated midway between the wheel wells, one crib can be built just behind the front wheel well and the other just ahead of the rear wheel well. If the person is close to a wheel well, however, one crib may have to be built under a corner of the vehicle on the other side of the wheel well.

While these rescuers get into position:

- Instruct the fourth team member to position the lifting toe of the jack under the side of the vehicle as close to the balance point as possible, but with consideration for the patient's location.

The balance point is the point where the car's weight will be equally distributed on both sides of the lifting toe.

If the ground under the vehicle is soft:

- Direct the rescuer to rest the jack base on a jack plate or two or three pieces of cribbing laid side-by-side. The jack plate or cribbing will spread downward forces over a wider area and will thus prevent the jack base from sinking into the soft ground.

When everybody and everything is ready:

- Have the rescuer slowly operate the jack to lift the side of the vehicle.
- Direct the two rescuers with cribbing to build cribs as the side of the vehicle lifts.

As the side of the vehicle goes up:

- Direct the rescuer who is lying at the patient's side to wiggle into position where he can clearly see into the space developing between the victim's body and the body of the vehicle.

If he informs you that the patient is not impaled by an object projecting from the underside of the vehicle:

- Direct the jack operator to continue lifting the side of the car until there is several inches of space between the patient and the underside of the vehicle.

When rescuers have the final layers of cribbing in place:

- Have the jack operator reverse the operating mechanism and lower the side of the vehicle the short distance onto the cribs.
- Have the rescuer at the patient's side remove the jack and any cribbing that has been used as a jack base.

If the rescuer who is at the patient's side sees that the person is impaled by a projecting object:

- Stop operating the jack until he is in position ready to apply a bulky dressing.

This is a ticklish situation, one of the few times when removing an impaled object is justified. While it is in place, the object may be preventing the flow of blood from severed vessels. To simply lift the side of the car until the object pulls free may be disastrous. Bleeding may be so severe that the person will die before you can get him out from under the vehicle.

Cutting an impaled object in this situation is out of the question. Even if there were room to operate a hacksaw, there would probably be no room for someone to support the impaling object. Movement of the object caused by the sawing motions could easily worsen damage to blood vessels.

When the rescuer is in place with a bulky dressing:

- Have the jack operator lift the side of the car until the rescuer underneath tells you that the object is a good distance out of the wound.

Keep in mind that the side of the car will drop down a short distance when the car is lowered onto the cribbing. The distance between the impaling object must be greater than the distance that the car will drop.

While the rescuer underneath works to control bleeding:

- Have the other team members complete the cribs.
- Have the jack operator lower the side of the car onto the cribbing, then remove the jack and anything used for a jack base.
- Prepare to move the person onto a long spine board with a rope sling (covered in Phase Eight).

Needless to say, the rescuer who is maintaining pressure on the wound will have to continue doing so during the removal operation.

An important point: If the patient is situated so close to the front or rear wheel that removal will be difficult, have rescuers remove the wheel. This is where a folding lug wrench will come in handy, or better yet, a powered impact wrench.

USING TWO HI-LIFT JACKS

When the edges of the fenders are not corroded, two Hi-Lift jacks can be placed at each fender opening. Two rescuers operate the jacks simultaneously to assure an even lift while other rescuers build cribs under the vehicle (Figure 6.56).

USING A HYDRAULIC RESCUE TOOL

A hydraulic rescue tool can also be used to lift the side of a vehicle. The preliminary steps are the same as described earlier: Prevent forward and rearward motion of the vehicle with wheel chocks, and build cribs under the side opposite the one to be lifted.

While one rescuer is getting into position at the patient's side, and while other rescuers are preparing to build cribs:

- Have the tool operator build a solid base of cribbing under the lifting point to minimize the space between the ground

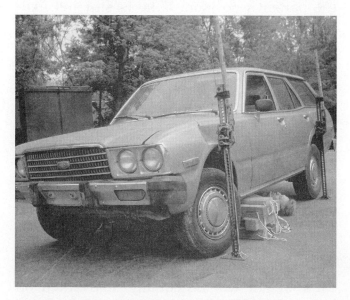

FIGURE 6.56   Using Two Hi-Lift Jacks

and the bottom of the car. The cribbing will also spread downward forces over a wider area—an important point when the ground is soft.

When everything and everyone is ready:

- Direct the tool operator to position the tool at a right angle to the vehicle.
- Have him operate the controls and spread the arms just to the point where the jaws are contacting the cribbing and the bottom of the vehicle.

Proper positioning of the tool is important. If the arms are not precisely vertical, the tool can slip while supporting the vehicle.

When you are satisfied that the tool will not slip:

- Carry out the lifting/cribbing procedure.

USING HIGH-PRESSURE AIR BAGS

When air bags are used to lift the side of the car, as when other lifting devices are used, the preliminary steps are preventing forward

and rearward motion with wheel chocks and building cribs under the opposite side.

- Have two team members lay a solid base of cribbing under the lifting point, not so much for spreading downward forces but to take up space between the ground and the bottom of the vehicle.

Depending on how far the side of the vehicle must be lifted, laying a solid base of cribbing under the lifting point may eliminate the need for a second air bag.

- Instruct the third team member to position the air bag so the center of the bag is directly under the lifting point.
- Tell the controller operator to inflate the bag and lift the side of the vehicle while the other rescuers build the cribs (Figure 6.57).

When the cribs are in place:

- Direct the controller operator to deflate the bag.
- Have rescuers remove it and the solid base of cribbing laid as a base for the bag.

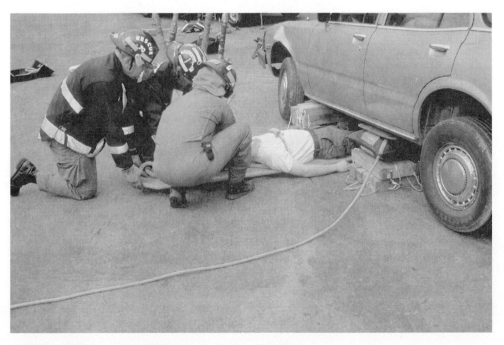

FIGURE 6.57   Using High-Pressure Air Bags

If you have to use two bags to lift the side of the vehicle, as when you don't have enough cribbing to place under the bags, or when you must lift the vehicle a considerable distance, be sure to position the bags so the top bag is centered precisely over the bottom one. This is an important step. Bags that are not centered can slip when supporting a load.

PHASE SEVEN

Caring for Life-Threatening Conditions

INTRODUCTION

Emergency Medical Service providers have various levels of training. While many levels are designated, the most common titles are First Responder, EMT-Basic, EMT-Intermediate, and EMT-Paramedic. For the sake of consistency, and to assure that we recognize all who provide medical care in the pre-hospital setting, we refer to these individuals as Medics.

How important is proper care for a patient's spine? An injury to the spine can result in a patient spending the rest of his life as a paraplegic or quadriplegic confined to a bed or a wheelchair. You will see some

patients with spinal cord damage as a direct result of the accident, while others will have damaged vertebrae but an undamaged spinal cord. Don't underestimate the threat to patients in this second category. The fragile spinal cord can be injured by even small movements of damaged vertebrae. And never lose sight of the fact that, for all practical purposes, the parts of the central nervous system do not regenerate and that a severed spinal cord cannot be surgically repaired. Therefore, the consequences of improperly moving a patient who has a spine injury, or allowing the patient to move, can be devastating!

Anyone who has sustained a violent mechanism of injury, significant injury above the collar bone, or a blow to the head that has resulted in a changed level of consciousness must be presumed to have a spine injury. He must be immobilized in a neutral, in-line position before being moved. This means that when a patient in a vehicle could have a spinal injury, he must be properly immobilized. No if's, and's, or but's!

SOME FACTS ABOUT THE HEAD AND SPINE

The next few paragraphs do not constitute a comprehensive lesson in anatomy and physiology. They present just a few things that you should know about the spine and what happens to it during an accident.

The head balances on top of the spine and the spine is supported by the pelvis. Ligaments and muscles form a web that sheathes the entire bony part of the column and holds it in alignment. The structure of the cervical spine allows the head a wide range of motion. The muscles in the back of the neck are very strong; they permit up to 60% of the range of flexion (bending forward) and 70% of the range of extension (bending backward) of the head with no stretching of the spinal cord. Even so, when there is sudden violent movement of the head because of acceleration, deceleration, or a blow to the body from the side, it can be likened to a bowling ball perched upon a relatively thin flexible stalk.

Although most of the vertebrae in the neck, back, and lower back are basically alike, the clearance between the cord and the vertebral foramen varies. The foramen are the holes in the rear portion of the vertebrae. In the lower portion of the neck, the spinal cord occupies about 95% of the spinal canal. In the area of the lower back, the canal is only 65% occupied by the cord. Therefore, in the cervical spine—in the neck, that is—the tolerance for safe movement beyond the normal range is limited.

Mechanisms of Injury

The spine can normally withstand forces of up to 1000 foot pounds, which is a pretty good jolt. However, forces generated in an accident can be well in excess of 1000 foot pounds. Even in a low-speed collision, the body of an unrestrained 150-pound passenger flying upward and forward can easily exert 3000 to 5000 pounds of force against the spine when the head is suddenly stopped by the windshield or roof.

A spinal injury can be caused by any mechanism that pushes the spine beyond its normal limits of motion or weight-bearing ability.

Axial Loading—sudden excessive compression—happens when the weight of a body is driven against the head, as when the head of an unrestrained passenger hits the windshield.

Violent or **Excessive Flexion, Excessive Extension,** and **Excessive Rotation** can cause bone damage, tearing of muscles and ligaments, and tearing of the spinal cord.

Lateral Bending—the sudden sideways thrust of the head—can more easily cause significant injury or fractures to the cervical spine since the head will tend to remain in place while the rest of the body is pushed out from under it. The range of acceptable lateral bending is much more limited than is that of flexion or extension.

Distraction—the opposite of compression—is a pulling apart of the spine. It can easily cause stretching and tearing of the spinal cord. Distraction can occur when the head of a restrained passenger flies forward as the result of a front-end collision.

Although any one of these violent movements can cause a spinal injury, spinal injuries usually result from several such movements.

The Effects of Injuries to the Spine

It is important that you understand and remember that an injury to the vertebrae may not cause any immediate damage to the spinal cord. Therefore, a patient may not have any paralysis (complete or incomplete), yet there may be severe spinal damage. In these cases, any movement of the patient may result in irreparable cord damage. It is quite possible that an injury that presents no signs or symptoms may still result in a spine that is so unstable that even minor normal movement can result in permanent damage.

A patient's ability to move his extremities or the absence of any numbness, tingling, and other usual signs of neurological damage indicates only that the cord is intact *so far*. It does not indicate an absence of spinal cord injury.

As a direct result of trauma, a patient can suffer:

- A complete or incomplete severing of the cord
- A pinching of the cord, with or without any vertebral displacement
- A stretching of the cord
- A compression fracture of the vertebrae
- A fracture of the vertebrae with comminuted "teardrop" bone fragments
- A displacement of vertebrae either minor or complete
- A bruise to the cord that can cause swelling and a reduction of the blood supply to the cord and/or hemorrhage
- Overstretching and other damage to ligaments and muscles, so that their normal ability to safely maintain vertebral alignment no longer exists

A cut or pinched cord can contribute to shock. The body's defense mechanisms that cause blood vessels to constrict are dependent on an intact central nervous system. If the cord is cut or severely damaged, vessels close to the surface of the body below the point of injury will not constrict. Instead, those vessels will remain dilated. The skin above the part of the body affected by the injury usually remains pink, warm, and dry, until the patient is at a very advanced level of progressive shock. The decreased volume of circulating blood resulting from cord damage and the lack of vasoconstriction below the point of cord damage is called spinal shock; it is an example of neurogenic shock.

Indicators of Spinal Injury

The nature and extent of damage to a vehicle is the most important indicator of possible spine injury; that's why so much emphasis was placed earlier on the rescue officer's need to carefully observe the vehicles during the assessment or size-up phase of operations. If a car looks like collision forces could have caused a spinal injury, then the occupants must be treated as if such an injury exists.

Spinal injury can be ruled out only by the lack of a mechanism of injury with forces strong enough to damage the spine or by X-ray. Therefore, you should assume that a patient has a spinal injury when:

- A vehicle has undergone violent movements, as determined from a witness, or by observation of the scene or the mechanism itself;
- A patient has a head injury accompanied by an altered level of consciousness;
- A trauma victim is unconscious;
- There is significant blunt injury to the head, face, or neck;
- A patient has been ejected from a vehicle;
- A motorcyclist has helmet damage.

Or when a trauma victim has:

- Pain with or without movement;
- Point tenderness in the areas of the spine;
- Deformity, or is guarding the head, neck, or back;
- Paralysis, partial paralysis, numbness or tingling; and/or
- Signs of dilation of the blood vessels.

Let's say it once more lest you forget: If it appears that a patient *may* have a spinal injury, care for him as if he *does* have a spinal injury.

MANAGING SPINAL INJURIES

The ultimate goal of pre-hospital spinal care is to completely immobilize a patient on his back on a long spine board or other rigid full-body device. However, this goal cannot be met until the patient is properly assessed; any problems with the airway, breathing, and circulation are corrected; the cervical spine is immobilized; and wreckage is removed from around the patient.

Let's assume that a medic has asked you to assist with the care for a patient. Your job will be to support the patient's head manually during the assessment and initial emergency care steps.

Initiating Manual Support

About the only time that a medic or rescuer can simply climb into a damaged vehicle, place his hands on the sides of a patient's head, and initiate manual support is when the patient is conscious, sitting perfectly upright, and holding his head in the normal anatomical position in a guarding effort. Rescuers usually find the head of a seated patient with the neck flexed chin to chest, hyperextended in a sniffing position, or tilted to one side or the other. The head of a patient lying on a seat or the floor of a car can be in any position within the range of motion. Thus in most accident cases, the head of a patient must be moved to the neutral in-line position before a cervical immobilization device can be applied.

The neutral in-line position can best be described as the normal anatomical position of the head and torso that a person assumes when standing and looking straight ahead. The chin is neither pulled in nor pushed forward. The head is held straight—not tilted or rotated in any direction. When you have the responsibility for manually supporting a patient's head, don't simply climb into the vehicle and place your hands over the patient's ears; you will not have sufficient control during the subsequent immobilization procedure. Instead:

- Take a position behind the front seat.

Depending on the height of the individual and your height:

- Either stand behind the seat with your feet on the floor of the car, or sit on the edge of the rear seat.

Obviously the best position from which you can maintain a patient's head in the neutral position is directly behind the individual. However, this may not be possible in every accident situation. There may be debris or another patient in the way. If this is the case, you will have to stand at the side of the vehicle.

When you are in position:

- Place your hands on the side of the patient's head with your fingers spread.
- Position the little finger of each hand under the angle of the mandible where they will support the head without holding the lower jaw shut.
- Stretch your thumbs slightly so they will rest against the back of the skull.
- Gently move the head into the neutral in-line position and hold it there.

Be aware that there are situations for which this procedure is not proper, such as:

- When the head must be moved in order to assure an open airway
- When the head is tilted to one side and the patient complains of increased pain on movement or the patient resists efforts to move his head
- When the rescuer detects resistance or "grating" on movement

These could be indicators of spinal column or cord injury. It is a rare occurrence when a trained medic will be required to stabilize the head in the position found rather than in the neutral position.

Let's say that you decide to move the patient's head to the neutral position. Depending on the style of the seat and the size of the patient:

- Either rest your forearms on the seat back or the headrest, or rest them on the patient's shoulders with your elbows pressed against your sides.

The hand placement and arm positions just described are ideal. You will be able to maintain the patient's head in the neutral position during the subsequent upper-body immobilization procedures; that is, with the neck neither flexed nor extended. Moreover, you will be able to prevent the patient's head from swaying side-to-side. If you have to stand behind the patient during the immobilization procedure, adjust the position of your hands so your fingers are pointed down slightly. Otherwise, your wrists may tire and you may inadvertently tilt the head down slightly while trying to get into a more comfortable position.

A patient's head can be maintained in a neutral position without any significant pulling or lifting. The term "traction" that was commonly used in the past has been replaced with the term "stabilization." Stabilization requires only enough force to maintain the head and neck in alignment. The goal is to support and stabilize the head and neck in their normal alignment, *not* to stretch them. Just enough pull should be exerted to remove the weight of the head from the axis and the rest of the cervical spine.

Once you have the patient's head in the neutral position:

• Maintain it in that position until the medic or another rescuer has applied a rigid cervical collar and taken over control of the head.

Applying a Cervical Collar

Let's say that another rescuer is maintaining the patient's head in a neutral position. The medic has asked you to apply a cervical collar while he moves to another patient.

A wide variety of cervical collars are available, ranging from soft foam collars to firmer foam collars to rigid plastic high-side "extrication" collars. However, only collars included in the last category should be used in vehicle rescue situations. Soft foam collars provide only 10% restriction of movement and are not suitable for use in the pre-hospital setting.

Two widely accepted and recommended collars for rescue operations are the Stifneck Extrication Collar manufactured by California Medical Products, Inc., and the Vertabrace Extrication Collar manufactured by Jobst Institute, Inc. Among the features of each brand are availability in several sizes, and color coding for convenience in sizing. The collars are radiolucent, and they have an opening for quick access to the wearer's trachea.

Using a Stifneck Extrication Collar

The Stifneck Extrication Collar is available in five sizes: tall, regular, short, extra-short, and pediatric. Selecting the proper size collar is important as too large a collar can cause hyperextension of the neck, while too small a collar will not provide proper support. Proper fit is also important. A patient's chin can slip down into a collar that is too loose, with the result being flexing of the neck. Moreover, too short a collar can act as a constricting band and put pressure on the wearer's airway and blood vessels that supply blood to the brain. Facial flushing and increased intracranial pressure can be caused by a cervical collar that is too tight.

Matching the height of the front of a collar to the distance between a patient's chin and the sternal notch is not a reliable way of sizing a cervical collar. A better way is to measure the distance between the horizontal plane of the patient's chin and the top of the shoulder where the collar will sit—a measurement that can be made with the fingers.

While your partner maintains the patient's head in neutral alignment:

• Hold one hand close to the side of the patient's neck with your fingers horizontal and together.
• Note how many fingers fill the space between an imaginary horizontal line that extends rearward from the bottom of the chin and the top of the shoulder.

- Select the collar with the same measurement between the black fastener and the bottom edge of the plastic encircling band, not the foam padding.

For example, if you can fit three fingers in the space between the line that extends rearward from the patient's chin and the top of the shoulder, select the collar on which you can lay the same three fingers between the black fastener and the bottom of the plastic collar.

Assembling and pre-forming the collar is the next step if the collar has been stored flat in its original container or folded rather than rolled.

- Grip the collar in your right hand with the thumb of that hand resting on the point where the front and back panels join and your fingers resting on the outer surface of the collar.

While you hold the collar with your right hand:

- Use the fingers of your left hand to push the black fastener through the round hole in the front panel of the collar (above and to the left of your right thumb). Doing so forms the chin piece.
- Continue to hold the front panel of the collar in your right hand, but now with your thumb on the foam padding and your first finger on the colored size marker that is fixed to the outer surface of the collar.
- Grasp the right side of the front panel with the fingertips of your left hand on the edge of the tracheal opening and your thumb against the left edge of the collar.
- Move the thumb of your left hand toward your finger tips to pre-form the collar.
- Flex the collar several times in this manner.

This pre-forming step simplifies securing the collar around the person's neck. If the step is

omitted, the Velcro surfaces may prematurely contact during application, with the result being improper tightening and inadequate immobilization.

When you have pre-formed the appropriate collar:

- Remove any jewelry that may become trapped when the collar is in place—earrings, necklaces, and so on.
- Push clothing away from the parts of the body that will be contacted by the bottom edge of the collar.

This last step is important. If clothing—especially heavy clothing—that is trapped by the collar edge becomes loose during subsequent immobilization, patient care, and transfer activities, the collar will become loose and effective immobilization will be lost.

- Initially position the collar by sliding it upward on the chest with your right hand just until the chin piece is supporting the patient's chin. Be careful! If you push the collar up too far, you will hyperextend the neck.

While you hold the collar with your right hand:

- Pass the back panel of the collar behind the patient's neck with your left hand.
- Gently pull free any long hair that is likely to be trapped under the back panel.
- Change hands so that you are holding the collar with your left hand and pulling on the Velcro tab with your right hand.
- Pull the tab until the collar is snug around the patient's neck and join the Velcro parts so that the edges of the hook and loop sections are aligned.

The collar must be pulled snug if it is to be effective. This can be accomplished by placing the finger tips of your left hand against the right side of the tracheal opening of the collar as a point of purchase, then pulling on the Velcro strap with your right hand until the desired tightness is achieved, then mating the Velcro parts.

If the collar is the correct size and properly applied, the patient's chin will come just to the outer edge of the chin piece. If the point of the chin does not at least cover the fastener at the mid-point of the chin piece, the patient's chin may slip off. This can be prevented by using a smaller collar or by tightening the applied collar until the chin is properly supported. On the other hand, if the patient's chin extends well beyond the end of the chin piece, a taller collar should be used for better support.

The extra-short collar was developed for obese and heavily muscled people such as athletes. Even so, this particular collar may not be suitable for some people, and an alternative immobilization technique may be needed.

Using a Vertabrace Extrication Collar

The Vertabrace Extrication Collar is available in five sizes: tall, regular, short, extra-short, and pediatric. Selection of the proper size collar is aided by a multicolored paper strip packed with each collar.

While another rescuer supports the patient's head from behind:

- Position the sizing guide alongside the patient's head so the bottom edge of the guide is resting on the uppermost surface of the patient's shoulder (the trapezius muscle).

Keeping the guide vertical:

- Align the colored end with the front of the patient's ear.
- Observe the colored area, along with the corresponding letter size that falls in line with the center of the ear opening (the concha). The color and the letter indicate the proper size collar.

Anatomically, the concha lies in the same plane as the lower margin of the occiput. For maximum support, each Vertabrace collar is sized to fit up against that bony protuberance.

The colored sizing guide is a convenient tool; however, its use alone should not be the only basis for selecting a particular size collar. Consideration should be given to the patient's upper-body dimensions. The next size shorter collar may be necessary for a large-boned or heavily muscled patient, or a patient who is wearing heavy winter clothing. A taller collar may better fit a thin patient.

Two steps are necessary before applying a Vertabrace collar: flipping up the chin support and pre-forming the collar.

- Hold the collar out in front of you with the chin support up and facing you. Your thumbs should be on each side of the tracheal opening and your fingers should be behind the collar.
- Pull your hands toward your body while you rotate your wrists outward. The chin support will flip up over the wall of the collar.

With the chin support up:

- Hold the collar in your left hand with your finger tips in the tracheal opening and the Velcro hook strip in the web between your thumb and first finger.
- Touch your thumb to your finger tips to roll—and thus pre-form—the collar.

Pre-forming partially shapes a rigid collar and makes application much easier. When storage space is no problem, some emergency personnel prefer to keep their rigid extrication collars rolled; that is, with the Velcro hook-and-loop sections joined. There is no need for pre-forming when collars are stored rolled.

When you have pre-formed the appropriate collar:

- Remove any jewelry that may become trapped when the collar is in place—earrings, necklaces, and so forth.
- Push clothing away from the parts of the body that will be contacted by the bottom edge of the collar.

While the other rescuer continues to support the patient's head:

- Slide the part of the collar that has the contact loop behind the neck.
- Position the chin support directly under the chin.

When the collar is in position, it's a good idea to tell your partner that you are about to fasten the mating parts. He can tighten his grip slightly on the patient's head and thus minimize movements associated with securing the collar.

While you hold the collar in place with your left hand:

- Use your right hand to draw the collar tight and press together the mating Velcro parts.

Finally:

- Look at the patient from the side to see that the collar is supporting the head in an in-line neutral position.

If it is not:

- Remove the collar and apply one of a more suitable size.

Using Pediatric Collars

Both the Stifneck and the Vertabrace pediatric collars have been designed to fit a wide range of children. Although they are generally intended for use on children older than three years, they have been used to immobilize the cervical spine of children younger than two years. The procedure for applying a pediatric collar is the same as for applying an adult model: The head is maintained in neutral alignment, the collar is pre-formed, and then applied so that the chin is correctly positioned in the chin piece.

Either a pediatric collar or an adult collar can be used on older children. A problem with using an adult collar to immobilize the cervical spine of a child is that when there is substantial overlap of the Velcro material, the end of the back panel near the loop material may contact the side of the child's head and cause lateral displacement. This can be prevented by cutting away a portion of the top and bottom of the back panel with shears.

Just as some children are well fit by an adult collar, some adults need a pediatric collar, especially older, small-framed individuals. Whichever of the cervical collars you elect to use, always remember that no collar by itself can adequately immobilize the cervical spine. Complete immobilization is possible only when a patient is rigidly secured head-to-toe on a long spine board.

Immobilizing a Patient's Head in the Position Found

Keep in mind that a patient's head should *not* be moved to an in-line neutral position, and a cervical collar should *not* be applied when:

- The patient's head is tilted to one side and he complains of increased pain on movement, or the patient resists moving his head.
- The rescuer detects resistance or "grating" on movement.

This does not mean that the patient should be removed from the vehicle without any sort of cervical support, however. While it will not be as effective as a cervical spine and immobilizing device, a short spine board can be used to immobilize the head in the position found.

USING A SHORT SPINE BOARD

The spine board used for this particular immobilization procedure should have a head-rest with scalloped edges or holes. Otherwise the cravats that will be used as a waist cinch will slip off. While one rescuer gets into position and manually supports the patient's head:

- You and the other rescuer roll the blanket tightly and form the six triangular bandages into cravats. Use tape or large rubber bands to maintain a neat, tight roll.

The blanket will be used as the immobilizing device and the cravats will be used to secure the patient to the spine board. Cravats are better suited to this procedure than straps because of their flexibility.

- Tie one end of one cravat around the headrest. Make sure that the cravat is seated within the indentations or holes in the board and that the knot is at the side of the headrest.
- Secure the second cravat to the spine board next to the first one in the same manner.

When the board is ready:

- Take a position on the seat next to the patient.
- Have your partner stand at the driver's door opening.

Because of the width of the spine board, insertion and placement of the board will be easier if the rescuer who is supporting the patient's head stands or kneels behind him rather than sits on the back seat.
When you are in position:

- Direct your partner to insert the bottom edge of the board behind the patient's back.
- Slide your hand into the void between the patient's buttocks and the seat back and grasp the nearest cravat.

As your partner moves the board into an upside-down vertical position:

- Pull the cravat from behind the patient.

Pulling the cravat as the other rescuer positions the board eliminates the need to disentangle the cravat after the board is in place—a possibly difficult operation.
When the board is in place:

- Carry the free ends of the cravats around the patient's waist as low as possible, preferably over the iliac crests.
- Join the ends of the cravats with a knot to form a snug waist strap.

The waist strap will hold the spine board in position during the rest of the immobilization procedure. If the headrest is left free and the board rotates after the patient's head is secured to it, neck movement is likely to result.
While one rescuer supports the head in the tilted position, and while the other rescuer supports the board vertically:

- Place padding behind the head and neck, and between the side of the head and the shoulder.

The padding behind the head and neck will prevent the head from being pulled back and the neck from extending when the head is secured to the board with cravats. Padding between the side of the head and the shoulder will maintain the head in the position found.

- Place the rolled blanket around the head and over the shoulders.
- Fill any obvious voids with padding.
- Lay a cravat over the blanket and shoulder of one side.
- Pass one end of the cravat behind the patient and under the armpit of the other side.
- Join the ends of the cravat with a knot tied over the chest just forward of the armpit.
- Repeat the procedure to secure the other end of the blanket to the patient's other shoulder. The tied cravats will have the appearance of an X.

Needless to say, the rescuer who has been supporting the patient's head will have to relinquish his hold while the blanket is being positioned. Once the blanket is in position, he can resume supporting the head by placing his hands on the blanket.

If the spine board has several openings close together on each side, it may be possible to pass the two cravats that are securing the blanket to the patient's shoulders behind the board and through the handholds. This will result in even more rigid stabilization.

- Pass the end of a cravat through the uppermost handhold opening on one side of the board, behind the board, and through the next lower opening on the other side from behind.
- Then pass the cravat over the rolled blanket and across the patient's forehead.
- Join the ends of the cravat in a knot tied close to the handhold.
- Repeat the procedure with the last cravat, starting at the uppermost handhold opening on the other side of the board. The cravats will form an X over the forehead.

This is makeshift immobilization, to be sure, but it is far better to rig a patient in this manner than to merely drag him from the vehicle with no cervical spine immobilization whatsoever. Needless to say, extra care will have to be taken when removing the patient from the vehicle.

EMERGENCY EVACUATION PROCEDURES

While the ideal way to remove a patient from a vehicle is to immobilize the cervical spine first, then immobilize the entire upper body, this is not always possible. Rapid evacuation is necessary when the vehicle is on fire or the threat of fire is high, when the atmosphere and/or the ground around the vehicle is contaminated by a hazardous material, when any other hazard poses an immediate threat to the welfare of victims and rescuers, or when the patient must be resuscitated.

Rapid evacuation is not the mere pulling of a patient from the wreckage and dragging him to a safe place. It includes quick but safe systematic preparation of the patient and movement onto a patient-carrying device in such a way that the chance of aggravating a spinal injury is minimized.

Following is a procedure that a team of rescuers can use to remove a patient from a vehicle quickly. As an example, let's consider that you have a patient who is the driver of the vehicle. You suspect spinal injury has occurred. You are in charge of the team. The first step is to assign someone to the task of manually supporting the patient's head.

- Have one rescuer enter the vehicle and from a position behind the driver, manually support the head in the in-line neutral position; then
- Have another rescuer apply a rigid cervical collar.

When the collar is in place and rescuer 1 has the driver's head firmly supported:

- Instruct rescuers 2 and 3 to push the driver's door beyond its normal range of motion.

Moving the door is important; it creates sorely needed working space at the side of the vehicle.

- Have rescuers 2 and 3 position the foot end of a long spine board on the seat next to the driver's left buttock—rescuer 2 at the right side of the board adjacent to the B-pillar, and rescuer 3 between the board and the door.
- You support the end of the board, or ask another rescuer or firefighter to do so.
- Direct rescuers 2 and 3 to ease the end of the board under the driver's left buttock.

This can usually be accomplished without moving the driver by pressing the end of the board down on the soft cushion and pushing the board into the resulting void. The board need not be pushed very far under the driver.

While rescuer 3 and you or another person support the board in place:

- Direct rescuer 2 to stand at the side of the vehicle and take over manual in-line immobilization of the driver's head from rescuer 1.

When the transfer is complete:

- Have rescuer 1 move to the front seat and place both hands under the driver's legs close to the knees.

While you (or another person) support the free end of the board:

- Have rescuer 3 lean over the board.
- Direct rescuer 3 to place his left hand in the driver's right armpit, and his right hand behind the driver's back where it will help to support the driver during movement.

While rescuer 2 supports the driver's head:

- Have rescuers 1 and 3 carefully rotate the driver on the seat until the right side of his right knee touches the front of the seat bottom.

This rotation just about moves the driver in line with the spine board.

When everyone is ready, and while rescuer 2 continues to support the head:

- Have rescuer 1 lift the driver's feet and legs onto the seat while rescuer 3 lowers the driver's upper body onto the board.

Close coordination between rescuers is critical. If rescuer 1 does not lower the driver's head at the same rate rescuer 3 is lowering the driver's body, the unsupported portion of the driver's neck will flex and the head will tilt forward into the chin-to-chest position. If rescuer 1 lowers the driver's head faster than rescuer 3 lowers the driver's body, then the unsupported portion of the neck will extend and the head will fall back into the sniffing position. Further injury to the cervical spine can result in either case.

When the driver's upper body is on the board, and while rescuer 2 continues to support the head:

- Direct rescuer 3 to place his hands in the driver's armpits.
- Direct rescuer 3 to slide the driver onto the board 6 to 12 inches at a time while rescuer 1 supports the driver's feet just above the seat.

The rescuer who is supporting the head must take care not to allow the back of the head to drop onto the board. A helpful hint is to gently "roll" the patient's shoulders back to the board by placing your hands on the shoulders and pushing them gently up and back. This maneuver usually aligns the head and back anatomically and lessens the potential that you will overpad the void between a patient's head and the board. For some individuals, a firm pad 1 inch to 1-1/2 inches thick must be placed between the back of the head and the spine board to keep the cervical spine in a neutral position.

If padding is immediately available, it can be placed under the head as the patient is lowered to the board and then slid with the head as the patient is moved. Lacking padding, the rescuer who is supporting the head can place his hand flat on the board under the head and move the hand as the patient is being slid into position.

When the driver is fully on the board:

- Have a rescuer place the necessary padding under the back of the head if it is not already there.
- Then have the rescuers pick up the board and carefully carry it to a safe place.

Careful movement is essential since the patient will not be strapped to the board until he is away from the immediate danger zone. A patient can also be pulled onto a long spine board with a 1-inch rope sling. The procedure is described in Phase Nine.

SUMMARY

Lifesaving measures are initiated by medical personnel during the seventh phase of a vehicle rescue operation. Rescuers can assist by manually supporting the head of a patient and applying a cervical collar. The assistance you can provide often allows for the medical team to care for two patients simultaneously.

There are very few conditions under which the head and neck of a patient cannot be maintained in a neutral position. Rescuers must be able to recognize those conditions and must be able to immobilize the patient's head in the position found.

A developing fire, the threat of an explosion, or the presence of a hazardous material will necessitate the rapid removal of a patient before he can be secured to an upper-body immobilization device. A trained team of rescuers can accomplish the task with a long spine board.

PHASE EIGHT

Disentangling Trapped Patients

INTRODUCTION

Disentangling patients from vehicles can be compared to eating an orange. Obviously you can't get to the fruit of an orange without making an opening in the skin, and you can't remove the fruit without removing most of the peel. Sure, you can pull fruit from the orange through a small opening in the skin, but you can't do so without damaging it.

So it is with vehicle rescue. You can gain access to patients through an opening made in a damaged vehicle, but the chances are good that you can't extricate them without injuring them or aggravating existing injuries unless you first remove the parts of the vehicle that are surrounding them.

There are three distinct parts to this eighth phase of a vehicle rescue operation: (1) protecting the trapped and injured patients from harm; (2) creating working space and exitways through which patients can be removed; and (3) removing mechanisms of entrapment from around the patients so they can be removed from the wreckage.

PROTECTING TRAPPED AND INJURED PATIENTS DURING DISENTANGLEMENT OPERATIONS

It's amazing how little consideration some emergency service personnel give to the need for patient protection during vehicle rescue operations. Yet in order to remove just one patient from a vehicle that has been damaged as the result of a single vehicle accident, rescuers may have to move a downed wire, extinguish a fire, plug a leaking fuel tank, cope with spilled fuel, stabilize the vehicle, illuminate dark work areas, make the roadways around the vehicle slip resistant, break the vehicle's side and rear windows, cut out the windshield, force open jammed doors, fold down B-pillars, sever roof pillars, fold back a section of the roof, sever the steering wheel, displace or sever the steering column, displace pedals, and displace the dash.

While rescuers are using any of dozens of sharp-pointed, sharp-edged, heavy, blunt, short- and long-handled, hand-operated and powered tools to accomplish these tasks, they can pinch, poke, prod, punch, puncture, abrade, lacerate, and incise a patient who may have already been lacerated by sharp metal and plastic edges, impaled by a sharp piece of debris, and cut by broken glass. Moreover, squad members may have to carry out the rescue operation under the broiling sun, or in numbing cold while being pelted by rain, sleet, or snow or a combination thereof! If you have such regard for your own welfare that you protect yourself from all of the mechanisms of injury that can be found at the scene, have an equal regard for the safety of the people who need your help. Protect them from not only mechanisms of injury but also the elements.

Protecting the Occupants of Vehicles from Mechanisms of Injury

Many rescuers believe that merely throwing a soft covering of some sort over patients during disentanglement operations is sufficient protection during disentanglement operations. This is not a good idea for at least two reasons.

While a woven fiber blanket, a disposable paper blanket, or a lightweight tarp may protect a patient from flying particles of glass and debris, none of these items will adequately protect him from forceful contact with a tool, a sharp metal edge, or a pointed object. Moreover, an already frightened patient may panic when his head is covered in this manner. Thrashing about wildly while trying to escape from under a covering can aggravate existing injuries and even cause new ones.

Every rescue unit should have a variety of items for affording patients head-to-toe protection during rescue operations.

Protecting a Patient's Eyes

Flying objects are common during aggressive disentanglement operations. Bits of metal often break off and fly when one steel tool is struck with another steel tool. Small metal particles are produced when vehicle components are cut with a saw. Even flakes of

paint can become dangerous objects when metal components are displaced and distorted. However, flying particles of glass pose the greatest threat to patients' eyes.

Regardless of how careful you are and what steps you have taken to minimize their spread, expect glass fragments to fly when you break side and rear windows and when you forcibly remove windshields. Eye protection for patients is a must.

USING SAFETY GOGGLES

It's important that you use the proper eye protection. Don't provide the patient with a fire helmet with a pull-down shield, or a pair of spectacle-type safety glasses unless you have nothing else available. While helmet shields and safety glasses will shield a patient's eyes from particles that strike head-on, they may not deflect fragments that approach from the side, and they will not protect the wearer's eyes from glass dust. Very finely divided glass fragments can be carried in a breeze for as much as 20 feet into a patient's unprotected eyes, and damage to the cornea can result if the particles are not removed quickly.

Remember: Glass is glass regardless of whether it is in the form of large shards or very small particles; and whatever its form, glass cuts.

If there are no injuries that will be aggravated by the frame or the elastic band of a pair of safety goggles:

- Carefully position the goggles over the patient's face (Figure 8.01).
- Quickly dress and bandage any open wounds to the remainder of the face to prevent contamination by flying glass particles.

Protecting an Unconscious Patient's Eyes

Untrained rescuers tend to minimize patient protection steps when patients are unconscious. They need more protection, not less! The eyes of an unconscious patient require special attention.

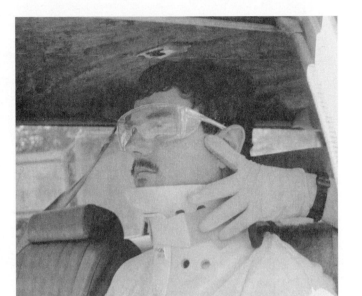

FIGURE 8.01 Goggles on Victim

If you discover that an unconscious patient's eyes are open:

- Gently hold both lids shut with a small piece of tape or an adhesive bandage before you put safety goggles on him. Remember that the eyes of an unconscious patient can dry and ulcerate quickly if they are left open, especially in a breeze.

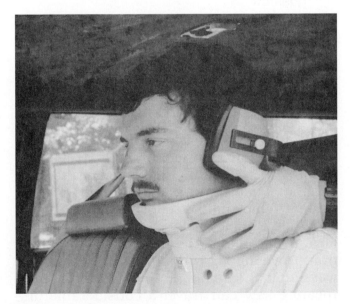

FIGURE 8.02 Earmuffs on Victim

Protecting a Patient's Ears

Flying particles of debris can enter unprotected ear canals as well as unprotected eyes during disentanglement activities. Moreover, unprotected external ears can be lacerated or even avulsed if they come in contact with tools or the sharp edges of vehicle debris.

You could have a rescuer hold a short spine board or other rigid device at the side of the patient's head while you are using tools nearby, or while you are breaking glass. However, chances are that both the board and the rescuer holding it will be in your way. A better way to protect a patient's ears is with an inexpensive device designed specially for the task.

USING INDUSTRIAL HEARING PROTECTORS

Inexpensive earmuff-style hearing protectors have rigid plastic oval-shaped cups at each end of a flexible head strap. Gel-filled cushions assure a snug fit against the sides of the wearer's head (Figure 8.02).

To fit a patient with an industrial hearing protector with minimum head movement:

- Spread the cups apart with both hands.
- Gently position the cups over the patient's ears. Be sure not to let them "clap" against the side of the face. The effect will be the same as clapping your cupped hands against the ears.

Industrial hearing protectors do more than protect the patient's ears from contact with tools or debris. They also shield the ears from the loud noises common to vehicle rescue activities; that is their original purpose. Even though they may be loud, the short-duration sounds of an air-operated chisel, a nearby gasoline-powered engine, or a steel tool repeatedly striking another steel tool or a part of the vehicle are not likely to cause permanent hearing loss. However, these noises can easily upset an already fearful person, and a sudden loud noise is likely to cause the patient to flinch or actually jump—reactions that may be harmful to an injured patient, especially one who has a cervical spine injury.

Protecting a Patient's Scalp and Skull

Don't neglect the rest of a patient's head after you have taken steps to protect his eyes and ears. Keep in mind that the scalp and skull are also quite vulnerable.

USING A HARD HAT

Every rescue unit should have several construction hard hats solely for the purpose of protecting the scalp and skull of patients during disentanglement operations (Figure 8.03).
    Before you put a helmet on a patient:

- Adjust the helmet suspension so it will fit over the headband of the hearing protector. A helmet that is too small will simply perch on top of the patient's head where it can be easily dislodged. When a helmet is too large, the suspension will not properly protect the patient.

When you cannot fit a patient with safety goggles, a hearing protector, and a helmet, at least protect his head and face by having another rescuer or a firefighter hold a rigid shield or a thick pad made of a folded soft covering between the patient and the potential mechanism of injury.

Protecting a Patient's Torso and Extremities

Contusions are likely even when a patient is struck lightly by a tool or other blunt object during a rescue operation. A forceful blow can aggravate existing fractures and even cause new ones. A sharp tool or sharp-edged piece of debris can lacerate unprotected soft tissues and contact with a sharp-pointed tool can result in impalement. Protecting a patient with a rigid shield can prevent these rescue-related injuries.

USING A RIGID SHIELD

A wooden or aluminum spine board or a plywood or particle board panel affords excel-

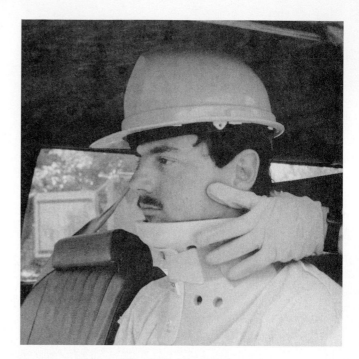

FIGURE 8.03   Hard Hat on Victim

lent shielding against contact with tools and debris.
    To protect a patient while forcing open or removing a door:

- Have another rescuer hold the board between the patient and the tool. The board should be partially supported by a seat or other solid structure, if possible.

When doors must be forced open and/or removed after a vehicle's roof has been folded back or removed, it may be possible to insert a long spine board between the seat and the B-pillar for patient protection (Figure 8.04).
    A short spine board can also be used to protect the driver and front seat passenger when a reciprocating saw is being used to sever roof pillars in preparation for folding back or removing the roof.
    When a hacksaw is used to sever roof pillars, the frame of the saw keeps the blade from traveling far when the blade leaves the work after the final cut. The blade of a reciprocating saw can travel a considerable distance after the final cut is made, especially if

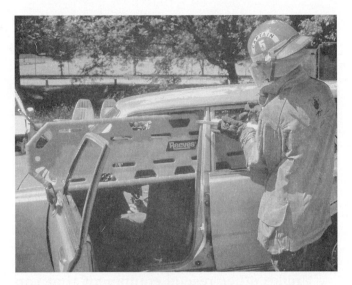

FIGURE 8.04   Spine Board to Protect Victim

the operator is really bearing down on the motor housing. A pointed, moving saw blade can severely lacerate a patient's unprotected chest, arms, or abdomen.

To protect a driver or passenger from contact with a reciprocating saw blade:

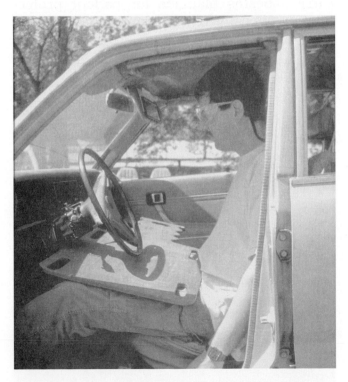

FIGURE 8.05   Short Spine Board to Protect Victim

• Have another rescuer hold the spine board or other rigid shield between the saw and the patient in such a way that the board will take the full impact if the saw breaks free from the work.

Removing a section of a vehicle's steering wheel with a reciprocating saw does not usually pose a threat to the driver, nor does removing the steering wheel altogether by severing the spokes. In most cases, the motor housing of the tool can be held steady with the blade pointing away from the driver. On the other hand, severing the steering column of a vehicle with a reciprocating saw can be dangerous to an unprotected driver.

The "ideal" way to sever a steering column with a reciprocating saw is to hold the tool so the edge of the blade is against the underside of the column and then cut upward. Thus the blade will always be moving away from the driver, and another rescuer can pull up on the column to prevent the saw blade from binding in the cut. Cutting a column in this manner is not always possible, however. If debris or the patient prevents you from holding the saw in a position from which it will cut upward, you will have no alternative to holding the saw so it cuts down.

Considerable downward force is required to move the blade of a reciprocating saw through the components of a steering column. Because of limited working space and an awkward position you may have to take at the side of the driver, balance is likely to be a problem. If the blade exits the column while you are bearing down on the motor housing, the blade may contact the driver's thigh or leg and cause injury.

To protect the driver's legs while severing a steering column with a reciprocating saw:

• Have another rescuer hold a short spine board or other rigid shield flat against the driver's thighs (Figure 8.05).

If the rigid shield cannot be positioned in this manner, as when the driver is obese:

- Either use a smaller device such as a board splint or even a folded immobilization vest; or
- Remove the steering wheel and hold the shield at an angle in front of the driver with the headrest pointed to the floor.

Provide some sort of protection even when you only have to sever part of the steering wheel with a bolt cutter or ratchet cutter.

If a rigid device can't be positioned between the driver and the tool:

- Have another rescuer support the tool with one hand to prevent its dropping into the driver's lap when the cut is made.

A rigid device such as a short spine board should be held in front of the driver when a steering column must be displaced.

While a spine board can be used to protect patients in many situations, there may be times when you won't be able to fit the board in the space available, or times when the board is needed for another task. In these cases, consider using some sort of covering that can be squeezed into tight spaces and/or molded around the patient.

USING SOFT COVERING MATERIALS

A turnout coat, wool blanket, disposable blanket, or lightweight tarp can be used to shield a patient from contact with tools and debris when a rigid device is not available. Do not simply cover the patient, however. One layer of a soft covering will do little, if anything, to deflect a tool.

To make a protective pad:

- Fold the covering as many times as you can without making a package too small to provide adequate protection.
- Have another rescuer hold the folded covering in front of the body part that is likely to be contacted if the tool slips.

The folded covering will not deflect a blunt tool, but it will absorb much of the striking force (Figure 8.06). A folded covering will also minimize the chance that a body part will be penetrated by a sharp tool or a sharp-pointed piece of debris.

Protecting Patients from Flames and Radiant Heat

Every rescue vehicle should have an aluminized rescue blanket that can be thrown over patients when a part of a vehicle is on fire, or when the threat of fire is high. An aluminized blanket can also be used to protect patients from radiant heat when an adjacent vehicle is on fire.

Unlike other rescue equipment that can be used for a number of operations, an aluminized blanket should be used only for protecting patients from flames and radiant heat. Using one for a ground cover can cause an aluminized blanket to become dirty, and heaping tools onto an aluminum blanket can cause the coating to flake off. In either case, the ability for the blanket to reflect radiant heat is then sharply reduced.

An important point: Some rescue units still carry asbestos blankets for patient protection. An asbestos blanket can shed fibers that

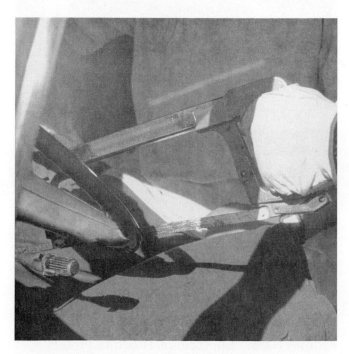

FIGURE 8.06   Folded Blanket to Protect Victim

are known to be harmful to a patient's health. Moreover, these blankets absorb a great deal of heat when they are exposed to flames or radiant heat. If a heated asbestos blanket is wet with water from a hose line, the resulting steam can fatally scald anyone underneath the blanket. It is for these reasons that asbestos blankets should be discarded.

Protecting Patients from Dusts and Mists

Cement, flour, and silica are examples of powdery materials that might be spilled from a bulk carrier as the result of a vehicle accident. A huge cloud of powder can settle on the scene after the crash, and if there is a strong breeze, clouds of powder can swirl around the wreckage during rescue activities. Inexpensive disposable dust masks will protect the respiratory passages of patients and rescuers against nontoxic dusts and mists. The masks can be easily slipped over a patient's head even if there are scalp or facial wounds.

Protecting Patients from Smoke and Noxious Fumes

If a vehicle catches fire or if a hazardous commodity is released, clouds of irritating smoke, noxious fumes, and toxic gases can swirl around the scene. A short exposure to nontoxic smoke and fumes may be more of a nuisance than a health hazard. However, continued exposure during a lengthy extrication procedure can sicken trapped patients. Retching, vomiting, and movement during an attempt to get away from the source of irritation may cause patients to aggravate their injuries. Thus it may be necessary to provide patients with fresh air when it appears that disentanglement and removal operations will be lengthy. A self-contained breathing apparatus will supply fresh air, but space limitations and the difficulties of getting a patient into the face mask make the use of a breathing apparatus impractical.

An appliance normally associated with firefighting activities—the smoke ejector—can be used to great advantage at locations of vehicle accidents. This device can be used either to move smoke or fumes away from a vehicle or to move fresh air into the vehicle.

If smoke is entering the vehicle from only one side:

- Instruct rescuers or firefighters to place the fan near an open window so fresh air will be forced through the vehicle against the drifting smoke.

If the vehicle is in the path of the smoke:

- Have rescuers stand away from the vehicle and attempt to deflect the cloud with fresh air from the fan.

A smoke ejector can be suspended from a stepladder or the combination step-to-straight ladder that is carried on many rescue and firefighting vehicles. Some rescue units carry a corrugated extension tube for use with a smoke ejector. This "elephant trunk" enables rescuers to place the fan at a distance from the wreckage where the air is clearer. When used with a tarpaulin, fresh air from a smoke ejector will create a positive pressure inside an accident vehicle until the hazard is eliminated (Figure 8.07). Occupants are protected from the intrusion of smoke and fumes just like firefighters are protected by a self-contained, positive pressure breathing apparatus.

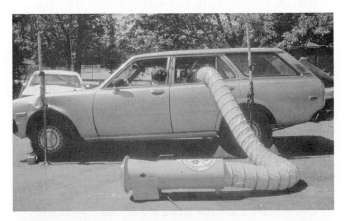

FIGURE 8.07   Smoke Ejector with Tube in Rear Window

Care must be exercised when using a smoke ejector to provide the occupants of vehicles with fresh air during cold-weather operations, especially when their clothing is wet. Wind chill and water chill will quickly lower body temperatures.

Protecting Patients from the Elements

Cold, rain, sleet, and snow do more than merely add to a patient's discomfort. When normal body processes are disrupted as the result of injury or shock, changes in temperature can cause a patient's condition to deteriorate quickly. While steps to protect a patient from the elements may not be necessary when he can be removed from a damaged vehicle quickly, such steps should certainly be undertaken when disentanglement and removal are likely to be lengthy.

Protecting Patients from Cold

Following are several ways unprotected patients can lose body heat:

Radiation from unprotected body parts is the leading cause of heat loss. An unprotected head is responsible for the especially rapid loss of body heat. At 40° F, an uncovered head can radiate away up to one half of the body's total heat production. At 5° F, up to three-quarters of the body's total heat protection can be radiated away from an uncovered head.

Conduction—the transfer of heat from a warm object to a cold object—causes a loss of body heat wherever an unprotected body part touches a cold surface. Heat is lost quickly where a bare arm contacts a door, for example.

Convection—the movement of warm air away from a warm body—also results in the loss of body heat. Three factors contribute to heat loss through convection: a brisk wind, exposed skin surfaces, and insufficient clothing.

Water Chill contributes to heat loss when a patient's clothing is wet. The thermal

conductivity of water is 240 times as great as that of still air. This means that wet clothing can extract heat from the human body up to 240 times faster than can dry clothing. Dry clothing holds an insulating layer of warm air next to the skin; wet clothing does not provide that protection. Instead, it conducts heat away from the body much faster than it can be produced.

Wind Chill aggravates heat loss due to convection. If there is no wind at all, convection will not be a major cause of heat loss from trapped and injured patients. But when there is a combination of wind and a low temperature, body heat is lost quickly, and if the wind chill factor is low enough, exposed skin areas will be in danger of freezing.

The *evaporation* of sweat is also responsible for the loss of body heat. Even *breathing* contributes to heat loss. A person breathes in cold air but breathes out warm air.

Remember: Cold can kill rapidly if steps are not taken quickly to prevent the loss of body heat. This is what is likely to happen to a patient as hypothermia develops:

99° F   Shivering begins. As the core temperature continues to drop, shivering becomes intense.

95° F   Violent shivering persists. A conscious patient may have trouble speaking.

90° F   Shivering decreases and strong muscular rigidity begins. Muscular coordination is affected; erratic or jerky movements are produced. If the patient is conscious, thinking is less clear. General comprehension of the situation is dulled. There may be total amnesia. Nonetheless, the patient is generally able to maintain the appearance of psychological contact with the surroundings.

85° F   The patient becomes irrational. Contact with the environment is lost and the patient drifts into a stuporous state. Muscular rigidity continues. Pulse and respirations are slowed.

80° F The patient becomes unconscious and does not respond to the spoken word. Most reflexes cease to function. Heartbeat becomes erratic.

78° F Cardiac and respiratory centers of the brain fail. Ventricular fibrillation occurs. Probable edema and hemorrhage in the lungs. Death.

PREVENTING THE LOSS OF BODY HEAT

Heat loss can be prevented in many ways. Consider the steps that you might take as a rescuer ordered to protect a patient from the effects of cold.

If the patient's clothing is wet:

- Cover him with an impervious material before covering him with a blanket. An aluminized survival blanket (not a rescue blanket) or an unfolded trash bag will work like a wet suit and hold in body heat.
- Then cover the patient with a wool or synthetic fiber blanket, or a disposable paper blanket to prevent heat loss due to radiation and air movement. Wool blankets are best because body warmth is trapped by the fibers.

If you have to use a lightweight tarp to prevent the loss of body heat:

- Fold it so that air can be trapped between the layers.

If to do so will not aggravate any existing injuries:

- Prevent heat loss by conduction by tucking the blanket between cold surfaces and body parts.

This last step is especially important when a patient is lying on cold ground. Body heat can be lost very quickly when a patient's entire back surface is in contact with cold ground.

After you provide whatever head protection is necessary (safety goggles, hearing protectors, and hard hat):

- Cover the patient's head with a towel and tuck the towel under the blanket.

To prevent the loss of body heat through respirations:

- Secure a thermal mask over the patient's mouth and nose. This inexpensive disposable item will warm inhaled air.

If it is raining or snowing:

- Ask someone to hold an umbrella over the patient during the disentanglement operation.

If another person will be in the way of the rescue effort or will be in danger:

- Provide the patient with an outer covering of a waterproof material such as a lightweight tarp or a large unfolded trash bag.

USING FLOODLIGHTS AS A SOURCE OF WARMTH

The 300- or 500-watt incandescent bulb floodlights that are usually carried on a rescue vehicle for illumination give off a tremendous amount of heat. When properly used, they can warm the interior of a vehicle.

- Have rescuers or firefighters hold the lights in such a way that they will illuminate and, to a degree, heat the work area.
- Be sure that the lights do not shine directly in the patients' or the rescuers' eyes, and that they are not held too closely to the patients.

Having people hold the lights is better than positioning them stationary. Movement will be easier if the lights get in the way of squad members during the rescue operation.

Protecting Patients from the Sun

Heat, like cold, can be harmful to patients. Too much heat in any form can quickly upset the body's temperature-regulating mechanisms and even cause death. Steps should be taken to shield a patient from direct sunlight on a hot day. Shading the patient's head is especially important. Vital nerve centers for breathing and circulation lie close to the surface of the head, and arteries that supply the brain with blood lie close to the sides of the neck.

To shield a patient from direct sunlight on a hot day:

- Don't cover the patient; to do so may quickly raise body temperature.

Instead:

- Have another rescuer or a firefighter shield the patient's head with a large umbrella during disentanglement and removal operations (Figure 8.08).

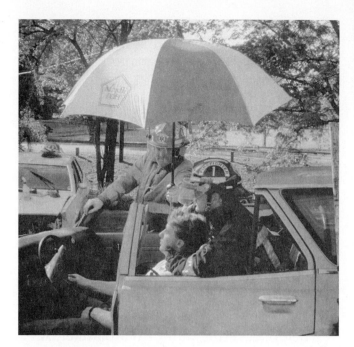

FIGURE 8.08   Umbrella

CREATING WORKING SPACE AND EXITWAYS THROUGH WHICH VEHICLE PATIENTS CAN BE REMOVED

In Phase Six we talked about gaining access to the interior of the vehicle. Now that we are inside, we must create working space for both treating the patient and removing same. Widening door openings and disposing of the doors altogether are a preliminary to removing the roof in most cases. In order to keep a flow going, we will repeat some of the steps discussed in Phase Six, naturally with more emphasis on disassembling the vehicle.

Once the patients have been properly protected, steps can be taken to create working space within the vehicle and exitways through which patients can be removed.

A vehicle's doors can severely impede the efforts of rescue squad personnel. Displacing doors or removing them altogether serves three purposes: (1) It creates working space next to the door openings; (2) it makes openings in the vehicle through which rescuers can reach mechanisms of entrapment; and (3) it creates pathways through which rescuers may be able to remove patients.

Widening Door Openings

The undamaged front doors of passenger cars will usually open about 45 to 50 degrees, while undamaged rear doors will normally open about 60 degrees. The resulting openings are usually wide enough for drivers and passengers to enter and exit the vehicle without difficulty. The doors of a damaged vehicle may not open nearly as wide, and even if they do, there may not be room to kneel at the side of a patient. A 200-pound rescuer trying to fit within a 30 degree space between the door and the door sill of a car is akin to trying to stuff 15 pounds of something into a 10-pound bag. It doesn't work! Nor will there be room to position a long spine board or other patient-carrying device at a right angle to the side of the vehicle during the patient removal procedure.

Working space at the side of a vehicle can be created either by manually or mechanically moving the doors beyond their normal range of motion or by removing the doors altogether.

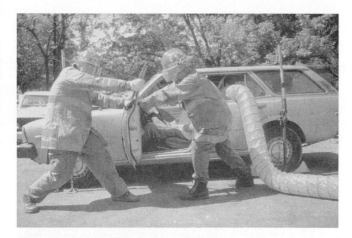

FIGURE 8.09   Manually Moving Doors

Manually Moving Doors

If the hinges are not damaged, it may be possible to move a door beyond its normal range of motion without having to set up any mechanical equipment. Don't just stand behind the door and attempt to move it with a series of pushes, however. Doing so may create movements sufficient to rock the car even though it has been rigidly stabilized.

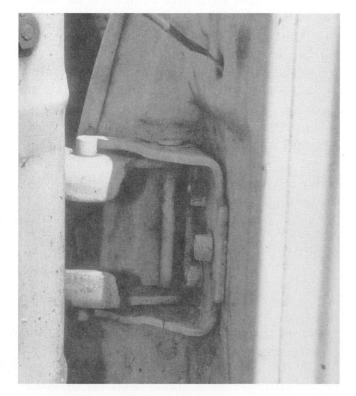

FIGURE 8.10   Stamped Hinge

- Stand next to the inner side of the door in a position where you can push.
- Direct another rescuer to take a position next to the outer skin of the door where he can pull (Figure 8.09).

On your signal:

- Together exert one combined pushing-pulling effort, then stop.

After a brief pause to allow the vehicle to come to rest:

- Repeat the push-pull effort and stop.
- Check your progress and repeat the procedure as many times as necessary to move the door the desired distance.

A word of warning: Examine the hinges before you attempt to move a door beyond its normal range of motion, either manually or mechanically. Note whether they are stamped or cast. Stamped hinges are irregularly shaped and have rounded edges and a smooth finish (Figure 8.10). Cast hinges have square edges and appear grainy (Figure 8.11).

You can usually push a door with stamped hinges all the way back to the fender of the vehicle. However, a cast hinge may break when it passes the 90 degree point. Be sure that your feet and the feet of your partner are not in a place where they can be injured if a door with cast hinges breaks during a movement effort.

Mechanically Moving Doors

It may be necessary to use tools that afford a mechanical advantage when doors are damaged to the extent that they cannot be manually moved beyond the normal range of motion.

USING A HAND WINCH AND A CHAIN OR STRAP SET

When equipment is in short supply during operations at a multiple-vehicle rescue operation, a chain or cable hand winch can be used by itself to pull a damaged door past the 90 degree point. The fixed hook of the winch can be secured to a bumper or other part of the vehicle, and the lip of the door can be snagged with the running hook. However, a hand winch is best used in conjunction with a chain or strap set. Following is a procedure that you and a partner can use to displace a door with a hand winch.

To create an anchor point for the hand winch:

- Pass the running hook of the long rescue chain around the axle or other rigid structure under the vehicle on the far side.
- Capture the standing part of the chain with the running hook and work out any slack from the resulting loop.
- Carry the free end of chain out from under the vehicle and around the bumper to the hood.

While your partner rescuer supports the anchor chain in place:

- Position lengths of cribbing under the chain wherever it might become snagged, and where sheet metal might be dimpled when forces are applied by the hand winch.

Finally:

- Adjust the length of the anchor chain with the grab hook so the ring or oval is resting on the hood, and join the chain with the fixed hook of the hand winch.

An important point: Take care in creating an anchor point in this manner when you see that a shock-absorbing bumper has been damaged. While it seldom happens, there is always the chance that a damaged bumper will unexpectedly spring forward. Instead of working at the front of a vehicle that has a damaged shock-absorbing bumper, work from the side and loop the chain around the axle just behind the wheel assembly.

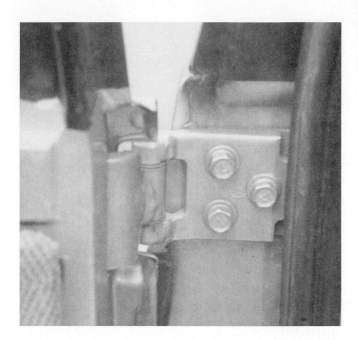

FIGURE 8.11   Cast Hinge

To create an anchor point with a rescue strap:

- Pass the end of the strap that has the small steel triangle around the axle or other rigid structure under the far side of the vehicle.
- Pass the small triangle through the slot of the choker triangle and draw the resulting loop tight around the anchor structure.
- Carry the free end of the strap from under the vehicle, around the bumper, and up to the hood.

While your partner maintains tension on the strap:

- Position cribbing under the strap wherever it is likely to contact sharp metal edges when under tension.

When the cribbing is in place:

- Join the fixed hook of the hand winch to the triangle of the strap.

Be careful! While a nylon web strap is extremely strong, it can be easily cut by a sharp metal edge.

To create the pulling point at the door:

- Loop the chain or strap around the door and join the ends.

There are many ways to secure a chain or strap around a door. However, the easiest way to form a pulling point is simply to lay the chain or strap in the notch formed by the outside corner of the door body, and then in the lip that exists at the lower outside corner of the door. Don't connect the moving hook of the hand winch to a pull handle or wrap a chain or strap around the vertical part of the window frame.

If the chain is not long enough to loop around the door in the manner just described, lay the chain in the notch formed by the window frame and the door body and catch the lower edge of the door with the slip hook.

While your partner supports the chain or strap looped around the door:

- Pull the chain or cable from the hand winch.
- Connect the moving hook of the hand winch to the ring of the chain or the triangle of the strap.

When the pulling system is complete (Figure 8.12):

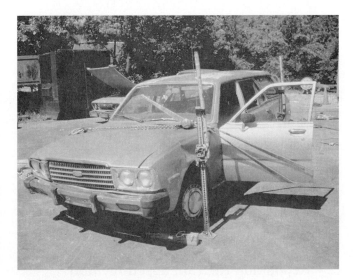

FIGURE 8.12 Moving a Door with Strap Set and Chain Come-along

- Warn your partner to keep clear of the door if it has cast hinges; then operate the hand winch to move the door the desired distance.

If you don't need the hand winch for another operation:

- Leave the winch hooked up in place. It will prevent the door from moving back to its original position when pulling forces are no longer being exerted.

If you need the hand winch and the door tends to close after the winch line has been removed:

- Secure the door in the wide open position with an elastic shock cord or a length of rope.

At this point, a few words about the safe use of hand winches are appropriate. There is seldom a problem moving a door with a hand winch. However, displacing a steering column or the front seat of a vehicle can be difficult, even with a 2-ton hand winch.

Rescuers sometimes attempt to gain additional leverage for difficult pulling jobs by sliding a "cheater bar" (a 5- to 6-foot length of 2-inch pipe kept on the rescue truck especially for the purpose) over the operating handle of the hand winch. To do so creates forces far in excess of the rating of the winch and may cause the winch mechanism to fail.

AN ALTERNATE RIGGING TECHNIQUE

There may be times when you will have to rig an anchor chain on the same side of a vehicle as the door that must be moved, as when the far side is badly damaged or when it is not accessible. A complication of this rigging procedure is that the hand winch is likely to slide off the hood and fender as it is pulling the door back.

To eliminate this problem:

- Drive the pike of a forcible entry tool into the fender so the head of the tool becomes a stop block for the hand winch.

When you are ready to move the door:

- Hold the shank of the forcible entry tool with one hand while you operate the winch handle with your other hand (Figure 8.13).

USING A HYDRAULIC HAND PUMP AND RAM ASSEMBLY

A 4- or 10-ton hydraulic jack can be used to move a damaged door when the jack kit has the necessary extensions. A lot of the time that is often lost while guessing the length of the ram assembly that is needed for the job can be eliminated by carrying a small steel tape measure in the hydraulic tool kit.

While your partner holds the door in the maximum open position:

- Measure the distance between the point on the door against which pushing forces will be exerted and the part of the vehicle's body against which the base of the ram assembly will be positioned (the junction of the B-pillar and door sill, for example, or the forward seat support).

Keeping the ram assembly low allows you to utilize strong points of the door and car vehicle body. It also minimizes the possibility that the ram assembly will drop onto an occupant if it slips during the pushing effort.

When you have the measurement:

- Assemble the ram with the necessary extensions and suitable ends.
- Have your partner position the ram assembly in the door opening and support it while you operate the hydraulic jack to move the door the desired distance.

Expect at least two problems when you use a hydraulic jack and ram assembly for this operation. Because of the rather short movement of the ram, you may have to remove the assembly and add extension pieces to it or place lengths of cribbing behind the pushing points. When you do, there may be

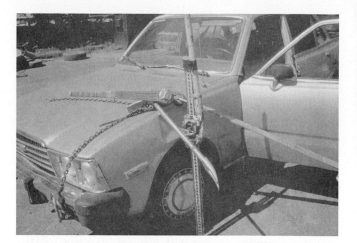

FIGURE 8.13   Moving a Door with Strap Set and Chain Come-along on the Same Side

a tendency for the door to move back to its original position.

To keep the door open:

- Catch the edge of the fender well with the running hook of a rescue chain.

Depending on the length of the chain:

- Either pass the other end of the chain around the outermost vertical part of the window frame and secure the grab hook to a link, or pass the free end of the chain around the door body and catch a link with the grab hook.

If you do not have a chain but have cribbing:

- Jam one or two lengths of cribbing or a combination of cribbing and wedges into the opening between the door and the body of the vehicle between the hinges, or position a piece of cribbing between the bottom of the door and the door sill in the manner of a buttress.

When you have extended the ram with additional sections (or positioned cribbing at the pushing points):

- Reposition the ram assembly and continue to widen the door opening.

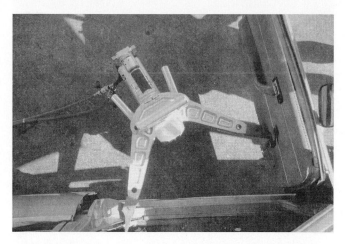

FIGURE 8.14   Widening a Door Opening with Hydraulic Spreader

USING A HYDRAULIC RESCUE TOOL

Pushing a door beyond its normal range of motion with a full-size hydraulic rescue tool can be accomplished quickly after the door has been forced open.

While another rescuer holds the door in the fully open position:

- Position the tool between the side of the floor pan and the bottom of the door.
- Spread the arms to move the door the desired distance (Figure 8.14).

The edges of the jaws are usually sharp enough to bite into the side of the floor pan and the door padding.

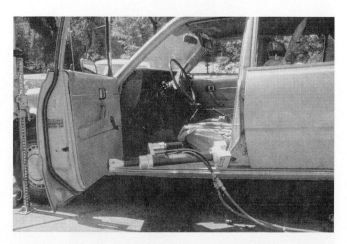

FIGURE 8.15   Widening a Door Opening with Hydraulic Ram

USING A HYDRAULIC RAM

A hydraulic ram can usually be used to move a door to a point greater than 90 degrees. While another rescuer holds the door in the fully open position:

- Position the ram between the junction of the B-pillar and the side of the floor pan and the door bottom.
- Extend the ram to push the door beyond its normal range of motion (Figure 8.15).

A smaller ram can be held with the cylinder base against the side of the floor pan and the face of the ram against the door bottom while another rescuer holds the door in the fully open position. The angled edges of the ram base and pushing face are usually sharp enough to prevent the ram from slipping while it is being extended.

If a smaller ram slips, the jaws of the spreading tool can be pinched against the side of the floor pan and used as a base for the ram.

Maintaining the Door in the Fully Open Position

Car doors often have a tendency to close for a short distance after they have been forced open beyond their usual range of motion.

To keep doors fully open:

- Catch the edge of the door and the edge of the near fender well with the S-hooks of a heavy-duty elastic shock cord.

Obviously, a rope or chain can be used for the task. However, a rope has to be knotted, and a chain may be needed for another (and more important) operation. A cargo strap can be installed as quickly as you can capture suitable anchor points with the S-hooks.

Removing Front Doors Altogether

Consider removing the front door of a vehicle altogether when you must reach the lower body of a trapped patient, or when you need all the working space possible at the side of the vehicle. The task can be accomplished quickly and easily by either breaking or severing the hinges.

REMOVING A FRONT DOOR BY BREAKING THE HINGES

The forces available at the tips of a hydraulic rescue tool are more than sufficient to either separate or break door hinges. Yet rescuers often spend a great deal of time struggling with the procedure. They have not learned that the secret of early success is placing the tips where they will push against rigid structures, not merely upset or punch through sheet-metal surfaces.

Your position and that of your partner or other helper should be carefully considered when breaking door hinges with a hydraulic tool. A door can be easily supported and its movements can be easily controlled when hinges are severed with a reciprocating saw or an air-operated chisel. But when hinges are broken with a hydraulic rescue tool, stored energy causes a door to spring away from the vehicle when the hinges separate or break, sometimes with considerable force.

Instead of having another rescuer stand near the door and support it while you operate the tool:

- Have the rescuer secure a 10-foot web strap to the window frame (or other suitable structure).
- Then have the rescuer take a position at the other end of the strap and exert a continuous pull while you operate the tool and break the hinges.

While the rescuer maintains tension on the strap:

- Break the hinges, the top one first (Figure 8.16).

The door will remain upright when the top hinge breaks. When the bottom hinge breaks, your partner will be able to pull the door away as soon as it separates from the body of the vehicle. The length of the strap will prevent his being struck by the door.

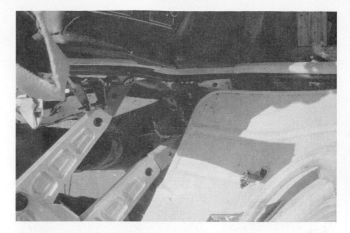

FIGURE 8.16   Breaking Hinges with Hydraulic Spreader

An important point: A great deal of trouble has been experienced by rescuers attempting to break the hinges of some new intermediate- and smaller-sized cars with hydraulic rescue tools. Positioning the tool has been found to be difficult, and when the hinge sections are joined with rivet-like fasteners instead of pins (Figure 8.17), rescuers have been exposed to the danger of flying chunks of steel. When it is necessary to remove doors that have this type of hinge, you might accomplish the task quicker and more safely by severing the hinges with hydraulic shears, a reciprocating saw, or a heavy-duty air-operated chisel than by trying to break them with a hydraulic spreader tool.

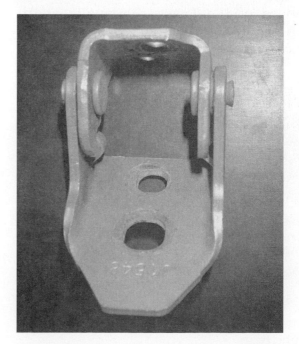

FIGURE 8.17   Hinge Rivets

REMOVING A FRONT DOOR BY SEVERING THE HINGES

Both cast and stamped hinges can be severed with either a reciprocating saw or a high-pressure air-operated chisel. Be sure that the saw has a 6-inch high-speed, shatterproof blade.

Using a Reciprocating Saw. The door should first be pushed well beyond its normal range of motion for this operation. If it is not, there may not be room to work safely.

While another rescuer holds the door in the fully open position and lubricates the blade throughout the cutting operation:

- Cut the top hinge from the top down.

If there is enough room that the point of the blade will not bottom out:

- Hold the shoe of the saw against the hinge to keep the blade from bucking.

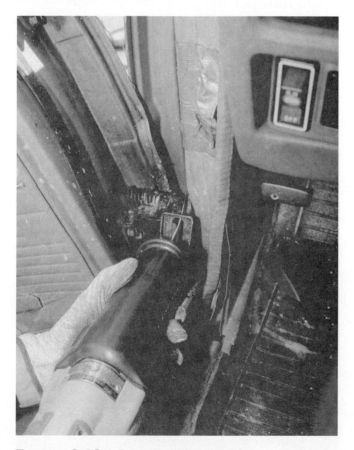

FIGURE 8.18 Severing Hinge with Reciprocating Saw

Depending on the manner in which the door is constructed, it may not be possible to hold the sole plate of the saw against the hinge without the point of the saw bottoming out. If bottoming out is a problem:

- Hold the body of the saw firmly with one hand while you hold the handle and operate the trigger with your other hand. Keep the sole plate just far enough from the hinge to prevent the point of the blade from striking something.

The more rigidly you hold the saw, the less likely it is that the blade will buck.

While you cut through the top hinges:

- Direct the rescuer who is holding the door to maintain a slight downward pressure on the door to keep the blade from binding.

When the top hinge is cut:

- Have the rescuer pivot the door downward on the hinge to give you additional working space.

While the rescuer supports the door and applies downward force:

- Sever the bottom hinge from the top down (Figure 8.18).

Together:

- Carry the door away from the vehicle.

Using an Air-Operated Chisel. A high-pressure air-operated chisel (one that operates at pressures up to 250 psi) is needed for this operation. Air guns that operate in the 90 to 120 psi range are not sufficiently powerful. The cutting procedure is essentially the same as that suggested for a reciprocating saw. However, lubrication is not necessary.

- Sever the upper hinge from the top down while another rescuer supports the door in the wide open position.

When the upper hinge is cut:

- Have the other rescuer force the door down to give you better access to the lower hinge.

While the rescuer continues to support the door:

- Sever the lower hinge.

Together:

- Carry the door away from the vehicle.

While you shouldn't have a problem severing stamped hinges, you may have to adjust the regulator to supply air to the gun at the highest pressure possible when attempting to sever cast hinges. Be aware that even then you may not be able to sever this type of hinge.

If cutting is difficult and it appears that severing a cast hinge will be either a lengthy operation or impossible, abandon the cutting operation and displace the door instead of moving it. Never spend time on what may be a non-productive task when you can accomplish the objective with an alternative procedure.

Removing Rear Doors Altogether

Just like the front doors, the rear doors of a four-door sedan can be manually or mechanically moved beyond their normal range of motion. But even when a rear door is moved to the 90 degree point, it is likely to interfere with rescue efforts. So rather than merely displacing rear doors to provide working space at the side of a car, remove them by disassembling, severing, or breaking the hinges.

REMOVING REAR DOORS BY UNBOLTING THE HINGES

The hinge bolts of the rear doors of a great many cars are fully exposed when the front doors are open. In some luxury models, the "dress-up" plastic panel that conceals the hinges can be easily removed with a forcible entry tool.

Let's say that you have a socket wrench set, or an air-operated or electric-powered impact tool with a set of heavy-duty deep sockets. Before you commit to unhinging the rear doors:

- Examine the hinges.

If you see a hex-head bolt (actually a machine screw), a hex-head bolt with a Phillips recess, or a round-head bolt with a Phillips recess, you can probably unhinge the doors. If you see a threaded stud projecting through the hinge from behind, you will not be able to unhinge the door.

If the hinges have bolts that can probably be removed:

- Select the proper socket. Remember that some cars have SAE fasteners, others have metric fasteners, and still others have bolts with Phillips recesses.

While your partner supports the door:

- Remove the bolts one by one (Figure 8.19).

When all the bolts have been removed:

- Together, carry the door away from the vehicle.

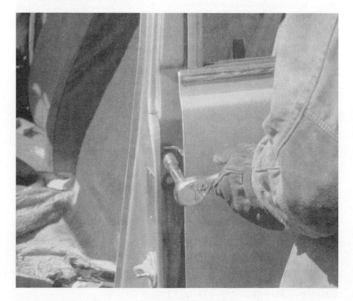

FIGURE 8.19   Unbolting Rear Door

Lest you think that disassembling rear doors will be so easy all of the time, be warned that such is not the case. You may have to distort the forward-facing lip of the door to reach the rear door hinge bolts of some cars. This can be done easily by catching the lip in the slot of the claw end of a forcible entry tool and prying outward. With other cars you may have to install a universal adapter on the wrench or impact tool to properly seat the socket on the bolt heads.

REMOVING REAR DOORS BY SEVERING THE HINGES

If you don't have a socket wrench set or an impact tool and deep sockets, but you do have a reciprocating saw or an air-operated chisel, you can remove the rear doors of a four-door passenger car by severing the hinges. Follow the procedure suggested for severing front door hinges.

REMOVING REAR DOORS BY BREAKING THE HINGES

If you have a hydraulic rescue tool, all you need to do to dispose of the rear doors of a four-door sedan is to break the hinges in the manner suggested for removing front doors. Be sure to follow the safety suggestions made earlier.

Disposing of the B-Pillars of a Four-Door Sedan After the Rear Doors Have Been Removed

With the front and rear doors gone, all that remains at the side of a four-door sedan are the B-pillars. But even relatively thin B-pillars sometimes get in the way of rescue operations, so why not get rid of them as well?

USING HAND TOOLS AND POWERED TOOLS

Before you do anything else, examine the pillar itself and the junction of the pillar with the floor pan of the vehicle. If the pillar appears to lack significant bulk and it meets the floor pan at a right angle, you can probably displace it downward without difficulty. On the other hand, if the pillar appears massive and the base curves inward (toward the interior of the vehicle), you will not be able to displace it unless you notch the base. Heavy pillars are quite common in older luxury cars. The same applies to displace the B-pillar of a four-door, hardtop sedan.

If you feel you can displace the pillar:

- Use a hacksaw, a reciprocating saw, or an air-operated chisel to sever the pillar just below its point of attachment with the roof.

While another rescuer holds the severed end away from the roof with his hands:

- Insert the small round end of a 51- or 60-inch pinch bar into the pillar.
- Together, pull the bar and the pillar down to the ground. Keep your hands as high on the bar as possible for maximum leverage.
- Finally, remove the pinch bar so it won't become a tripping hazard.

The heavy pillars of luxury cars can be displaced in this manner, but only after the base is weakened with an air-operated chisel or a hand-held ripping chisel. If all you have are hand tools, the small bit of working space gained by displacing the pillar may not be worth the time and effort.

If you have a reciprocating saw, a heavy-duty air-operated chisel, or hydraulic shears, you can dispose of most B-pillars altogether simply by severing them at the top and then close to the point of attachment with the floor pan.

Displacing Rear Doors and B-Pillars Together

Thus far we have discussed techniques for removing doors and displacing B-pillars separately. When you're working on a four-door sedan which has B-pillars that can be displaced, you can save time and effort by disposing of both at the same time. You can sever both the top and bottom of each B-pillar and remove the pillar and the door as a unit.

- Open the rear door as far as possible to create the maximum working space.
- Sever the B-pillar as close to the roof as possible with a hacksaw, a reciprocating saw, or an air-operated chisel, or take the top off of the low B-pillar found in a four-door hardtop, as shown in Figure 8.20.
- Close the door just to the point where the latch mechanism contacts but does not engage the safety bolt.

While another rescuer holds the door almost closed with one hand and pulls the cut end of the pillar away from the roof edge with his other hand:

- Insert the small end of a 51- or 60-inch pinch bar into the cut end of the pillar (Figure 8.20).
- Pull on the bar to bring the door and pillar down as a unit (Figures 8.21 and 8.22). You may have to notch the base of the pillar if it has a large curve, as in a luxury car.

The door and the pillar will be out of the way of subsequent rescue operations, and the door will serve as a reasonably stable work platform for EMS personnel who must work at the side of the vehicle (Figure 8.23), or it can be cut off.

Moving doors beyond their normal range of motion, or disposing of doors and B-pillars altogether, creates a great deal of working space at the side of an accident vehicle, but does not create working space *within* the vehicle. That comes from disposing of the roof.

Disposing of the Roof of a Vehicle That Is on Its Wheels

Removing all of the doors and both B-pillars of a four-door sedan affords almost unlimited access to at least the patients who are seated next to the doors. EMS personnel can apply cervical collars, conduct a proper head-to-toe survey, and even care for lower extremity injuries that are seldom discovered, let alone treated, until a patient has been removed from a wrecked vehicle.

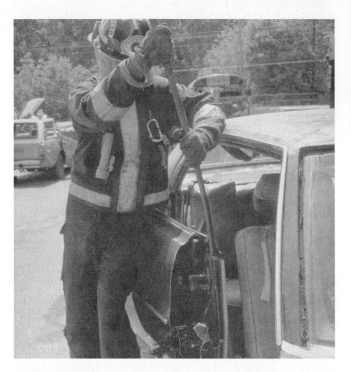

FIGURE 8.20   Inserting Long Bar in B-Pillar

What ambulance or rescue personnel can't do properly without carrying out one more procedure is immobilize a patient who is likely to have a cervical spine injury. That procedure is folding back or removing the roof of the vehicle. Granted, a patient can be secured to a short spine board or other immobilizing device while the roof of a vehicle is still in place. But

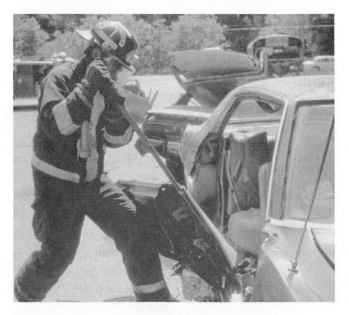

FIGURE 8.21   Pulling Down the B-Pillar

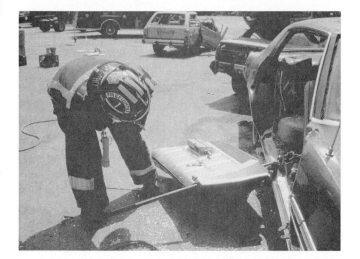

FIGURE 8.22   Pulling Down the B-Pillar

can it be done correctly with assurance that the device will not loosen and slip, when the patient is moved from the seat of the vehicle to a patient-carrying device? We think not.

Securing a patient to an upper-body immobilizing device is a two- or three-rescuer procedure. One rescuer must continually support the patient's head while the other rescuers position the device behind the patient and carry out the strapping procedure.

A medic at the side of a vehicle can kneel or crouch anywhere at the driver's side. There are no doors or a B-pillar to limit or interfere with his movements. The medic in the back seat does not have it quite so easy. He is crouched in an uncomfortable and per-

haps cramping position. If the roof were partially crushed, he would have to keep his head to one side at a level not much higher than his arms. When it is necessary to pivot the driver's upper body forward so the outside medic can position the immobilizing device, the inside medic will also have to move forward, perhaps to a position where he will lose his grip on the driver's head.

Consider the space available for the medics after the roof has been removed. While one works at the driver's side, the other is able to stand fully upright in a comfortable and sure-footed position. He can support the driver's head in the traditional manner (with his hands held horizontally), or by cradling the driver's head between his forearms while his hands are cradling the driver's shoulders in the manner of a yoke.

When it is necessary to move the driver's upper body forward so the outside medic can seat the immobilizing device, the inside medic will have to bend forward only at the waist while continuing to maintain the driver's cervical spine in proper alignment. If the outside medic needs to move the driver sideways just a bit to adjust the straps, the inside medic will be able to track his partner's movements exactly.

If the procedure can create much-needed working space, why don't more rescue personnel remove vehicle roofs? Some are concerned about liability, but more often than not the failure to act can be attributed to the belief that removing a vehicle's roof is a difficult and time-consuming procedure. It is neither difficult nor time-consuming, even when only hand tools are available.

The interior of a vehicle can be exposed in three ways: by folding back a section of the roof like the top of a convertible, by removing a section of the roof, and by removing the roof altogether. Your decision as to what technique to use will be influenced by the construction of the roof and the availability of equipment.

Folding Back a Section of the Roof

The vehicle is an older model, full-size four-door car that has wide pillars. You have stabilized the vehicle, opened the doors, and

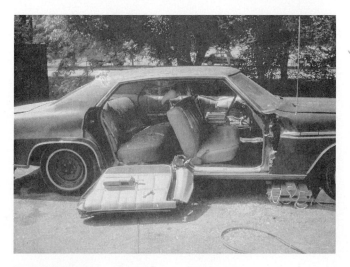

FIGURE 8.23   B-Pillar on Ground

removed the windshield; now you are ready to dispose of the roof. A medic is inside the vehicle supporting the driver's head. Because of the wide pillars, you have decided that the quickest way to expose the interior of the vehicle is to fold back a section of the roof.

USING HAND TOOLS

Two things can slow down a roof-removal operation when hacksaws must be used: chrome and plastic trim and the mastic material used to secure the windshield in its frame. It's difficult to start a cut in chrome, and windshield mastic can clog a hacksaw blade to the point where cutting is just about impossible. Thus an effort should be made to dispose of both the trim and the mastic.

- Assign two rescuers to each side of the vehicle.
- Have them use short pry bars to strip metal and/or plastic trim from around the A-pillars, then the B-pillars, and then the drip molding just ahead of the C-pillar (if any).

If the vehicle has a mastic-mounted windshield:

- Instruct the rescuer who strips the A-pillar to use the flat end of the pry bar to peel away about 2 inches of mastic where the cut will be made on each pillar.

When the roof pillars and the roof edges are stripped:

- Have one rescuer sever the A-pillar as low as possible with the hacksaw while the other rescuer supports the roof edge with a shoulder and lubricates the saw blade.

People who are not used to working with a hacksaw tend to cut metal parts with short strokes while holding the hacksaw frame with one hand. That's why it takes so long for some rescuers to cut through roof pillars. The proper way to cut is to hold the handle

of the saw with one hand and the forward portion of the saw frame with the other hand, and bear down on the saw while pushing the entire blade through the work, not just two or three inches. It's amazing how quickly even the heavy A-pillars of older cars can be severed when hacksaws are held in this manner (Figure 8.24).

Having a rescuer push up on the roof edge is important for two reasons. First, the upward force will cause the severed portion of the roof pillar to move away from the stub when the last cut is made, instead of dropping down and binding the saw blade. Second, the tool operator will be able to free the saw while his partner maintains the gap.

When the tool operators have cut through the A-pillars:

- Instruct them to move to the B-pillars and sever them as high as possible. Have the second rescuer on each side lubricate the saw blade and push up on the roof edge with a shoulder.

This instruction contradicts the one often given to rescuers to sever B-pillars as low

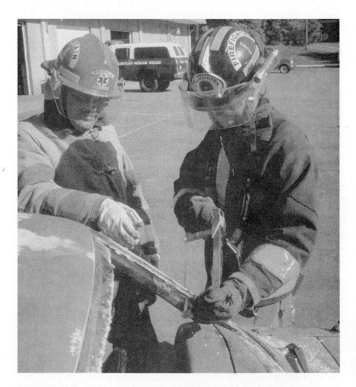

FIGURE 8.24   Correct Holding of Hacksaw

as possible so they are not in the way of the rescue operation. By cutting the B-pillar high, you will have a lever to use if you want to dispose of the post during subsequent operations.

- Tell the medic inside the vehicle what the squad members are about to do so he will be prepared for a slight movement of the vehicle.
- Then direct the tool operators to carefully climb onto the trunk of the car and then onto the roof.

While the second rescuers on each side lubricate the saw blades from a position on the ground:

- Have the tool operators each cut through the roof edge at a point just ahead of the C-pillar.

Two points need to be made about cutting into the roof edge ahead of the C-pillars: one about position and the other about the depth of the cut. The tool operators could stand at the side of the car and notch the roof edge. However, holding a hacksaw in this position is somewhat awkward, and they will have only the strength of their arms working for them. But if they kneel on the roof and hold the saw with both hands, they will have arm muscles plus upper-body weight providing the cutting force.

As for the depth of the cut, the tool operators will have to sever rather complex structures that give the roof strength and rigidity. To that end, they should hold the saw frame at a comfortable angle and cut until the top of the saw frame prevents them from cutting any more. They should then tilt the saw so the front end actually points into the vehicle and cut until they can't cut any more. This maneuver will assure severing even the heaviest roof structures.

At this time, cut the seat belts from their anchor points.

When all the roof pillars are severed and the roof edges are cut, have the rescuers fold back the cut section of the roof. Resist the

temptation to have a rescuer who is either standing on the trunk of the car or at the side of the vehicle pound on the roof with a sledgehammer to make a "hinge." It's not at all necessary, and usually accomplishes little more than causing an already frightened, injured patient to think that his time has come!

- Have one of the rescuers who cut the roof edge stand on the roof with his feet on the imaginary line that extends from notch to notch.
- Instruct him to press down with his feet to dimple the curved metal and thus form a hinge.

While this rescuer keeps his weight on the roof:

- Direct rescuers on each side of the car to pivot the severed portion of the roof upward.

When the rescuer on the roof has the front edge of the roof in his hands:

- Have him carefully step onto the trunk lid and lay the cut section of roof against the uncut part.
- Finally, have team members secure the folded section in place and shield the sharp edges of the severed pillars.

If the roof of the vehicle is wet (and thus slippery) or if for some other reason you don't feel that it will be safe for a rescuer to stand on the roof, have two rescuers stand at either side of the car supporting a pike pole between them. Have them press the pole into the roof to dimple the metal while other rescuers fold the cut section back.

If the procedure for using hand tools to fold back a section of a vehicle's roof sounds easy, that's because in most cases, it *is* easy. Barring any problems, four rescuers should be able to fold a section of roof back in the manner just described in less than two minutes.

USING HYDRAULIC SHEARS

The procedure is essentially the same as just described. After removing or cutting the windshield, have the tool operator sever the roof pillars first (Figure 8.25), then notch each roof edge ahead of the B-pillar or C-pillar (Figure 8.26).

Be sure that the tool operator holds the shears so the blades are at a right angle to the work. While this may seem to be an inconsequential instruction, it's an important tip. Shears or any other cutting tool held at an angle to the work have to cut more metal and can jam easier than when they are held at a right angle. When a hacksaw is used, more metal to cut means more effort to expend.

Needless to say, a section of a vehicle's roof can be folded back after similar cuts are made with a reciprocating saw or an air-operated chisel. If you have either of these tools, however, you can create even more working space in the vehicle by either removing a section of the roof or removing the roof altogether.

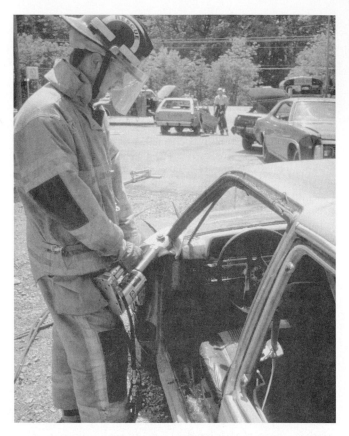

FIGURE 8.25 Severing A-Pillar

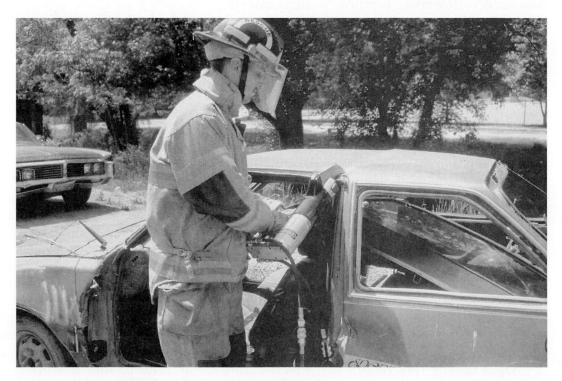

FIGURE 8.26 Notch Roof Ahead of B-Pillar

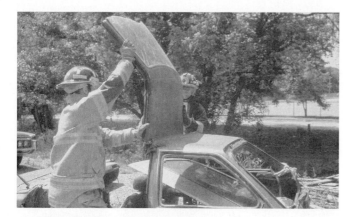

FIGURE 8.27 Folding the Roof

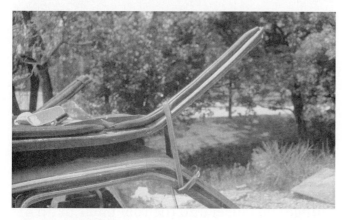

FIGURE 8.28 Using Cargo Hooks for Tiedown

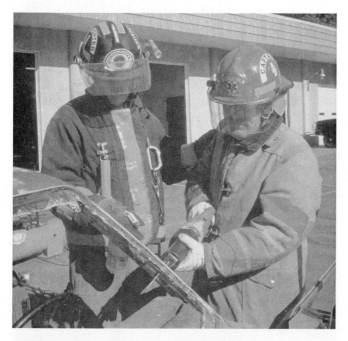

FIGURE 8.29 Severing A-Pillar with Reciprocating Saw

PREVENTING THE RETURN OF A FOLDED ROOF SECTION

While it may seem an unlikely event, strong winds have blown back folded roof sections onto rescuers and victims, especially when the roof section was left in a near vertical position after being cut. To prevent blow-back:

- Have rescuers fold the roof section all the way back (Figure 8.27).
- Then have them secure the folded roof section in place with a length of rope, a chain, or a heavy-duty elastic cargo strap that has S-hooks (Figure 8.28).

Using Elastic Shock Cords. Shock cords are included on the suggested equipment list in Phase One just for this task. A rescuer needs only to clip the S-hook of one end of the cord to the roof edge or other projection, stretch the cord, and snag the edge of a fender well or the bumper with the S-hook of the other end.

Removing a Section of the Roof

The advantage of removing a section of roof instead of folding it back is that you don't have to go through the steps of dimpling the roof, making the fold, and securing the folded section in place. A disadvantage is that a sharp metal edge remains after the section is removed. Two tools are well suited to the task: the reciprocating saw and the heavy-duty air-operated chisel.

USING A RECIPROCATING SAW

Four rescuers are needed for this procedure: one to operate the saw, two to support and move the roof section, and one to act as the safety person.

- Position one rescuer on each side of the vehicle.
- Have those rescuers support the roof section and lubricate the saw blade while the tool operator severs the A-pillar (Figure 8.29) and the B-pillar (Figure 8.30).

- Tell the safety person to stand behind the tool operator where he can see the saw blade.
- Have the tool operator position the saw blade at a right angle to the roof edge just ahead of the C-pillar with the shoe of the tool contacting the roof.

While the rescuer who is supporting the roof lubricates the saw blade:

- Direct the tool operator to cut through the roof beam and the roof to approximately the midline of the roof (Figure 8.31). Then have him withdraw the saw blade and repeat the operation on the other side of the vehicle.

After cutting the remaining A-pillar and B-pillar:

- Instruct the tool operator to cut through the roof beam and the roof itself until the blade meets the first cut.
- Have the other rescuers cut the seat belts at the anchor point, and carefully lift the cut roof section from the vehicle and carry it away from the wreckage (Figure 8.32).
- Finally, have the team members shield the sharp edges of the pillars and the remaining roof section with duct tape and/or hose sections (Figure 8.33).

USING AN AIR-OPERATED CHISEL

The sequence of events is essentially the same as when using other tools, but the cutting techniques are slightly different. Following are suggestions that you might find helpful when you are the tool operator of a rescue team.

When you have the cutting equipment assembled:

- Install a curved chisel in the tool holder of the air gun.
- Then sever the first A-pillar.

A common mistake of a rescuer who is not experienced in the use of an air gun is to

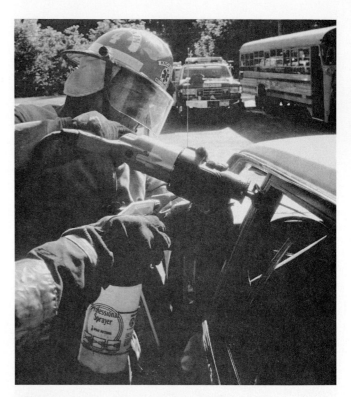

FIGURE 8.30 Severing B-Pillar with Reciprocating Saw

plunge the chisel into the roof pillar in an attempt to cut as much metal as possible at one time. As a result, the chisel usually becomes firmly lodged in the pillar, and the rescuer uses up much of the air supply by operating the gun in an effort to free the chisel by vibration.

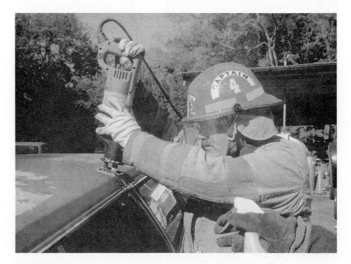

FIGURE 8.31 Cutting the Roof with Reciprocating Saw

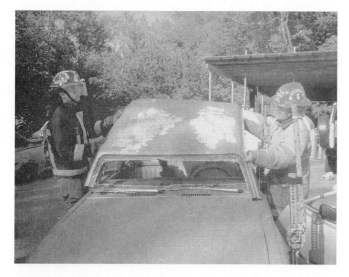

FIGURE 8.32   Remove the Roof

Instead of forcefully driving an air-operated chisel deep into a roof pillar, first make a cut that is about half the width of the chisel through one side of the pillar. Then make a similar cut on the other side of the pillar. Finally, drive the chisel through the remaining central portion. Even though the procedure has three steps, severing the roof pillars in this manner is faster and uses less air than the "plunge and get stuck" method.

When you have severed the A-pillar:

• Move down the side of the car and sever the B-pillar in the same manner (if there is a B-pillar) while another rescuer supports the roof edge.

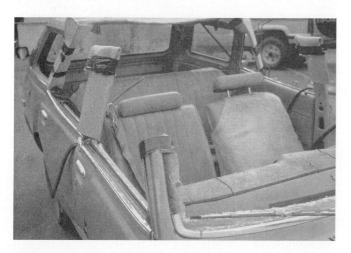

FIGURE 8.33   Cover Cut Pillars

• Then cut through the edge of the roof at a point just ahead of the C-pillar.

Instead of climbing onto the roof as you may do when cutting with a hacksaw or reciprocating saw, make the roof edge cuts from a standing position. You'll have better control of the chisel, and the operation will be safer (Figures 8.34 and Figure 8.35).

If you kneel on the roof and cut with a reciprocating saw, you continually pull the saw toward you. When using an air gun from a position at the midline of the roof, you must push the gun forward to make the cut. If the chisel slips from the work when it reaches the roof edge, you might lose your balance and topple headfirst from the roof.

To cut through the sometimes complex structure of roof beams without difficulty, first cut through the sheet-metal skin. Then make successively deeper cuts until the entire roof beam is severed.

When you have severed the A- and B-pillars and the roof beam on one side:

• Move to the other side of the car.
• Have another rescuer stand at the side of the car and support the roof edge with his hands.
• Then sever the A- and B-pillars and the roof beam on that side of the vehicle.
• Replace the curved chisel with a panel cutter.

While changing the chisel may seem unnecessary, it's an important step. Unless you carefully control the curved chisel (which is difficult to do), it will continually plunge through the roof and perhaps become stuck. You'll spend more time freeing the chisel and repositioning it than cutting. You won't have this problem with a panel cutter; the bullpoint or "T" part of a panel cutter will ride on the surface of the roof while the cutting edge severs the metal.

• Next, climb onto the trunk of the car and kneel on the portion of the roof that will remain intact after the forward section has been removed.

- Cut through the sheet metal of the roof between the severed roof beams.

When you have finished cutting between the notches:

- Replace the panel cutter with the curved chisel and cut the stamped stiffener that lies just below the roof (if a stiffener is present).
- Finally, direct your helpers to cut the seat belts at the anchor point and carefully lift the cut roof section from the vehicle and carry it away.

Removing the Roof Altogether

When you're confronted with the problem of creating working space in a vehicle full of patients, consider removing the roof of the vehicle altogether instead of simply folding it back or removing just a section. Thus you will eliminate a likely impediment to the care and ultimate disentanglement of rear seat patients.

The roof of a small vehicle with narrow C-pillars can usually be removed with a hacksaw. A reciprocating saw, an air-operated chisel, or hydraulic shears is necessary when the vehicle has wide C-pillars.

USING A RECIPROCATING SAW OR AN AIR-OPERATED CHISEL

A- and B-pillars are cut in the manner described earlier. Cutting C-pillars can be a little tricky. Again, here are some suggestions for properly using cutting tools.

If you are using a reciprocating saw:

- Position the blade on the forward edge of the C-pillar with the shoe of the tool resting tightly against the metal.
- Then cut toward the rear of the vehicle on an angle. This will avoid any seams running straight through the post. Always cut to the closest glass, thus the least metal.

Be sure to keep the tool shoe pressed firmly against the metal as you cut through the

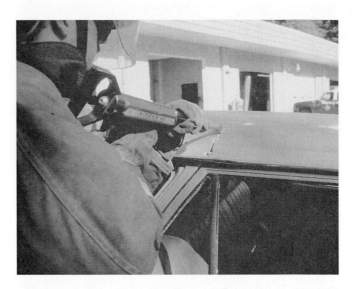

FIGURE 8.34 Cutting the Roof with Air-Operated Chisel

C-pillar. By doing so, you will prevent the blade from bucking and bending, and if the pillar is thick, from bottoming out.

If you are using an air-operated chisel to sever a wide C-pillar:

- Install the panel cutter and make a three-sided flap in the sheet-metal skin before you do anything else.

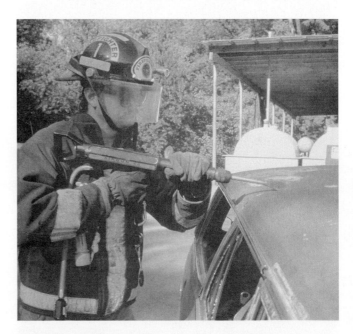

FIGURE 8.35 Cutting the Roof with Air-Operated Chisel

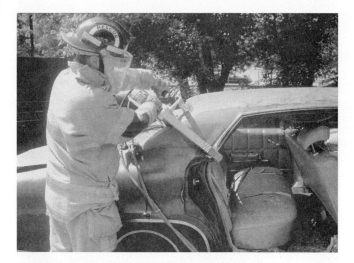

FIGURE 8.36   Squashing the C-Pillar

If you simply drive the curved chisel through the pillar, you may experience the problem of the chisel becoming stuck each time it breaks through the inner side of the pillar. Removing the chisel may be difficult because of the tendency of the sheet metal, plastic, and fabric trim to grip the shank of the chisel as it is being withdrawn.

By making a three-sided flap—actually a "window"—you eliminate the need to drive the chisel blindly through the pillar. You can cut

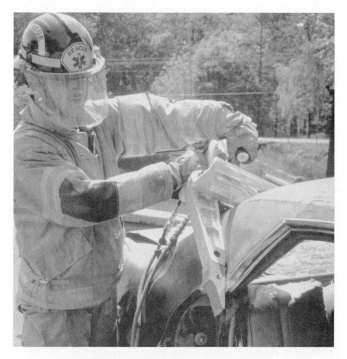

FIGURE 8.37   Squashing the C-Pillar

through the thick forward and rear portions of the pillar just as you would cut A- and B-pillars and then sever the remaining central portion.

USING HYDRAULIC SHEARS

Rescuers who have hydraulic shears may be intimidated by wide C-pillars—often to the point where they will forego any attempt to sever the pillars even though the space that will be available when the roof is removed altogether is really needed.

The wide C-pillars of some vehicles can be severed by making two cuts, one from the rear and one from the front of the pillar, and thus are seldom a problem. If the C-pillars of the vehicle that you are working on are too wide to sever with two cuts:

- First, open the hydraulic spreader a few inches and slide it onto the C-pillar until you bottom out. Activate the spreader until the pillar is squashed into a thin strip of metal (Figures 8.36 and 8.37).
- Then remove a pie-shaped wedge of metal by making two cuts in the rear edge of the pillar (Figure 8.38).
- Then remove a pie-shaped wedge of metal by making two cuts in the front edge of the pillar (Figure 8.39).

From a position at the side of the vehicle:

- Position the shears in the resulting V-shaped openings and sever the remaining metal (Figure 8.40).

Now let's do something different:

- Cut the seat belts at their anchor points. After cutting through all the pillars, lift the roof up *from the rear* and bring it over the front (instead of front to rear). The bottom of the windshield will rip loose, and the roof can be set on the hood upside down. It can then be completely removed from the work area. This method will eliminate hoisting glass over the patient(s) (Figures 8.41 and 8.42).

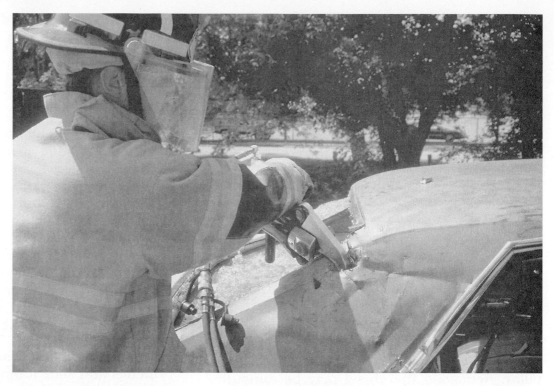

FIGURE 8.38   Removing Pie-shaped Pieces on Rear

Disposing of the Roof of a Vehicle That Is on Its Side

Problem: It's virtually impossible to immobilize a patient in the confines of the passenger compartment of a vehicle that is on its side, and it's extremely dangerous to pull a patient through a window or door opening, immobilized or not.

Solution: Dispose of the roof in any of a number of ways. You still may not be able to immobilize the patient because of the cramped quarters, but you will be able to remove him with a minimal amount of spinal movement.

There are several ways to dispose of the roof of a vehicle that is on its side. The roof can be removed altogether, but the steps of severing the roof pillars on the side of the vehicle closest to the ground can be difficult and time-consuming, especially when rescuers have only hand tools. There are faster and easier ways to create working space: (1) fold down the entire roof, (2) fold back a section of the roof, or (3) make a three-sided cut

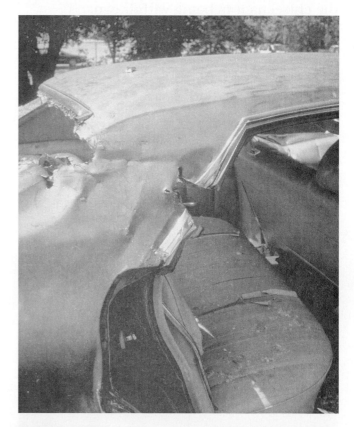

FIGURE 8.39   Removing Pie-shaped Pieces on Front

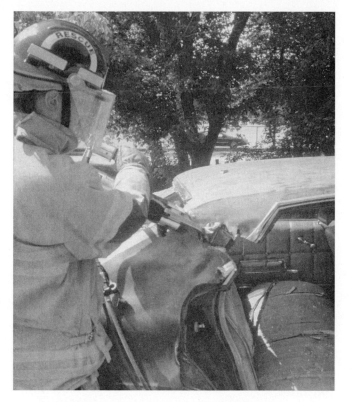

FIGURE 8.40   Severing Remaining Metal

in the roof and fold the resulting flap down. Which of these techniques is selected depends on how the vehicle is stabilized, the width of the C-pillars, and the type of tools available.

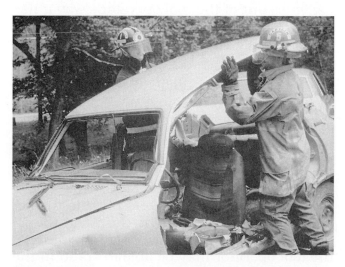

FIGURE 8.41   Removing Roof Over Front of Vehicle

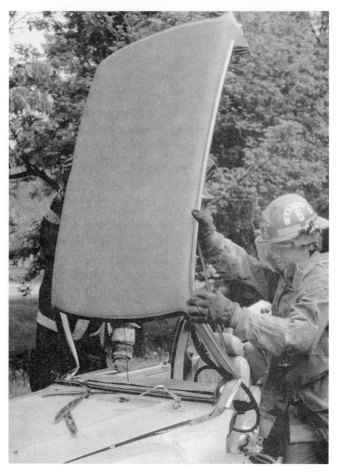

FIGURE 8.42   Removing Roof Over Front of Vehicle

Folding Down the Roof

This procedure creates the most working space and the largest exitway. The vehicle has been stabilized and a medic is inside the vehicle supporting and protecting the lone patient. The windshield and rear window have been removed.

- Instruct two rescuers to support the roof at the windshield and rear window openings.
- Assign the third rescuer to the tool.
- Have the fourth rescuer support the tool operator.

If the tool operator is using a hacksaw or a reciprocating saw:

- Have the fourth rescuer continually lubricate the saw blade during the cutting operation.

If the tool operator is severing the roof pillars with an air-operated chisel:

- Have the fourth rescuer keep the air hose out of his way.

If the tool operator is using hydraulic shears:

- Have the fourth rescuer keep the fluid lines away from the tool operator and the shears.

When everyone is in position:

- Have the tool operator sever the roof pillars.

Unless he is quite tall, the tool operator may have trouble holding the tool in proper position, especially if the car is a full-size model. Standing on a stepladder that has been placed next to the vehicle will enable the rescuer to handle the tool with a degree of safety. Working on the top of the vehicle (actually the side) is dangerous. If the tool twists while cuts are being made, the operator can be thrown from his perch.
When all of the pillars are cut:

- Cut the seat belts at their anchor points.
- Direct the rescuers who have been supporting the roof at the windshield and rear window openings to lower the roof to the ground carefully.

If the vehicle is small, this should be no problem. The roof should easily "hinge" at the points where the pillars on the opposite side are attached to the roof. If the vehicle is large and pulling the roof down becomes difficult, the tool operator can weaken the A- and C-pillars where they join the roof. It will seldom be necessary to cut through these pillars.
When the roof is folded down:

- Have rescuers protect the sharp pillar stubs. (The procedures are covered later in this section.)

There are two benefits to folding the entire roof down in this manner. First, the entire interior of the vehicle is exposed. Second, the roof section becomes a platform on which rescuers and EMS personnel can work—a clean platform when the surrounding ground is muddy or snow covered.

Folding Back a Section of the Roof

The following procedure can be used when you do not have a tool suitable for cutting a wide C-pillar. The vehicle must be stabilized with cribbing or other stabilizers placed under the A- and C-pillars. While the resulting opening is slightly smaller than the one created when the roof is folded down, it still creates working space around front and rear seat patients.

- Instruct the tool operator to sever the uppermost A- and B-pillars and then cut through the roof rail at a right angle just ahead of the C-pillar.
- Have one of the standby rescuers continually lubricate the blade if the tool operator is using either a hacksaw or a reciprocating saw.
- Have another rescuer keep the supply lines out of the tool operator's way if he is using either an air-operated chisel or hydraulic shears.
- Then have the tool operator sever the other A- and B-pillars and cut through the roof edge ahead of the other C-pillar.
- Cut the seat belts at their anchor points.

Severing the lowermost B-pillar may be troublesome because it is close to the ground and not easily accessible. If the medic inside the vehicle and the rescuers outside the vehicle can move the patient closest to the B-pillar without fear of aggravating injuries, the tool operator may be able to stand in the rear window opening and use the tool in the usual manner.

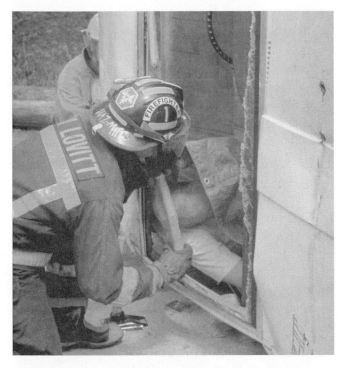

FIGURE 8.43 Protecting the Patient While Cutting

When all of the cuts have been made:

- Have one rescuer dimple the roof with his hip or shoulder while the other team members fold the cut section back.

Again, it is not necessary to kick the roof or beat on it with a hammer to create a hinge. Doing so only serves to upset patients.

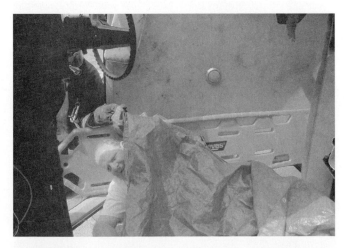

FIGURE 8.44 Protecting the Patient While Cutting

- Have rescuers secure the folded roof section in place with an elastic shock cord, a chain, or a length of rope secured to the bumper or another anchor point.
- Then have the rescuers protect the sharp severed pillar ends on both the roof section and the body of the vehicle.

If a reciprocating saw is used to sever the roof pillars, the tool operator can cut from one side of the roof to the other, and rescuers can remove the entire section of roof rather than folding it back. The operation will take about 15 seconds more.

Making a Flap in the Roof

This procedure must be used when a stabilizing jack will prevent folding the roof down or folding a section of the roof back. Making a flap does not create the working space afforded by the other techniques, but it does make an opening sufficiently large for the safe removal of occupants of both the front and rear seats. An additional patient protection step should be taken before the cuts are made.

- While the medic holds the patient a few inches from the roof's headliner, have two of the rescue team members pass a long spine board from the windshield to the rear window with the smooth side toward the patient.
- Have these rescuers hold the spine board in place while the tool operator makes the flap (Figure 8.43).

The spine board will serve two purposes. It will shield the patient from contact with the cutting tool, and it will serve as a backstop against which the patient can rest during the cutting operation (Figure 8.44).

When everyone is in position:

- Have the tool operator make the three-sided flap (Figure 8.45).

If the tool operator has a panel cutter and a short sledgehammer:

- Instruct him to make a starting hole in an upper corner of the roof at a point about 6 inches from each edge, then drive the tool straight down until the blade contacts (or is near) the roof beam.
- Have him replace the blade of the tool in the starting hole and make a horizontal cut to a point about 6 inches from the roof edge, then turn the tool and drive it straight down until the blade once more contacts (or is near) the roof beam.

If the tool operator has a reciprocating saw:

- Instruct the fourth team member to make a starting hole with the pike of a forcible entry tool.
- Then have the tool operator follow the same cutting route as just described— down, across, and down.

If the tool operator has an air-operated chisel:

- Have the fourth team member make the starting hole with either the point of the panel cutter or the pike of a forcible entry tool.
- Then have the tool operator follow the same cutting procedure.

There may be a tendency for the flap to drop down as the third cut is made. This can be prevented by having the fourth rescuer stand alongside the roof and keep the flap closed with his hand while the second and third cuts are made (Figure 8.46).

When the final cut is made:

- Have the tool operator put down the equipment and grip the upper edge of the flap with his gloved hands.

While the rescuer who has been supporting the flap dimples the sheet metal at the hinge point with his foot:

- Direct the tool operator to pull the flap down.

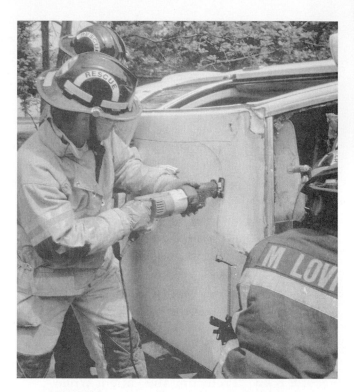

FIGURE 8.45   Cutting a Three-Sided Flap

- Have the rescuer who dimpled the metal press down on the flap at the hinge point with his foot to cause the flap to lie flat (Figure 8.47).

When the flap is down, and while the two team members continue to hold the long spine board in place:

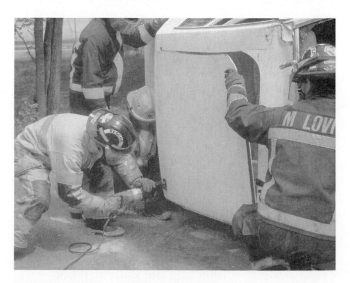

FIGURE 8.46   Holding the Flap

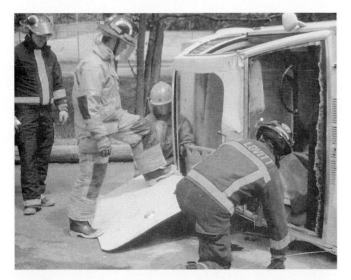

FIGURE 8.47 Dropping the Flap and Standing on It

- Have the tool operator and the fourth rescuer remove the roof stiffener, the headliner supports, and the headliner.
- Remove the patient (Figure 8.48).

Some cars have only a front-to-back stiffener, while others have a stiffener in the shape of a cross. Whatever the case, a stiffener can be cut with a hacksaw, a reciprocating saw, an air-operated chisel, or a cold

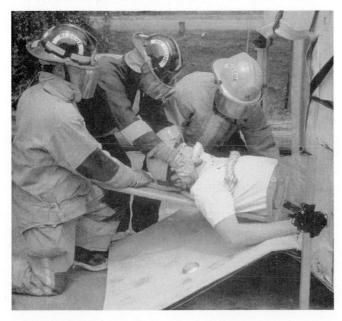

FIGURE 8.48 Removing the Patient

chisel. The headliner can be either cut away with a knife or simply ripped free by hand, and the headliner supports can be pulled from their sockets.

While creating a three-sided flap rather than a complete opening may seem strange, there are reasons for making a flap. To make a four-sided opening takes time, and working close to the ground is difficult. Moreover, the "hinge" of the three-sided flap is smooth, whereas the bottom edge of a four-sided cut will be sharp and dangerous.

When the tools just mentioned are being used for other tasks and speed in opening the roof of a car that is on its side is essential, a three-sided flap can be made with a can-opener type tool, a flat-blade screwdriver and a hammer, or a flat-blade ax and a sledgehammer.

Protecting Rescuers and Patients from Sharp Metal Edges

Making an opening in the roof of a vehicle and severing roof pillars invariably produce sharp metal edges. A severe laceration can result when an unprotected body part (rescuer's or patient's!) accidentally contacts one of these edges. Heavy clothing does not always protect the wearer from injury. The razor-sharp edges of a roof opening made with an ax can cut through even the heavy sleeves of a turnout coat.

Guarding the Sharp Metal Edges of Roof Openings

Regardless of the tool used, sharp metal edges are a common product when a three-sided flap is made in the roof of a vehicle. A can-opener type tool leaves edges that are both sharp and jagged. These edges can be shielded with lengths of scrap fire hose or duct tape.

USING SPLIT SECTIONS OF FIRE HOSE

Jagged edges (such as those made with a can-opener type tool) and badly burred edges require a more substantial shield. Short split sections of 1-1/2-inch fire hose (Figure 8.49) are excellent for the task. Simply slip the split sections of hose over the cut edges.

The rubber lining of the hose sections should grip the roof sufficiently for them to remain in place. However, if it appears that some of the sections are likely to move during subsequent disentanglement and removal activities, they can be secured in place with lengths of tape applied at a right angle to the cut roof edges.

USING DUCT TAPE

Two-inch-wide duct tape can be used to shield relatively smooth sheet-metal edges that are not badly burred. A fabric-backed tape should be used, not masking tape.

- Mask the entire roof opening by applying strips of tape to the outer surface of the roof so that half the width of the tape is adhered to the roof and the other half is available for turning under (Figure 8.50).

With your gloved hands:

- Fold the exposed part of the tape under and press it against the underside of the roof.

If the edge is slightly burred and you feel that the burrs will poke through the tape and become snagging points:

- Apply a second layer of tape over the first layer in the same manner.

Covering the Stubs of Severed Roof Pillars

The remaining stubs of severed roof pillars are often impediments to rescue operations, especially when the pillars were not severed close to the body of the vehicle. They are dangerous impediments when they are left bare. Unsplit sections of 2-1/2- or 3-inch fire hose make excellent shields (Figure 8.51).

- Slip a section of hose over each severed roof pillar (Figure 8.52).

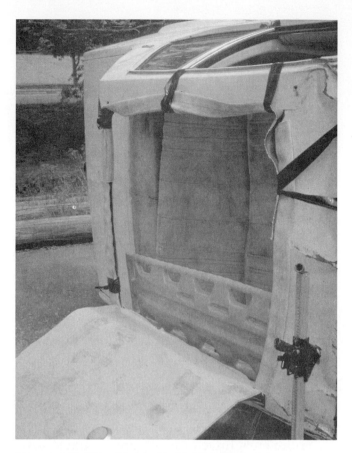

FIGURE 8.49   Using Split Fire Hose

If you do not have short sections of hose:

- Overlap several turns of 2-inch fabric-backed tape, starting an inch or so below the cut end of each pillar.

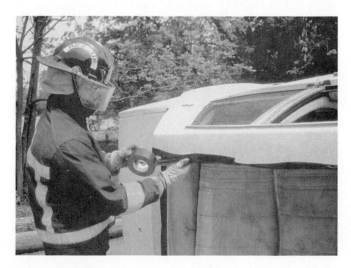

FIGURE 8.50   Using Duct Tape

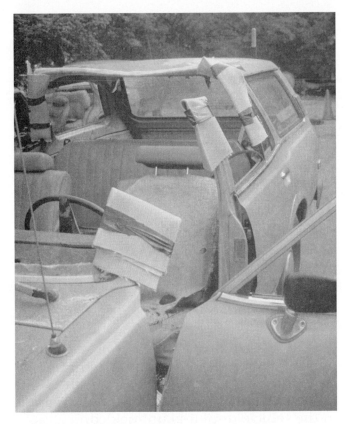

FIGURE 8.51   Using Unsplit Fire Hose

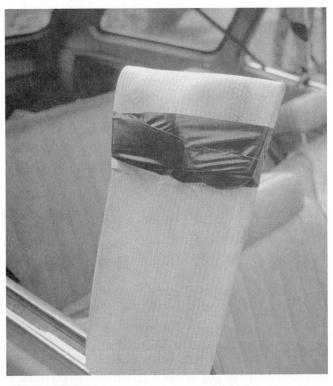

FIGURE 8.52   Hose Section over Pillar

- Spiral wrap the tape upward until the resulting cylinder or cone of tape extends several inches beyond the end of the pillar.
- Tear the tape from the roll.
- Squeeze the sides of the tape cylinder or cone together so the adhesive surfaces stick to each other and form a cap (Figure 8.53).

Remember: Shielding sharp edges will benefit you and your partner as much as the patients.

Some Thoughts from the Authors About the Suggested Roof-Removal Procedures

Fire, rescue, and EMS personnel are becoming increasingly worried about their liability for the procedures discussed thus far in this phase. Concern has reached the point where some rescuers may not be acting properly in the fear of being sued for damaging a person's vehicle.

How do you wreck a wreck? If a motorist drives his car head-on into a tree at 65 miles an hour, shortens his car by about two feet, and ends up with the motor on his lap but is still alive, the last thing you should be worrying about is further damaging his car!

Should a similar attitude prevail at accidents of lesser magnitude? We feel that if your training, experience, observations of the mechanisms of injury, and the patient survey cause you to suspect that a motorist has suffered a spinal injury, you have the license to remove as many of the vehicle components as necessary to assure the safe movement of the patient.

We asked insurance agents, insurance investigators, and officials of insurance companies what they thought about rescuer-caused damage. All agreed that their companies would much rather pay $25,000 for a totaled car than a million dollars or more in death benefits to the survivors of a patient who may have died as the result of the rescue effort, not the accident. One insurance investigator reminded us that it costs about

$2,500 to replace a roof removed during rescue operations, but it costs three quarters of a million dollars to put a patient through a spinal rehabilitation center—a trip that may not have been necessary if only the rescuers had removed the top of the vehicle in which the patient was injured.

We are not suggesting that you "trash" every vehicle, just that you carefully assess every situation. When you feel that you cannot safely move a patient from the wreckage, first remove the wreckage from the patient.

FREEING PATIENTS FROM MECHANISMS OF ENTRAPMENT

Problem: While these efforts have created working space and openings through which patients can be removed from the vehicles, they have not freed the patients from mechanisms of entrapment within the vehicles.

Solution: Remove wreckage from the patients so they can be removed from the wreckage.

After stabilizing a vehicle, removing the windshield and rear window, folding back the roof (or removing it altogether), and either widening door openings or removing doors, rescuers still may not be able to remove patients from a vehicle safely. Seat belts, the steering column, pedals, the front seat, and the dashboard may individually or in combination be mechanisms of entrapment.

Removing Seat Belts from Patients

While seat belts are seldom perceived as either mechanisms of injury or mechanisms of entrapment, they can be both. When a seat belt is buckled too high on the body, the abdominal organs and the great vessels can be squeezed against the spine if the vehicle suddenly decelerates. A diagonal shoulder belt that is worn alone (not in conjunction with a lap belt, that is) can be particularly dangerous. The wearer is subject to a variety of injuries to the upper body ranging from

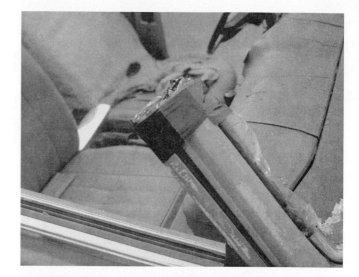

FIGURE 8.53 Duct Tape on Pillar

simple bruising to decapitation. While most vehicles have lap and shoulder belts that are buckled together, some older cars have only lap belts. As for being a mechanism of entrapment, a seat restraint will hold a patient in the vehicle until it is unbuckled.

In their efforts to help trapped and injured patients quickly, untrained rescuers sometimes unbuckle seat belts without regard for the consequences of their hasty actions. They fail to realize that when the tension of a seat belt is suddenly released, the wearer's upper body may twist, and if there is a shoulder girdle injury, broken bone ends may override. When the tension of a lap belt is abruptly released, bleeding from an abdominal injury may become profuse.

Some emergency care procedures—the application of a cervical collar, for example—can be undertaken while a seat belt is still in place. Other procedures cannot be accomplished properly—or in some cases at all—without first removing the seat belt. A sling and swathe cannot be applied when a shoulder belt is snug against the wearer's body. Unbuckling or cutting the belts is the answer, but before you do so, be sure that someone is available to support the patient in position.

Some operational guidelines call for the positioning of cravats around a patient's body to maintain pressure on bleeding vessels when abdominal injuries are suspected. However, it may be better to leave a lap belt in place while carrying out the rest of the disentanglement operations, then to un-buckle or cut the belt just when you are ready to remove the patient from the vehicle. Follow the protocol established for your EMS system.

Unbuckling Seat Belts

As is the case with many other vehicle res-cue operations, there's a right way and a wrong way to do something as simple as un-buckling a seat belt. Don't just push the re-lease button with your finger. If the belt is under a great deal of tension, the ends will fly apart and pressure on the lower abdomen imposed by the seat belt will be released in a split second. Instead:

- Hold the buckle end of the belt with one hand, and the mating part with your other hand.

When you have a tight grip on both parts of the belt:

- Depress the button with a thumb.
- Allow the parts to separate slowly.

A sudden deterioration of the patient's con-dition upon release from a seat belt will sig-nal an increase in abdominal bleeding. Be ready to take appropriate measures.

Cutting Seat Belts

While it's highly unlikely that the quick re-lease buckles of seat restraint systems will not operate after an accident, it's nonethe-less possible. When you find that you cannot unbuckle a seat belt in the usual manner, don't simply cut through the webbing and allow the parts of the belt to spring apart.

- Grip the belt tightly with one hand close to its roller mechanism.

While you grip the belt firmly with one hand:

- Cut the webbing with your utility shears, a seat belt cutter, or a very sharp knife at a point between your hand and the roller mechanism.

When the webbing is severed:

- Move your hand slowly to release tension on the wearer.

One final point about seat belts. Just be-cause the procedure appears early in this phase does not imply that unbuckling or cutting seat belts must always precede other disentanglement efforts. A combination shoulder and lap belt restraint system may hold the wearer upright in the seat while res-cuers and EMS personnel carry out other procedures. The "third pair of hands" that a seat belt offers will be welcome when there is much to do and few hands to do it.

Coping with the Steering Column

The steering apparatus of a vehicle can be a major impediment to proper patient care ef-forts. A steering wheel can prevent rescuers from effectively immobilizing a patient who may have a spinal injury. A steering column can prevent rescuers from quickly and easily freeing a patient's legs from mechanisms of entrapment under the dashboard.

The "Hollywood" approach to disposing of a vehicle's steering column (so-called because it is dramatic) is to virtually pull the column forward through the windshield opening with a hydraulic rescue tool. In reality, this pro-cedure is time-consuming, dangerous, and in most cases, completely unnecessary. The practice is dangerous for several reasons. Pieces of metal and plastic invariably break away and fly for a considerable distance when a steering column is displaced forward. Tilt-and-telescoping steering columns have been known to break apart when displacing forces were applied. And when the steering columns of some late-model cars are moved with de-vices that store energy (air bags, hydraulic rescue tools, and cable winches), universal joints can fail.

In one instance of universal joint failure during an attempt to displace the steering column of a car with air bags, the upper portion of the steering column pivoted on its point of attachment to the underside of the dash, described an arc at the end of the pulling strap, broke loose from the strap, and landed on the ground about 40 feet in front of the car! If someone had been sitting unprotected behind the steering wheel, he probably would have been disemboweled and killed.

Displacing a steering column is often unnecessary; some more easily accomplished steps may be all that are necessary to create working space in front of a patient.

However, never say never! Tonight may be the run that calls for moving the column itself. The tool of choice here is the Colum-Master. It was developed just for this job (though it will do others). Rather than pulling at a 90 degree angle to the load, the lifting arm of the tool raises the steering column *straight up*, thereby eliminating the dangers associated with hydraulic spreaders, rams, come-alongs, and air bags.

The set up procedures are as follows:

- Remove the windshield or roof or both.
- Place the Colum-Master on the vehicle with the hooks toward the front end, directly in front of the steering column. The U-channel or foot should overlap the bottom sill of the windshield (Figure 8.54).
- Raise the lifting arm until it reaches its stop.
- Adjust the slide tube by pulling the small lever to release the inner tube. Pull the inner tube to its fullest length. The spring will lock it in place.
- Wrap the column with 6 feet of chain as close to the dash as possible. Use your department standard operating procedure wrap. This is not critical, as long as it is secure.
- Push down on the lifting arm when hooking the chain to it. The adjustable arm should rise about 1 foot. This helps to remove the slack out of the setup.

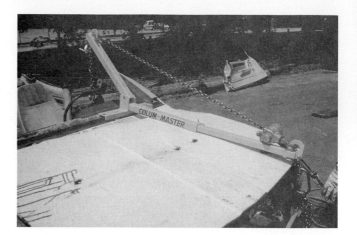

FIGURE 8.54   The Colum-Master

- Hook the second chain (12 feet) onto a solid point under the vehicle.
- Hook the chain onto the adjustable arm while pushing down on it.
- Hook the pulling device between the eye loops on the lifting arm and the adjustable arm. Note that we used a 3/4-ton chain come-along (Figure 8.55). It is lightweight and has more than enough strength to do the job.
- Have your safety person in a position to watch the lower limbs and any unwanted motion on the column or dash.
- Always place a long or short spine board in front of the patient before jacking.
- Start the lifting operation. Remember, jack the column only enough to free the victim (Figure 8.56). If you need an inch, you do not go two.

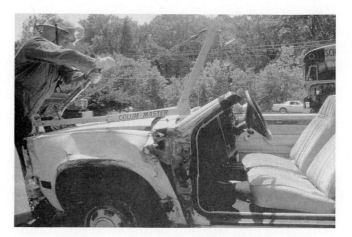

FIGURE 8.55   Using a 3/4-Ton Come-along

• In performance testing of this tool, we took the column to its maximum (Figure 8.57).

Notice in Figure 8.58 that the dash rolled all the way across. The column did not tear loose as it was being pulled up. It certainly is not recommended to go to this extreme, but it did prove to be far superior and safer than any other method. Tests on other model vehicles proved equally effective.

• After release of the patient, release the tension slowly and reverse the order for breakdown.

Shortening the Column

The first step is to adjust a tilt-and-telescoping steering column if the vehicle has one. Tall motorists often drive with the seat all the way to the back and the steering wheel of a telescoping column in the fully extended position; thus they have maximum legroom. While some motorists drive with the steering wheel of a tilting column in the fully raised position, others drive with the steering wheel depressed almost to the level of the seat. As the saying goes: There's no accounting for taste!

Before doing anything else to create working space in front of an injured driver:

• Determine whether the vehicle has a tilt-and-telescoping steering column.

If the vehicle has a tilt-and-telescoping wheel:

• Disengage the friction-locking mechanism.
• Push the steering wheel into its fully retracted position.
• Then operate the adjustment lever and tilt the wheel up as far as it can go.

The steering wheel of General Motors' tilt-and-telescoping steering column moves in and out 2 inches, and up and down 4-1/2 inches. While pushing the wheel all of the way in and tilting it all of the way up may not create enough room for rescuers to secure

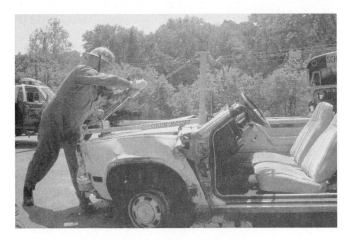
FIGURE 8.56   Lifting the Column

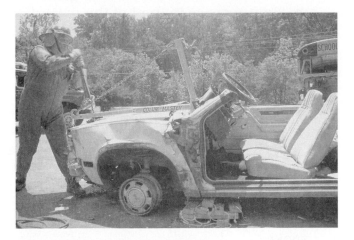
FIGURE 8.57   Maximum Lift

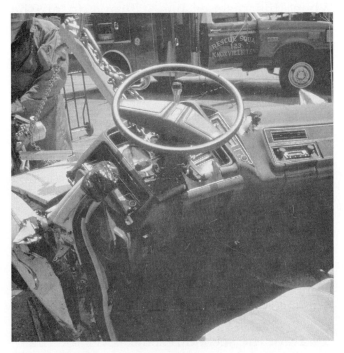
FIGURE 8.58   Dash Rolled

the driver in an immobilization device, it will make the wheel more accessible for subsequent steps.

Moving the Seat Backward

Moving the front seat backward usually takes only seconds and may create as much as 8 or 9 inches of working space between the driver and the steering wheel. Even in head-on collisions, the seat adjustment mechanism usually remains intact and the seat tracks are left undamaged.

If the vehicle has motorized seats and you have left the electrical system intact, moving the front seat backward may be a matter of simply operating a switch. If the vehicle has a manually adjustable bench seat, use the following procedure after making certain that all required packaging of possible spinal injuries has been completed.

While a medic or rescuer supports the patient from behind or at the side:

- Kneel at the driver's door opening.
- Direct another rescuer to kneel at the passenger door opening.

While you operate the seat adjustment lever with one hand and push on the front of the seat with your other hand, and while the other rescuer pushes on the front of the seat on his side:

- Carefully slide the seat back.

Always work together with another rescuer to move a manually adjustable bench seat. If you attempt to move the seat alone, chances are that the seat will angle on the tracks and become virtually immovable. The spring action can also cause a spine-wrenching effect if you are not careful.

Removing a Section of the Steering Wheel

When it's not possible to move the front seat backward, or when moving the seat does not provide adequate working space in front of an injured driver, removing a section of the

steering wheel should be the next step. Before you remove a section of a steering wheel, however, make sure that the patient is protected by a rigid shield and firmly supported by other rescuers.

Using a Saw

Either a hacksaw or a reciprocating saw can cut through the plastic covering and the soft steel core of a steering wheel without difficulty.

After protecting the patient:

- Rotate the wheel, if possible, to gain maximum space in front of the patient when you remove a portion of the rim.

If the wheel has only two spokes:

- Rotate it so the spokes are horizontal.

Next:

- Direct a second rescuer to take a position on the seat next to the driver.
- Have him reach across the wheel and grip the rim about two inches below the spoke.

When this rescuer has a firm grip on the wheel:

- Sever the rim at a point just below the spoke.
- Have a third rescuer lubricate the saw blade while you make the cut.

When you have finished the cut:

- Pass the saw over the steering column to the second rescuer.
- Reach across the wheel and grip the distant rim at a point about 2 inches below the spoke.

While you support the wheel and the third rescuer lubricates the saw blade:

- Have the second rescuer sever the rim at a point just below the spoke.

When he has finished the cut:

- Remove the severed portion of the wheel.

At this point you may be wondering why two rescuers should go to the trouble of one making just one cut and then passing the saw to the other. Cutting the closest part of the rim while standing at the side of the vehicle is no problem. When the tool operator leans across the wheel to cut the distant rim, however, he may move slightly off balance. If he slips and drops the saw onto the driver's legs, the blade can cause injury, or striking his legs with either the saw or a hand can aggravate a fracture.

Needless to say, both rescuers can stand at the side of the vehicle when it is not possible for someone to sit on the seat next to the driver.

Using a Bolt Cutter

The steering wheel of most vehicles can also be cut with a bolt cutter. A problem is that the plastic covering may make the wheel too thick to cut with even a 42-inch tool. When this is the case, portions of the covering must be removed to expose the steel core.

While another rescuer is taking a position on the seat next to the driver:

- Rotate the steering wheel, if possible, so that you will create the maximum working space by cutting away a section of the rim.
- Then use vise-grip pliers or channel-locking pliers to break away a section of the plastic rim covering just below the spoke closest to you.

When you are finished:

- Pass the tool to the other rescuer and have him do the same.

From your position at the side of the vehicle:

- Grip the rim of the steering wheel in the jaws of the cutter but do not make the cut just yet.

- Have the other rescuer reach across the wheel and support the head of the cutter with one hand while he supports the wheel with his other hand.

When the other rescuer is in position:

- Sever the rim by bringing the handles of the bolt cutter together smoothly.

Having someone support the head of the tool in this manner is important. If you attempt to operate the cutter alone, chances are that when the rim is severed, the head of the cutter will drop onto the driver's legs with sufficient force to aggravate an injury or cause a new one.

When you have severed the part of the rim closest to you:

- Pass the tool either over the steering column or behind the driver's seat to your partner.

While you support the portion of the rim that will be removed with one hand and the head of the cutter with your other hand:

- Have your partner make the cut.
- Remove the severed section of rim.

Some rescuers advocate making just one cut with either a saw or a bolt cutter and then bending the offending section of rim out of the way. The question that must be asked is "Will the bent section of rim really be out of the way, or will it become an even greater impediment to subsequent disentanglement operations?" As long as you are making one cut, why not make two? The job will take only a fraction of a minute more, and you will be rid of the piece of rim altogether.

Removing the Steering Wheel Altogether

Unless a steering wheel has massive spokes, removal is seldom difficult and is preferred over simply removing a section of the rim. Use a hacksaw or a reciprocating saw to cut through the spokes close to the hub.

Do not try to disassemble the wheel from a steering column even if you have a suitable wrench. While you may be able to remove the retaining nut without difficulty, you probably will not be able to pull the wheel from the column without a tool designed specially for the task.

Severing the Steering Column

There may be times when you will not be able to employ any of the techniques suggested thus far. You may not be able to move a motor-operated seat because the vehicle's electrical system has been damaged or purposely but permanently disabled, and you may not be able to move a manually adjusted seat because of damage to the operating mechanism or track. For any of a number of reasons you may decide that even removing the steering wheel will not provide sufficient working room for proper patient care.

To an untrained individual, severing a steering column sounds like a difficult and lengthy task. It really is not. Although a steering column may appear massive (and thus formidable), it may consist of nothing more than some concentric metal tubes around a 3/4-inch diameter soft steel shaft, all enclosed in a plastic shell.

You should be able to sever a steering column with a hacksaw in less than 2 minutes or with a reciprocating saw in about half that time. With either tool, you can dispose of a steering column in far less time than it takes to rig the equipment needed for displacement.

Be aware that not every steering column can be severed. The diameter of the column must be less than the distance between the blade and the frame of your hacksaw, or less than the length of the blade of a reciprocating saw. If you feel that you can sever the column of an accident vehicle with the tools at hand, do so in the following manner.

- First disconnect the battery from the vehicle's electrical system.

This important step must not be overlooked. As the blade moves through the column, it will sever wires that lead to and from the horn button, the turn signal control, the ignition switch, and, in some cars, the cruise control box, the windshield wiper controls, and the headlight and parking light switch. At the very least, the horn may blow and scare you!

After protecting the patient with some sort of rigid barrier:

- Get rid of as much plastic and metal as possible with a ripping chisel or a cold chisel. Most cars will then be down to the column itself and a few component parts. If the wheel or column is in a position so that you cannot pull up on the saw, make sure the victim is well protected (Figure 8.59).
- Have another rescuer take a position either on the seat next to the driver or on the hood of the vehicle.

While this rescuer lubricates the saw blade and presses down or pulls up on the wheel to prevent the blade from binding:

- If at all possible, it is preferable to pull up on a reciprocating saw away from the victim (Figure 8.60).
- Sever the column at the narrowest point accessible to the saw blade (Figure 8.61).

As you approach the end of the cut, the other rescuer will have to release some (but

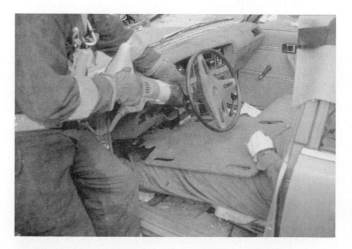

FIGURE 8.59   Protecting the Patient While Cutting Column

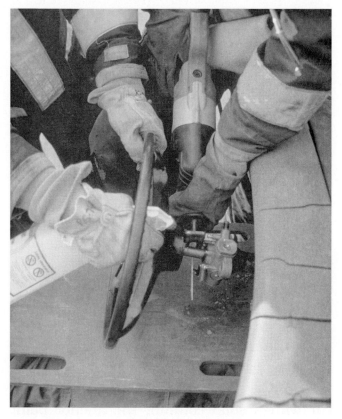

FIGURE 8.60 Pulling Up on Reciprocating Saw

not all) of the downward or upward force on the wheel so he doesn't lose control and drop the wheel assembly when the column is finally severed (Figure 8.62). Notice the size of the actual column without the cosmetic plastic!

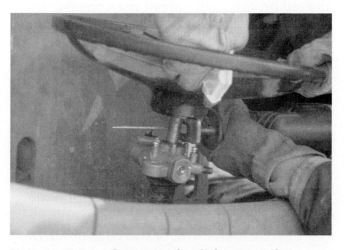

FIGURE 8.61 Severing the Column at the Narrowest Point

Displacing the Steering Column from Outside the Vehicle

Even though the techniques just described are faster and safer, there will undoubtedly be times during your career when you will have no choice other than to displace a steering column, as when:

- A manually adjustable seat cannot be moved because of damage to the tracks;
- A motorized seat cannot be moved because of damage or because the vehicle's electrical system has been disconnected; or
- Debris prevents the use of a hacksaw or reciprocating saw to sever the column.

Displacing a steering column involves much more than simply securing one chain or strap to an anchor point, securing a second chain to the steering column, and then pulling the ends of the chains or straps with a hand-operated or powered tool.

The procedure includes protecting the driver and then rigging a pulling system that consists of:

- A sufficiently strong chain or strap that is secured to a reliable anchor point underneath or adjacent to the vehicle;
- An equally strong second chain or strap that is properly wrapped around the steering column;
- Cribbing that is arranged so it will prevent the collapse of vehicle components when the chains or straps are under tension;
- Cribbing or some other device arranged so that it will provide lift for the chain or strap that is wrapped around the column, and at the same time allow the chain or strap to move freely;
- A pushing, pulling, or lifting tool that will develop sufficient force to move the column the desired distance; and
- A firm base of cribbing for the tool.

Following are suggestions as to how you might rig the three tools most commonly used to displace steering columns: the hydraulic rescue tool, the hydraulic ram, and the chain or cable hand winch. But first, a word about safety.

Protecting the Driver

Even when it is done correctly, displacing a steering column can be a dangerous operation to the trapped driver, other passengers, and rescuers. Glass fragments can separate from broken windshield edges, and bits of metal and plastic debris can fly for a considerable distance as the dash assembly collapses. Thus definitive patient protection steps are essential. Do not simply drape a tarp or blanket over the driver, or have rescuers hold a tarp or blanket in front of him. Neither will provide adequate protection. Instead:

- Have rescuers or firefighters hold a rigid shield in front of the patient during the entire displacement operation.

Note: A long or short spine board can also be used.

If there are any doubts in your mind that the shield will adequately protect the driver:

- Provide additional protection with a helmet, safety glasses, and hearing protectors (if those items are not already in place).

Creating a Suitable Anchor Point

Since considerable force will be exerted on the pulling system, the anchor chain must be secured to a component underneath the vehicle that is not likely to deform and fail during the column movement operation. The axle assembly is usually the most reliable anchor point.

All of the following anchor problems are associated with the use of hydraulic spreaders, rams, and come-alongs. The Colum-Master can always be anchored in line. Where to secure the anchor chain or strap depends on the type of column that must be displaced. If the vehicle is a rear-wheel drive

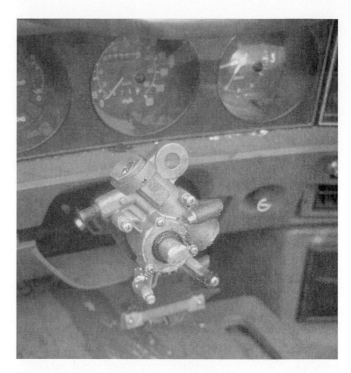

FIGURE 8.62   Severed Column

car with a solid column, the anchor point should be in line with the column so a straight pull can be made.

A different arrangement is necessary for a front-wheel drive vehicle. The pull must be made in such a way that the chance of the column separating from the universal joint near the driver's legs is minimal. After a great deal of experimentation, it has been found that the safest way to move the jointed column of a front-wheel drive vehicle is to make a diagonal pull from an anchor point that is located on the right side of the vehicle.

If you are using either a 1/4-inch rescue chain or the heavy chain that is part of a hydraulic rescue tool set:

- Wrap the slip hook end of the chain (the 12-foot chain if you have a rescue chain set) around the anchor point and capture the chain with the hook. Be sure that the point of the hook is facing down.
- Adjust the chain as necessary to remove any slack and assure an even pull.
- Carry the free end of the chain over the bumper to the hood of the vehicle.

If you are using a rescue strap set:

- Pass the smaller triangle of the longest strap around the anchor point and through the slot of the larger triangle to form a choker.
- Adjust the choker as necessary to remove any slack and assure that the choker fits snugly around the anchor point.
- Carry the free end of the strap over the bumper to the hood of the vehicle.

When the anchor chain or strap is in place:

- Have another rescuer or a firefighter hold the free end of the chain or strap to prevent it from slipping from the hood.

Sometimes there are just not enough people for tasks like the one just identified. If you find that this is the case while you are setting up equipment for displacing a steering column, catch the free end of the anchor chain or strap with the S-hook of an elastic cargo strap that you have hooked to the windshield frame, the rearmost edge of the hood, or another convenient point. The cargo strap will have enough "give" to allow you to position cribbing under the anchor chain— the next step in the operation.

Whenever you are creating an anchor point in preparation for displacing a steering column, remember the admonition made earlier in the section that dealt with widening door openings. If the vehicle has a damaged shock-absorbing bumper, work from the side of the vehicle and loop the chain or strap around the axle just behind the wheel.

While it is the technique most often used when it is necessary to displace a steering column, there is no law that says you must always create the anchor point underneath an accident vehicle. If you cannot work safely at the front or side of the vehicle, or if debris prevents you from reaching a strong component, rig the chain or strap to an anchor point away from the vehicle, like another accident vehicle, the bumper of a wrecker, or the towing eye of a rescue vehicle or fire apparatus.

Preventing the Collapse of Front-End Components

When an older car has a massive bumper, front end, and hood assembly, there is usually no problem of sheet-metal collapse when the anchor chain or strap is simply laid over the bumper and leading edge of the hood.

Newer, smaller cars do not have such strong front ends, however. When pulling forces are exerted on the anchor chain or strap during a column displacement, the chain or strap is likely to "sink" into the front end unless something is used to prevent the sheet metal from collapsing. While the displacement of front-end components by an anchor chain or strap is often viewed as nothing more that a nuisance, it can seriously slow a rescue operation. Forces that should be moving the column are lost as front-end components collapse, and rescuers are required to reposition the pulling tool and adjust the chains or straps.

A cribbing ladder works well. Loose cribbing can be placed between the chain and strap and components that are likely to collapse. When front-end damage is such that a cribbing ladder or loose cribbing will not provide the necessary support, 4-foot lengths of 4- by 4-inch lumber will spread forces exerted by the chain or strap over a wide area.

Joining the Pulling Tool to the Anchor Chain or Strap

Because of the spread of the arms of full-size hydraulic rescue tools, and the overall length of hydraulic rams and hand winches, it is essential that the tool is joined to the anchor chain or strap just behind the leading edge of the hood.

When one of the hydraulic rescue tool chains is used as an anchor chain, there is no requirement for shortening. A link close to the leading edge of the hood can be captured with the grab hook that is part of the shackle that is attached to the tool arm (or to the base of the ram if a hydraulic ram is being used to displace the column).

When a 12-foot rescue chain is used in conjunction with a hand winch or another hand-operated tool, the chain should be shortened by means of the grab hook so that the ring or oval of the chain is situated just behind the leading edge of the hood. Thus there will be ample space for the hand winch on the hood.

The triangle of the longest strap of a three-piece rescue strap set will lie just behind the leading edge of the hood of a full-size car when secured to an anchor point under the vehicle. When the strap is secured to the undercarriage of a smaller car, it may be necessary to position loose cribbing between the strap and the front of the vehicle to assure that the triangle lies close to the hood edge.

As soon as the anchor chain or strap is properly in place:

- Join it to the pulling tool.

If you are using a hydraulic rescue tool:

- Spread the arms of the tool to their widest position, if necessary.
- Position the tool on the hood of the vehicle with the grab hooks roughly in line with the anchor chain or strap and the steering column. Be sure that the shackle pins are installed with the pull ring down and that both of the grab hooks are facing up.
- Capture a link of the anchor chain (or the triangle of the strap) at a point as close as possible to the leading edge of the hood.

If you are using a hydraulic ram:

- Fully open the ram, if necessary.
- Position the tool on the hood of the vehicle in line with the anchor chain or strap and the steering column. The base of the ram should be adjacent to the anchor chain or strap. Be sure that the grab hooks are both facing up.
- Capture a link of the anchor chain (or the triangle of the strap) at a point as close to the leading edge of the hood as possible.

If you are using a hand winch:

- Capture the chain ring or the triangle of the strap with the fixed hook of the winch. Be sure that the hook is facing up.
- While you operate the winch, have another rescuer pull out enough chain or cable to reach the steering column.

The next step is to secure a chain or strap to the steering column.

Wrapping the Steering Column

How the second chain or strap is rigged to the steering column is influenced by the construction of the column and type of chain or strap.

If you are going to use the heavy chain that is part of a hydraulic rescue tool set to displace the standard column of a rear-wheel drive vehicle:

- Simply wrap the end of the chain around the column and capture the standing part with the slip hook.
- Lay the free end of the chain on the dash and hood.

This is the traditional (and quickest) way to secure heavy rescue tool chain to a steering column. Just where the wrap is made on a standard, non-jointed column is of little consequence since the available pulling force is far greater than that needed to displace the column.

The smaller link, lighter-weight chain that is usually used in conjunction with a less powerful hand winch should be rigged in such a way that maximum leverage is available.

If you are going to displace the standard, non-jointed column of a rear-wheel drive car with a hand winch and you have a 6-foot rescue chain:

- Lay the chain over the column just behind the hub of the steering wheel.
- Cross the two resulting "legs" of chain under the column.

- Carry the ends of the chain around the front of the wheel spokes from underneath to a point between the wheel and the dash.

Depending on how much chain is needed, either:

- Capture the links of the chain with the slip hook at a point just above the hub of the steering wheel; or
- Capture the ring of the chain with the slip hook.

In either case:

- Adjust the wrap as necessary to remove any slack in the chain and assure an even pull.

While another rescuer keeps the chain taut:

- Capture the ring of the chain with the running hook of the hand winch.

Either the medium or short strap of a three-piece rescue strap set can be similarly rigged for maximum leverage when a standard, non-jointed column of a rear-wheel drive vehicle is to be displaced with a hand winch. If the turn signal lever will be in the way of rigging the strap, simply break the lever off at its base.

- Lay the midpoint of the strap over the column just behind the hub of the steering wheel.
- Carry the ends of the strap around the front of the wheel spokes from underneath to a point between the steering wheel and the dash.
- Capture both triangles with the running hook of the hand winch.

A column that has a tilt-and-telescoping steering wheel should be rigged in such a way that the chance of the wheel separating from the column at the tilting joint is minimal.

If you are going to displace the column with a hydraulic rescue tool or a hydraulic ram:

- Wrap the slip hook end of the chain around the column as low (close to the dash) as possible.

This will assure that the pulling force is exerted below the tilting joint.

If you are going to displace the column with a hand winch and you have a 6-foot rescue chain:

- Lay the midpoint of the chain over the column just ahead of the dash.
- Make one full wrap.
- Cross the ends of chain under the column.
- Carry the ends around the spokes of the steering wheel from underneath to a point between the steering wheel and the dash.
- Capture the slip hook end of the chain with the grab hook of the other end.

While another rescuer supports the chain:

- Adjust the chain as necessary to remove slack and assure an even pull.
- Capture the chain ring with the running hook of the hand winch.

This rigging will not prevent the failure of the tilting joint during column displacement, but by its cradling action, it will minimize the chance that the wheel will forcefully separate from the column.

Providing Lift and a Smooth Surface for the Pulling Chain or Strap

While all of the rigging may be in place at this time, the column displacement system is not yet complete. Some means must be provided to change the angle of the pulling chain or strap so that it does not dig into the soft dash or otherwise have its movement impeded. A chain that is simply laid across the dashboard of a car can become so deeply imbedded in the dash that a hydraulic tool must be used to free it after the column displacement operation. Cribbing that is laid in the manner of railroad tracks works well.

If the upper surface of the dash and the rear portion of the hood are relatively undamaged:

- Lay two lengths of 2- by 4- by 18-inch cribbing on the dash, one on each side of the pulling chain or strap with the end of each piece of cribbing flush with the edge of the dash.

Then:

- Position one or more lengths of cribbing across the "tracks." Use as much cribbing as is necessary to get the necessary lift.
- Lay the chain or strap across these lengths of cribbing.

Complete the pulling system either by capturing a link of the chain with the other grab hook of the hydraulic rescue tool or ram or by removing slack from the chain or cable of the hand winch.

Longer lengths of 4- by 4-inch lumber can be used to advantage when damage to the hood is such that the proper placement of 2- by 4-inch cribbing is impossible. A 2-foot length of 4- by 4-inch stock will provide the necessary lift.

An easily made appliance is the half-wheel. When the upper surface of the hood and the rear portion of the hood are not badly deformed, the appliance can be positioned without cribbing.

Providing a Solid Base for the Pulling Tool

If the hood of the vehicle is buckled as a result of the accident, or if buckling occurs during the column displacement, folds of metal may interfere with the operation of the pulling tool. It is not unusual for the arms of a hydraulic rescue tool to "gather" sheet metal as they close, and then squeeze the metal into a mass that prevents the arms from closing all the way.

Likewise, dimpled sheet metal can gather under the movable part and the base of a hydraulic ram. Dimpled sheet metal under a hand winch can prevent the movement of the drum of a cable winch and can impede the movement of the operating handle of a chain winch.

Strategically placed lengths of cribbing will prevent the further buckling of the sheet metal and will place the pulling tool above the hood where it can operate freely. A length of 4- by 4-inch lumber, for example, will serve as a smooth runway for the arms of a hydraulic rescue tool while at the same time keeping the shackles and chains above possible snagging points.

Checking the Pulling System

Whenever several pieces of equipment are assembled in a number of steps to perform a certain task, a final check should be made to see that the system is ready for operation. So it is when rigging equipment is used to displace a steering column. If cribbing has slipped out of place, much of the pulling force will be expended on removing the slack from a chain or strap rather than on the column displacement. If the anchor chain has slipped from its point of attachment, there will be no pulling force whatsoever exerted on the column. Therefore, quickly check the pulling system from anchor point to column wrap. Ask yourself these questions as you do:

- Is the anchor chain or strap properly in place around or connected to a rigid structural member?
- Is the cribbing that was positioned to prevent the collapse of front-end components properly in place under the anchor chain or strap?
- Is the pulling tool in position on the hood so that it will make a straight pull?
- Is the pulling tool properly joined to the anchor chain or strap?
- Is cribbing properly arranged under the tool so that buckling of the hood will not interfere with the pulling operation?
- Is the tool properly joined to the pulling chain or strap?

- Is the steering column properly wrapped with the pulling chain or strap?
- Are other rescuers or EMS personnel adequately protecting the driver?

If your answer to any of these questions is "no":

- Make corrections or adjustments as necessary.

If the system is intact and ready:

- Get into position to operate the pulling tool.

Posting an Observer

From a position at the passenger side of the vehicle (if you are operating a hydraulic rescue tool or ram) or at the front of the vehicle (if you are operating a hand winch), you will not be able to see any more than the top of the steering wheel. You will not be able to see how the column reacts to the pulling effort, nor whether the pulling chain or strap is remaining in the proper position. Moreover, you may not be able to determine when the column has been displaced the desired distance.

Rather than work blind:

- Have another rescuer stand at the side of the vehicle where he can clearly see the steering column and where you are able to see him.

Needless to say, the rescuer should be knowledgeable in the displacement technique and should be able to recognize problems immediately as they develop. You and he should be familiar with various hand signals.

While you are operating the tool:

- Watch the rescuer, not the column, and react immediately to his hand signals.

Some rescuers elect to cover the steering column and adjacent dash assembly with a tarpaulin prior to operating the pulling tool.

While a tarp will undoubtedly protect rescuers and victims from the bits of debris that often break away and become airborne during a column displacement operation, it will also prevent anyone from watching the column and seeing potentially dangerous conditions develop. There should be no worry about flying bits of debris if rescuers are wearing a full set of protective gear and patients are protected by rigid shields.

Operating the Tool

Displacing a steering column with a hydraulic rescue tool or a hydraulic ram involves nothing more than standing by the side of the vehicle and operating the controls in the prescribed manner.

If fully closing the arms or retracting the ram does not move the column the desired distance:

- Spread the arms.
- Disengage the pulling chain from the grab hook.
- Pull the chain taut.
- Recapture the pulling chain with the grab hook.
- Operate the controls to close the arms and move the column.

The ideal position for operating a hand winch is just behind the winch where you can exert a straight, in-line pull with a combination of arm, back, and leg muscles. But if there is any doubt in your mind as to the integrity of a damaged shock-absorbing bumper, you will have no choice other than to operate a hand winch from a position at the side of the vehicle. Moving the operating handle of a hand winch from this position is difficult, however; it gets increasingly harder to push the handle sideways as the requirement for pulling force increases. To gain efficiency, have another rescuer stand at your side and, working together, move the handle. Your combined strengths should be sufficient to move the column the desired distance.

ALTERNATE TOOLS FOR DISPLACING A STEERING COLUMN

While hydraulic rescue tools, hydraulic rams, and hand winches are the tools most commonly used to displace steering columns from positions outside of vehicles, they are by no means the only tools that can be used. A Hi-Lift jack, a number of hydraulic tools, and even a bumper jack can be used to move a column.

Since these are lifting and pushing devices, a slightly different setup is required. Rescue chains are secured to an anchor point and the steering column in the manner suggested for use with a pulling tool. Instead of being joined to the tool, however, they are joined to each other to make a solid chain from anchor point to steering column. Cribbing is placed in the manner suggested earlier to prevent the collapse of front-end components and to give lift to the pulling chain.

A solid bed of cribbing is placed on the hood where the pushing device will be located. The crib has to be large enough and sturdy enough to prevent the hood from collapsing when pushing forces are exerted downward. Two lengths of 4- by 4-inch lumber that extend from one side of the vehicle to the other make an excellent rigid base.

The Hi-Lift jack and bumper jacks are excellent tools; they exert far more force than is necessary to displace a column, and enough lift to move the column the desired distance without adding to the cribbing base.

A small hydraulic ram such as the Mini-Ram can be operated in the vertical position on a solid base of cribbing.

A hydraulic hand pump and cylinder assembly can also be used to displace a steering column. If a set of attachments is available, a V-block or wedge head can be secured to the end of the ram to assure contact with the chain during the pushing effort. If there are no attachments, a length of cribbing must be used to keep the face of the ram in line with the chain. If the hydraulic hand pump and cylinder are part of what is known as a maintenance and rescue set, they can be used in conjunction with a chain puller to displace a steering column.

Any of a number of general-purpose hydraulic hand jacks ranging in capacity from 3 to 100 tons can be used to displace a steering column.

A problem common to all three of the hydraulic devices is that the stroke—the distance that the ram moves, that is—is short. The stroke of the Mini-Ram is slightly less than 8 inches, and the stroke of the 12-ton general-purpose hydraulic jack is just over 5 inches. If the initial pushing effort is not sufficient to displace the column the desired distance, it will be necessary to retract the ram, add cribbing to the base, and extend the ram again. This can be a time-consuming procedure.

Displacing the Steering Column of a Front-Wheel Drive Vehicle

These facts are known about the steering column of front-wheel drive vehicles:

- The universal joint that is on the driver's side of the firewall can break when a pulling force is exerted close to the steering wheel.
- When the joint fails, the column can pivot forcefully on the point of attachment with the dash. The disjointed column becomes a lever, and the point of attachment to the dash becomes a fulcrum.
- A forcefully pivoting column can inflict injury to even a protected driver and rescuers.

Given these facts, it stands to reason that if the pulling force needed to move a column can be exerted at a point between the universal column and the point of attachment to the dash instead of at the wheel end of the column, the chance of the universal joint failing is just about nonexistent. This manner of movement can be accomplished on *some* vehicles with a Hi-Lift jack and a 12-foot rescue chain. Note the emphasis on the word "some." The procedure has not been successful on all front-wheel drive vehicles because of complex dash assemblies.

If you have no other choice than to displace the steering column of a front-wheel drive car, look at the dash assembly. If it appears that you can accomplish the following procedure, try it! You will know in a minute whether you are going to be successful.

The first step is to make pathways for the rescue chain. From a position on the hood of the vehicle:

- Drive the wedge end of a 51-inch pinch bar through the top of the dash just to one side of the steering column. Have another rescuer sight the path that the bar will take so that it passes rather than strikes the column.

Driving the bar through the dash may take considerable force. You may be attempting to push it through gauge assemblies, wiring, metal stiffeners, and defroster ducts. If you are unsuccessful in driving the pinch bar through the dash:

- Abandon the procedure and attempt to create working space in front of the driver in another way.

If you are able to punch through the dash:

- Sweep the end of the pinch bar in a circular motion to widen the resulting tunnel. It should be large enough for the slip hook of the rescue chain to pass through; then
- Make a similar tunnel on the other side of the column.

When both tunnels are open:

- Drop the slip hook of the rescue chain through one tunnel.
- Have another rescuer pass the hook around the underside of the column and up through the second tunnel.

If the tunnels are large enough, the other rescuer should be able to push the hook partway through, and you should be able to reach in far enough to catch it. Be careful! There are likely to be sharp edges inside the tunnel. If the tunnels are not large enough for your hand, fashion a hook from a length of wire and fish the hook up through the hole.

When the chain is around the column and both ends of the chain are within reach:

- Join the slip hook end of the chain with the grab hook of the other end to make a loop.
- Adjust the chain so the ring is at the top of the loop. The top of the ring should be 9 to 12 inches above the top of the dash when the loop is taut.

While another rescuer holds the chain ring and keeps the loop taut:

- Make a solid base for the lifting tool. Put down two layers of 2- by 4-inch cribbing, one laid on top of the other at a right angle, or two lengths of 4- by 4-inch cribbing side-by-side. One side of the base should be just behind the junction of the cowl with the dash.
- Position the jack so the base is on the cribbing and the lifting toe is in line with the chain ring.

While you hold the body of the jack with one hand and the other rescuer supports the chain ring:

- Operate the jack handle and raise the lifting toe to the point where the other rescuer can slip the chain ring over it.

When the ring is in place:

- Operate the jack until the column is moved the desired distance.

Displacing the Steering Column from Inside the Vehicle

While most column displacement operations are accomplished outside the vehicle with a pulling, pushing, or lifting tool situated on the hood, there may be times when you can move a column with the pushing force of a hydraulic tool held situated inside the passenger compartment.

If you have a small ram such as the Mini-Ram:

- Position the ram between the driver's legs and make a vertical push against the underside of the column.

A base of cribbing will prevent the ram from pushing through the floor pan if it is badly rusted, and the V-block attachment will assure that the ram does not slip from the underside of the column.

If you have a 30-inch ram:

- Position the ram with the base of the unit against the bottom of the door frame and push the column up and to the right.

The sharp edges of the ram base should keep the tool from sliding rearward as pushing force is exerted. As with the small ram, the V-block attachment will assure firm contact with the underside of the column.

If you have a hydraulic hand pump and cylinder assembly:

- Add extensions, a base plate, and a V-block to the cylinder, as necessary, and position the assembly either between the driver's legs or at the driver's left side with the base plate on the bottom of the door frame.

If you have a hydraulic rescue tool and there is room to work (as when both of the driver's legs are on the right side of the steering column):

- Position the tool nearly vertical so that when the arms are spread, one tip will push against the floor and the other arm will push against the underside of the column.

A base of cribbing will be needed to prevent the sharp point of the tip from pushing through the floor pan, especially if the underside of the vehicle is severely rusted.

If you have a Hi-Lift jack and there is room to position the jack between the driver's legs, or if both of the driver's legs are on the right side of the column:

- Position the jack vertically on a base of cribbing and operate the handle to move the column.

Put down a layer of cribbing even though the base of the Hi-Lift jack is much larger than the base of the other tools. Some floor pans are so rusty that even the 35-square-inch base of the Hi-Lift jack will push through. It's better to spend half a minute making a base of cribbing than many minutes extricating a jack that has broken through the floor pan, then putting down a layer of cribbing, then repositioning the jack and trying again.

The overhang of the padded dash over the instrument cluster of some cars may prevent positioning the jack so the lifting toe is close to the point of attachment of the column to the underside of the dash. A notch in the overhang will accommodate the body of the jack. The notch can be cut easily with a hacksaw or keyhole saw.

"Blowing Out" the Front End

Being a vehicle rescue manual, we would be remiss if a list of different methods for removing the wreckage from the patient were not mentioned and discussed in length. However, there is one method to remove everything in front of the front seat patient in one action that is far superior and quicker than many individual tasks. That is, "blowing out" or moving forward the entire front of the vehicle.

After assuring the vehicle is properly stabilized and the patient(s) are adequately protected:

- Move the doors forward beyond their operating range or remove them altogether.
- Remove the roof.
- With the hydraulic shears, reciprocating saw, or hand hacksaw, cut a slot on a

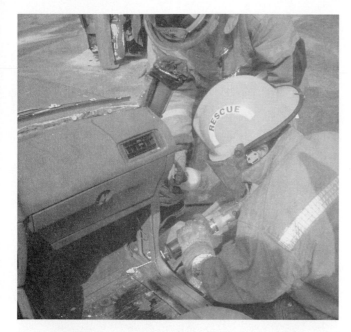

FIGURE 8.63   Cutting the Base of the A-Pillar with Reciprocating Saw

diagonal toward the front of the car, at the base of the A-pillars (Figure 8.63). Cut as far as possible on unibody-constructed cars. Do not attempt to cut the frame on framed cars, only the body. Figure 8.64 shows cutting with a reciprocating saw while Figure 8.65 shows use of the hydraulic cutter. Figure 8.66 illustrates the finished cut.

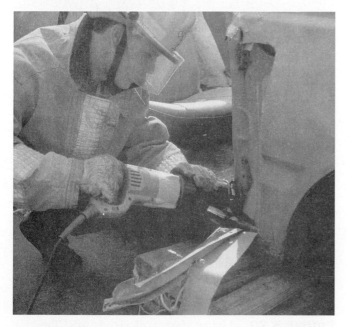

FIGURE 8.64   Cutting the Base of the A-Pillar with Reciprocating Saw

- If you are using only hand tools, place a notch-style bumper jack or a Hi-Lift jack with the base against the bottom of the B-pillars and the lifting lip under the front door hinges (Figure 8.67). By jacking both sides simultaneously, the diagonal slots will rip open, allowing the front end to move forward because of the out and downward motion. This will cause the floor to lift as the wheels tilt down. Crib under the A-pillars as you jack.

Only move the front end out as far as it takes to remove the patient. If you need an inch, do not go two inches! Remember the cardinal rule in rescue; never exceed what is needed. To do so may result in injury or death.

- If you are using hydraulic rams, set them up in the same fashion (Figure 8.68). If you experience the base of the rams punching through the B-pillars, reinforce it with a homemade or commercial sill box or use railroad tie plates, which work well for this task (Figures 8.69 and 8.70).
- Always place cribbing in the slots as they open. This will prevent them from closing up if something happens to the jack or rams (Figure 8.71).
- You can also use the spreader to push the front end out (Figures 8.72 and 8.73).

Freeing a Driver's Foot from Entrapment by a Pedal

When vehicles had clutch and brake pedals with shafts that passed through the floorboard, it was not unusual for drivers to have at least one foot trapped as the result of a front-end collision. The problem is not as severe today, since clutch pedals and brake pedals are usually suspended from a pivot point in the vehicle. Nonetheless, you may respond to an accident and discover that a driver's foot is trapped by a pedal or that a pedal will interfere with the movement of an injured foot. Several techniques can be used to deal with troublesome pedals.

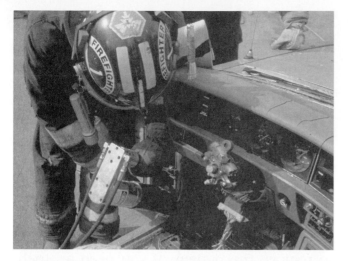

FIGURE 8.65   Cutting the Base of the A-Pillar with Hydraulic Cutter

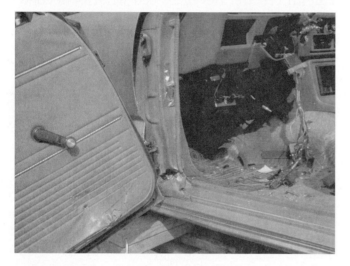

FIGURE 8.66   ■ Finished Cut

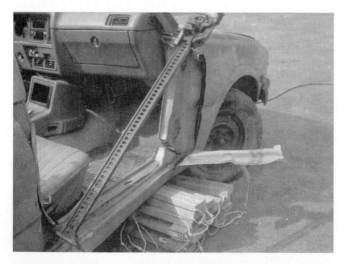

FIGURE 8.67   Jacking Front End Out with Hi-Lift Jack

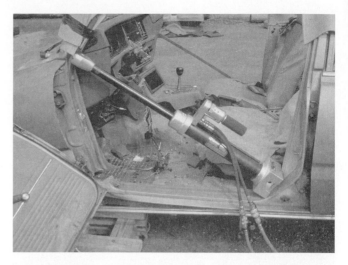

FIGURE 8.68   Jacking Front End Out with Hydraulic Ram

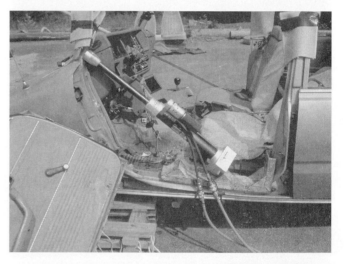

FIGURE 8.69   Using Hydraulic Ram and Sill Plate

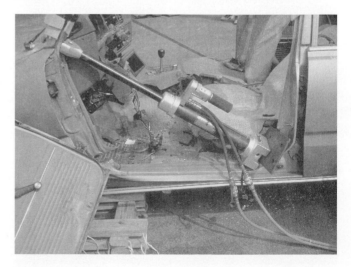

FIGURE 8.70   Using Hydraulic Ram and Tie Plate

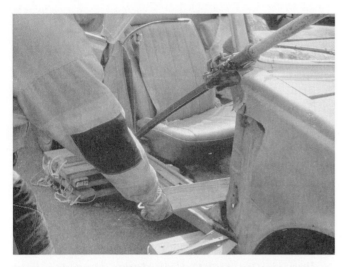

FIGURE 8.71 Placing Cribbing in Slot

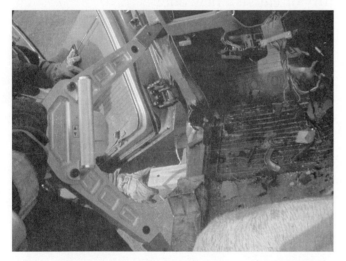

FIGURE 8.72 Using the Spreader to Push Out Front End

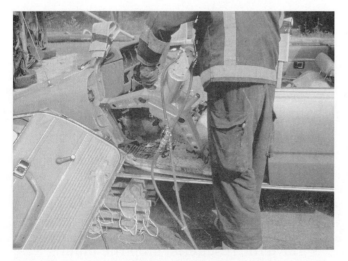

FIGURE 8.73 Using the Spreader to Push Out Front End

Disassembling the Pedal

If damage to the firewall is not severe, you may be able to pull the pin from the pivot point with pliers and simply move a brake pedal out of the way.

Removing the Driver's Foot from the Shoe

More often than not it is a driver's shoe that is trapped by a brake pedal, not the foot. If the edge of the pedal has creased the leather or fabric at the point where the toes join the instep, the person may not be able to withdraw the foot. This is especially true when the edge of the pedal is pressed into a work shoe just behind the steel toe cap.

Before you initiate any equipment setup procedures:

- Examine the shoe carefully with the aid of a light.

If the edge of the pedal does not appear to be pressed so deeply into the shoe that it has injured the foot:

- Use pocket shears or aircraft snips to cut away the rear portion of the shoe.

Make cuts from the top of the foot opening down, and from one cut to the other at the level of the sole. The shoe should have the appearance of a clog or shower sandal when you remove the cut section of leather. The farther forward you cut the shoe, the easier it will be to withdraw the foot.

When the rear of the shoe is cut away:

- Carefully try to ease the foot from the shoe (if to do so will not aggravate an injury to the foot or leg).

If you are unable to slide the foot from the shoe, or if you hesitate to do so in fear of aggravating an injury, you will have to take steps to dispose of the pedal.

Severing the Pedal

If the pedal does not have the massive stamped shaft that is common to many older luxury cars, and if there is sufficient working space, severing the pedal shaft should be no problem. A low-profile hacksaw such as the Klein Tools Mini Hack Saw is an excellent tool for the task. It will fit in a space too small for a hacksaw or a reciprocating saw. Remember that good lighting and lubrication are essential when using a saw close to a body part in a tight space.

While another rescuer maintains constant upward force on the pedal from a position at the driver's right side, thus relieving pressure on the foot:

• Sever the shaft from behind.

If you attempt to sever the shaft by cutting from the top down in the usual manner, the pulling force exerted by the other rescuer will cause the saw to bind as the cut progresses. If you cut the pedal from behind, the upward force on the pedal exerted by the other rescuer will tend to separate the cut material as the saw blade passes through the shaft.

Displacing the Pedal

If you can't disassemble the pedal from its pivot point or cut a portion of the shoe away or sever the pedal, you may be able to displace the pedal with a length of chain.

Using a Chain

Displacing a pedal with a length of rope is a disentanglement technique that has been used for many years. A common practice was to secure one end of the rope to the pedal and the other end to the window frame of the right front door, then to pull the door open. The procedure usually worked with all but massive pedal shafts.

Today, doors are usually removed or at least moved beyond their normal range of motion long before any attention is given to pedals, and squad members are less inclined to use rescue rope for this task. Nevertheless, the job can be accomplished with a length of 1/4-inch rescue chain, and

with an advantage: There is no need to form the end of the chain into a loop as there is with a length of rope!

Don't simply drop the slip hook of the rescue chain over the pedal shaft and give a yank, however. First:

• Examine the pedal and the foot with the aid of a light.
• Visualize the path that the pedal will take when it is displaced.

Determine whether the left lower corner of the pedal will drop down when the shaft is pulled to the right. If it does, even for just half an inch, it may aggravate an existing injury or cause a new one.

If you feel that to displace the pedal to the side will not be a problem:

• Have another rescuer pass the slip hook to you from a position at the right side of the vehicle.
• Drop the slip hook over the pedal shaft with the throat of the hook facing down.

While you support and protect the foot:

• Instruct the rescuer (or rescuers) to exert a slow pull on the chain.

If you see that the left lower corner of the pedal will clear the foot:

• Have the rescuer(s) continue to pull on the chain until the pedal is moved the desired distance.
• Instruct the rescuer(s) to secure the chain on the stub of the A-pillar or another convenient anchor point to keep the pedal from returning to its original position.

If you see that the left lower corner of the pedal will not clear the foot without contacting it:

• Have the rescuer(s) stop the pulling effort.

- Disconnect the hook from the pedal shaft and prepare for another procedure.

USING A HAND WINCH

A chain or cable hand winch is the tool most commonly used to displace a pedal when the techniques that have been discussed thus far are unsuccessful or not possible. The hand winch is set up in exactly the manner suggested for displacing the steering column.

Needless to say, other tools can be used to displace a brake pedal when working space is available, including a powered or hand-operated hydraulic rescue tool, a hydraulic hand pump and cylinder assembly, and even a small hydraulic ram. Be extremely careful when using any of these tools; patient protection steps of the type suggested for other rescue procedures may not be possible because of the extremely limited working space.

Disposing of the Front Seat of a Passenger Car

A patient can end up on the floor ahead of the front seat of a vehicle as the result of either diving there when the crash seemed inevitable or being thrown there upon impact.

One technique for removing a patient from the floor ahead of the front seat of a vehicle has been used for years. Three or four people stand behind the front seat (or crouch, if the roof has not been removed or folded back). They lean over the seat back, grasp the patient's clothing, and lift him like a sack of potatoes onto a spine board that has been laid on the seat bottom.

This technique is far better than dragging a patient by his shoulders or feet through the space between the seat bottom and the base of the A-pillar, to be sure. But by today's standards of pre-hospital care, the procedure is totally unacceptable except in the direct circumstances when speedy removal is essential to survival. If one of the rescuers loses balance or if the

patient's clothing tears, the patient will drop back onto the floor with disastrous results.

However, if the front seat of a vehicle can be moved partially out of the way, or better yet, removed altogether, rescuers can roll the patient directly onto a long board while keeping the spine in proper alignment.

Deciding on the Technique

The decision to remove or displace the front seat of a vehicle is usually influenced by the availability of equipment and the type of seat. If you have a hydraulic rescue tool or a heavy-duty air-operated chisel, you would do well to dispose of the seat altogether and thus create unrestricted working space within the vehicle.

If you have only a hand winch and a rescue chain or strap set, you can displace one side of the seat backward far enough to allow the easy removal of the patient with a rope sling and a long spine board.

Protecting the Patient

A problem common to seat removal and displacement operations is that both can be dangerous to the trapped patients. Pieces of metal and plastic can become dislodged and airborne, strong springs can break loose and inflict injury, tools can slip, and the patient can be bumped by rescuers carrying out the procedures. Accordingly, patient protection should be accomplished in three steps.

- Rescuers or EMS personnel should apply a rigid cervical collar if there is sufficient working space at the patient's head, and one rescuer or medic should support the head throughout the disentanglement operation.
- Other rescuers or EMS personnel should cover the patient with a lightweight tarp or disposable blanket to provide at least minimal shielding from flying debris.

- Two rescuers—one on each side of the vehicle—should hold a long spine board firmly in place between the patient and the front of the seat bottom throughout the removal or displacement procedure. The board will shield the patient from contact with tools or debris and at the same time prevent him from rolling toward the rear of the vehicle when the seat is moved.

Removing the Seat

It would be great to say that one technique can be used to remove the front seat of all vehicles. This is not possible, however, for there are solid bench seats with non-moving backs, solid bench seats with folding backs, bucket seats, 50-50 split seats, 60-40 split seats, manually adjustable seats, motor-adjustable seats, four-way adjustable seats, six-way adjustable seats, and even seats that are adjusted by a computer to fit a particular driver. While it doesn't sound at all scientific, or even professional, it might be said that the best way to remove the front seat of a vehicle today is to try something, and if that doesn't work, try something else and keep trying until you get the job done!

The one type of seat that can usually be removed with ease is the manually adjustable bench seat that has either a rigid or folding back. There are probably a number of tools that can be used to remove this type of seat, but the ones most commonly used are the hydraulic rescue tool and the heavy-duty air-operated chisel.

Using a Hydraulic Rescue Tool

A bench seat can be removed by using a hydraulic rescue tool in one of two ways: moving the seat backward until it breaks free of the track, or lifting the seat from the track.

To move the seat backward on its track:

- First remove the rear seat bottom, if possible.

The rear seat bottom will probably not interfere with moving the front seat back, but doing so will create that much more working space within the vehicle for emergency care and patient packaging activities.

Removing a rear seat bottom usually involves nothing more than pushing the lower edge of the seat bottom in about 12 inches from each side until a metal rod is disengaged from a simple latch.

When you have disposed of the rear seat bottom:

- Operate the seat adjustment lever, and with the help of another rescuer at the other side of the car, push the front seat back as far as it will go (if this has not already been done).

This step is often overlooked. A manually adjusted seat's position on the track is maintained by a spring-operated plunger seated in a notch in the track. If the seat is in any of the forward positions when pushing force is exerted by the rescue tool, it is liable to jerk backward as the plunger disengages from the notch and may become jammed on the track.

When the seat is all the way back:

- Position cribbing against the base of the A-pillar to take up some of the space between the pillar and the seat bottom. Leave just enough room for the tips of the rescue tool.

Two lengths of 4- by 4-inch cribbing or four lengths of 2- by 4-inch cribbing are generally sufficient for a full-size car. If speed is not that important, take a moment to make a solid bundle of the loose cribbing with a couple of wraps of duct tape. To do so will eliminate the need for a rescuer to hold the cribbing in place; it will also eliminate the possibility of the loose cribbing turning into a jumble if the pushing force is slightly off center.

When the cribbing is in place:

- Position the tool with one tip against the bundle of cribbing and the other tip against the bottom of the seat front at a point close to the corner.

Positioning the tip against the seat bottom in this manner is important; you want to move the seat back on the track. If you position the tip under the seat, you will tear the track from the floor, probably along with a section of the floor pan.

When the tool is in position:

- Operate the controls and move the seat back slowly (Figure 8.74).

Be prepared for a sudden—almost explosive—movement of the seat. It may move just a bit at first, and then stop until the tool exerts sufficient force to break it from the track.

When the seat is free of the track:

- Continue to move the seat back with the tool until the spring that helps with the

seat adjustment is exposed (Figure 8.75).

While you hold the seat in position:

- Have another rescuer use side-cutting pliers or a bolt cutter to sever the spring wire at its point of attachment with the floor. The spring will fly toward the rear of the vehicle (Figure 8.76).

When the one side of the seat is completely free of the track:

- Repeat the procedure on the other side; and
- Remove the seat from the car.

Lifting the seat with a hydraulic rescue tool is another technique for removing the front seat of a vehicle, but it's one of those "damned if you do, damned if don't" procedures.

If you position the tips of the tool between the rocker panel and the bottom of the seat in an effort to separate the seat from the

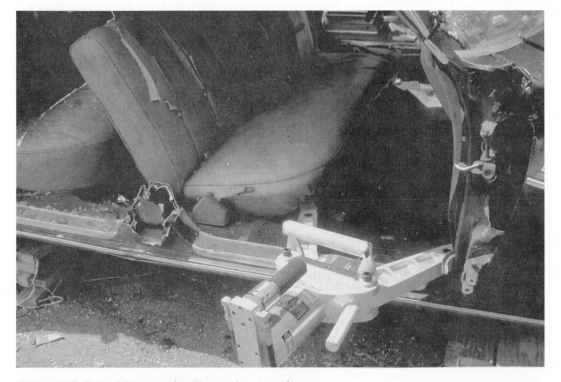

FIGURE 8.74 Moving the Front Seat with Hydraulic Spreader

track, the energy stored in the arms of the tool and the springiness of the seat bottom will probably cause the seat to fly up from the track when separation occurs. When the patient is properly protected and other rescuers are aware of the likelihood of this happening, the violent separation is usually more disconcerting than dangerous. If you elect to use this technique, position the tips of the tool under the forward half of the seat bottom so that if violent separation occurs, the seat will move backward rather than forward.

Working the tips of the tool under the seat track by means of a series of opening and closing movements will enable you to pull the seat track from the floor and thus minimize the chance of a violent movement. The procedure is not without its own peculiar problem, however. The pushing effort may not result in the seat track being pulled from the floor, but rather in the creation of a flap of floor pan to which the seat track is attached. If this happens, you will have to use shears, an air-operated chisel, or another cutting tool to cut the flap before rescuers can remove the seat.

So . . . take your pick of the two techniques if you elect to lift the seat in order to remove it. Whichever one you try, remember that you will have to cut the seat adjustment springs before you can remove it from the vehicle.

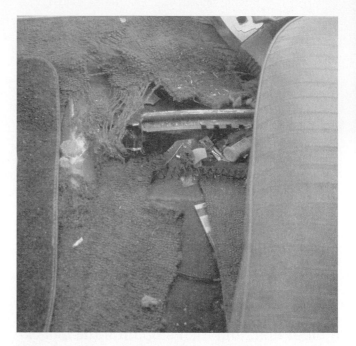

FIGURE 8.75 Exposing Seat Spring

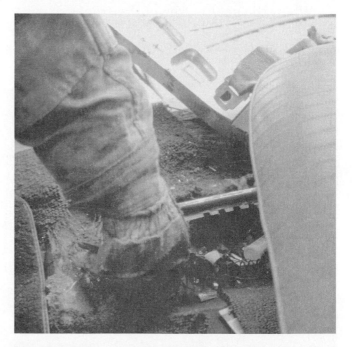

FIGURE 8.76 Cutting Spring

Packaging Injured Patients for Removal and Transfer

INTRODUCTION

The ninth phase of a vehicle rescue operation begins when squad personnel have created exitways in the wreckage and disentangled patients from mechanisms of entrapment.

Injured patients cannot simply be pulled from a vehicle; to do so could seriously aggravate injuries and negate all of the good work done by the rescue squad up to that point. Instead, the patients must be packaged so that existing injuries will not be worsened during removal and transfer activities.

When there are sufficient EMS personnel on the scene, there may be nothing for you to do at this point in the rescue operation other than to provide continuing scene support. But in multiple-casualty situations when EMS personnel are busy, you may be asked to assist medics with patient-packaging activities or even to package patients with the assistance of other squad members.

Following are suggestions for the use of several often-used upper-body immobilization devices. Regardless of the particular device that is carried on your rescue unit, heed these six warnings as you immobilize the upper body of a patient who has a known or suspected spine injury.

- Complete your initial assessment of a patient's back, scapulas, arms, and clavicles before you immobilize him. You will not be able to examine these body parts once the patient is secured to a spine board or other immobilization device.

- Push the bottom edge of the short spine board or other immobilizing device down against the seat cushion. If you fail to do this, the device may shift while the patient is being removed from the vehicle. As a result, segments of the spine may be compressed.

- Do not use a chin cup or chin strap to secure a patient's head to a short spine board. A cup or a strap may prevent the patient from opening his mouth if he has to vomit.

- Do not pull the abdominal strap so tight that it causes injury or impedes respiration in a patient who is breathing only with his diaphragm.

- Do not position strap buckles directly over the sternum. They will interfere with hand placement if CPR becomes necessary.
- Do not place padding between the cervical collar and the spine board. In those rare instances when padding must be used to maintain the head in neutral alignment (as when an extremely heavy person is the patient or when the patient has a preexisting spinal deformity), place the padding behind the head.

IMMOBILIZING ADULTS WHO MAY HAVE A CERVICAL SPINE INJURY

Let's say that you and another rescuer have been assigned the task of immobilizing an injured driver. Disentanglement efforts have provided plenty of working room. You can work at the driver's side since the door has been pushed beyond the normal range of motion. The front seat has been moved all the way back, and the steering wheel will not be an impediment to the packaging operation. It's gone! The roof has been folded back, so your partner is able to stand upright behind the patient while supporting the head in neutral alignment. The driver has a rigid cervical collar in place.

Preparing the Patient

When you are ready to package the driver, don't just tilt him forward and insert the immobilizing device behind him. First:

- Remove his glasses (if he is wearing eyeglasses) and remove everything from his shirt and jacket pockets.

This seems like an inconsequential step. However, objects in a person's shirt or jacket pockets, especially bulky objects, can seri-

ously interfere with strapping operations. Next:

- Tell your partner what you are going to do so that he can continue to support the patient's head.
- Grip the driver's hips with your hands and carefully slide him forward on the seat 2 or 3 inches.

This important step is often overlooked by EMS and rescue personnel. If you simply tilt the driver's upper body forward at the waist, you probably will not be able to position the lower edge of the immobilizing device against the seat cushion as it should be. And even though the straps appear tight when you complete the packaging, the board may shift when you attempt to move the patient. If it does, the board's immobilizing effect will be lost.

Using a Short Spine Board

The short wood spine board that has been carried in ambulances and rescue vehicles for many years is rapidly being replaced by any of a number of vest-type devices. Nonetheless, every rescuer should still be able to immobilize an injured patient with a short board during multiple-casualty situations when all the vest-type devices are in use and only short boards are left.

While your partner continues to support the patient's head in neutral alignment:

- Angle the board and insert the head end between your partner's arms.
- Rotate the base of the board to a position between the patient and the seat back.
- Adjust the position of the board so that it is vertical with the midline of the board and in line with the patient's spine.
- Slide the board down until the lower edge is resting on the seat cushion.

The next step is to rig the lower torso strap.

- Use one hand to hold the buckle of a 9-foot strap against the patient's abdomen in line with the board's lower handholds.

With your other hand:

- Pass the end of the strap around the edge of the handhold on one side of the board.
- Carry the end through the handhold opening, up and over the patient's abdomen, and under the buckle to the opposite handhold opening.
- Pass the strap through the handhold opening.
- Carry the end of the strap around the handhold, up and over the patient's abdomen, and through the buckle.
- Buckle the strap snugly across the patient's abdomen.

The chest straps are rigged next. With one hand:

- Hold the buckle of the second 9-foot strap high on one side of the patient's chest, just below the clavicle.

With your other hand:

- Pass the end of the strap around the upper handhold on the same side and through the handhold opening.
- Carry the end of the strap under the buckle and across the patient's chest to the lower handhold on the other side.
- Pass the end of the strap through the handhold opening and around the handhold.
- Carry the end of the strap back across the chest and through the buckle.

Using both hands:

- Buckle the strap snugly across the patient's chest.
- Secure the patient's chest to the board by threading the third strap through

the handhold openings in the manner of an X.

- Fill any void between the person's back and the board with multi-trauma dressings, gauze pads, or soft roller bandage. Pad under the buckles.

Finally:

- Adjust the straps, if necessary, to assure that the patient is held snugly against the board.

This particular strapping technique offers an advantage over other methods. Since the ends of the straps are not passed from handhold to handhold behind the board, there is no need to move the board (and thus the patient) during the immobilization procedure. The next step is to secure the patient's head to the spine board.

While your partner continues to support the head:

- Snugly wrap 6-inch soft roller bandage three or four times around the patient's forehead and the headrest portion of the spine board.

The lower edge of the bandage should be just above the eyes, and the wraps should angle down from the forehead to the notches in the board.

- Wrap the bandage snugly three or four turns around the cervical collar and the headrest portion of the spine board.

To finish securing the head:

- Tape the end of the bandage to the last turn, or simply tuck the end under the last turn.

Cravats or tape can also be used to secure the patient's head to the board. Tape? Yes, tape! You can use wide adhesive tape or the 2-inch-wide fabric-backed duct tape that has so many other uses during a vehicle rescue operation. While it may sound strange, taping a patient's head to an immobilizing device is about the surest way to prevent possibly harmful movements.

To prevent the patient's arms and legs from moving during the subsequent removal operation:

- Place suitable padding between the patient's knees and tie his legs together with a cravat or several turns of roller bandage.
- Tie his wrists together with a cravat or several turns of roller bandage.

The patient is now packaged on the short spine board and ready for removal.

A short spine board is often difficult and sometimes impossible to use when a patient is on a bucket seat, the seat of a compact car or a seat with a deeply contoured back, or when wreckage interferes with positioning the board. A number of other devices are more suitable in those cases. Those that are uniquely different from each other are described here.

Using a Sherman Vest

Of all the upper-body immobilization devices, the Sherman Vest is the least expensive and the least complicated. Prepare the vest by removing the sliding headrest and accordion-folding the sides of the vest and the straps over the board. This will make positioning easier.

While another rescuer continues to support the person's head in neutral alignment:

- Angle the vest and insert the head end between your partner's arms.
- Rotate the lower portion of the vest to a position between the patient and the seat back.
- Adjust the vest until the midline of the vest is vertical and in line with the patient's spine, and push the vest down so that its lower edge is on the seat cushion.

Next:

- Join the lower straps snugly (but not tightly) across the patient's abdomen.
- Join one set of shoulder straps across the patient's chest, red to red or blue to blue.
- Then join the other set of chest straps.

When all three straps are in place:

- Be sure that all the straps are snug. Make adjustments, if necessary.

While your partner continues to support the patient's head:

- Slide the headrest over the top of the headrest.
- Position the headrest so the V is cradling the patient's head in an open airway position.
- Snugly wrap 6-inch soft roller bandage three or four times around the patient's forehead and the headrest portion of the spine board. The lower edge of the bandage should be just above the eyes, and the wraps should angle down from the forehead to the notches in the board.
- Wrap the bandage snugly three or four turns around the cervical collar.

To finish securing the head:

- Tape the end of the bandage to the last turn, or simply tuck the end under the last turn. Cravats can also be used to secure a patient's head to the Sherman Vest.

To prevent the patient's arms and legs from moving during the subsequent removal operation:

- Place a suitable padding between the patient's knees and tie his legs together with a cravat or several turns of roller bandage.
- Tie his wrists together with a cravat or several turns of roller bandage.

The injured patient is now packaged in the Sherman Vest and is ready for removal.

Using a Kendrick Extrication Device

The DYNA M.E.D. and the Ferno-Washington K.E.D. are the same devices. Dyna-Med is licensed to manufacture and market the device.

While your partner continues to support the patient's head in neutral alignment:

- Angle the device and insert the head end between your partner's arms.
- Rotate the base of the device to a position between the patient and the seat back until the midline of the device is aligned with his spine.
- Pull the leg straps down so that they are clear of the device, and position the device so it is snug under the patient's armpits.

Be sure the device is snug under the armpits. If it is not, it will slide up the torso during subsequent operations.
Next:

- Fasten the middle and bottom straps across the chest. They can be relatively tight without any impairment of chest movement.
- Fasten the middle and lower straps, but not so tightly that you cannot slide your fingers under them.

On each side of the body:

- Tie one end of a cravat to the handhold in the back of the vest.
- Pass the cravat over the shoulder; and
- Secure it to the top chest strap.

This step assures that the device will not slide down the torso while the patient is being removed from the vehicle.
Next:

- Pass the leg straps under the patient's legs and cross them at the crotch. Use

caution when positioning leg straps to avoid causing discomfort or injury to the external genitalia.
- Pass each strap to the opposite side of the patient and connect them to the appropriate fasteners.
- Secure the patient's head to the device with the Velcro head straps, self-adhering bandage, or tape.
- Fasten the top strap.
- Assure that all the straps are snug. Make adjustments, if necessary.

On each side of the body:

- Tie one end of a cravat to the handhold in the back of the vest.
- Pass the cravat over the shoulder; and
- Secure it to the top chest strap.

We have found this extra step helpful as it assures that the device will not slide down the torso while the person is being removed from the vehicle.

To prevent the patient's arms and legs from moving and perhaps interfering with the subsequent removal operation:

- Place padding between his legs and loosely tie them together with a cravat or roller bandage.
- Loosely tie the wrists together with a cravat or roller bandage.

The patient is now packaged and ready for removal.

Using Life-Support Products' Half Back Extrication/Lift Harness

The LSP Half Back is unique in that it can be used for the vertical movement of a spine-injured patient as well as for an upper-body immobilization device.

- Open the Half Back vest. Be sure the back stay is secured with the Velcro straps on the back of the Half Back.
- Remove the Velcro-attached head harness from the back stay, but do not

remove any straps from their pockets at this time.

- Position the Half Back behind the patient with the straps to the outside.
- Release the padded leg straps to expose the torso strap pockets on the patient's right side.
- Open the two torso strap pockets.
- Connect each color-coded buckle to the matching strap on the opposite side of the patient's chest. Leave the straps loose.
- Connect the other straps in the same manner.
- Adjust the shoulder straps to bring the sides of the vest up against the patient's underarms.
- Adjust the torso straps so the Half Back is snug against his torso.
- Remove a leg strap from the pocket on one leg pad and start the strap under his knee from the outside.
- Work the strap back and forth up the underside of the leg to the groin area using the webbing only to work the strap into position.
- Pull the foam-padded portion under the leg.
- Connect the buckle to the color-coded snap on the same side under the patient's arm, pulling the strap snugly.
- Repeat the procedure for the other leg.
- Disconnect the chin and forehead Velcro straps on the head harness.
- Place the patient's head in the foam V of the back stay.
- Move the foam V forward to meet the back of the patient's head.
- Hold the head harness by the two thin flaps with the Velcro facing toward the patient.
- Lay the center foam section of the head harness against the top of his head.
- Bring the two outer sections down on each side of the head and connect the Velcro flaps to the rear of the back stay so that the foam section is snug against the patient's head.

- Firmly adjust the forehead strap by using an arching motion over the patient's eyebrows so the head does not move.

When properly positioned, the forehead strap should connect to both outer sides of the foam head harness at the same angle. Be sure to hold the patient's head firmly in place to prevent movement when adjusting the forehead strap.

Finally:

- Adjust the chin strap snugly, but loose enough to allow the patient's mouth to open, if necessary.

IMMOBILIZING YOUNG CHILDREN WHO MAY HAVE A SPINAL INJURY

Thus far we have discussed procedures for using a variety of upper-body immobilization devices to package adults who may have a cervical spine injury. Unfortunately, many children are also injured in motor vehicle accidents. In fact, more than 1000 infants and children die in vehicle-related accidents every year, and tens of thousands more are injured.

Just as injured children in a pre-hospital setting should not be surveyed and cared for as "little adults," neither should injured children be immobilized in the same manner as adults, especially children 5 years old and younger. In a paper published in *The Journal of Bone and Joint Surgery*, John E. Herzenberg, M.D., Robert N. Hensinger, M.D., Dale K. Dedrick, M.D., and William A. Phillips, M.D., of the Section of Orthopedic Surgery, University of Michigan Hospitals at Ann Arbor, reported that using a standard backboard to immobilize the spine of an injured child may be dangerous.

The head of a young child is disproportionately larger than the rest of the child's body. An infant's head achieves 50% of adult size by age 18 months, while the chest requires 8 years to reach 50% of the size of an adult chest. Dr. Herzenberg and his colleagues found that when a young child is supine on a spine board, the neck may be flexed to the point where a cervical spine injury is aggravated. On the basis of their study, the doctors have recommended that children 5 years and younger be secured to a spine board in such a way that the cervical spine is in as near the neutral position as possible. A general rule of thumb for achieving that goal is to line up the external auditory meatus (the passageway that leads to the eardrum) with the shoulder. This can be accomplished by:

- Immobilizing the child on a spine board that has a recess for the occiput (the bulge of the back of the head); or
- Placing the child on a mattress that ends at the shoulders (the mattress being on a long spine board); or
- Placing a folded sheet or towel under the child's shoulder blades to lift the upper body slightly.

All these procedures will cause a slight extension of the neck that will result in proper cervical spine alignment and an open airway.

Using the Pedi-Immobilizer

The Pedi-Immobilizer is a device that can be used to immobilize a child (up to 60 pounds) who may have a spine injury. A very important feature of this device is the foam pad that can be placed under the child's shoulders to raise the upper body and thus place the spine in the neutral position.

A Pedi-Immobilizer can also be used to remove a child from a hard-to-reach place such as the floor of a car and to partially restrain an aggressive or hyperactive sick child.

As with any other procedure for immobilizing a patient who may have a spine injury, it is vitally important that a cervical collar be applied before the child is moved onto the immobilizer and that a rescuer maintain in-line manual stabilization until the child's head is secured in the immobilizing device.

While another rescuer maintains in-line manual stabilization on the child's head:

- Slide the Pedi-Immobilizer under the child until the head is centered between the Velcro pieces and the shoulders are even with the top part of the diagonal straps.

While the rescuer continues to maintain in-line stabilization on the child's head:

- Gently slide the foam pad under the child's shoulder blades.
- Check to see that the opening of the auditory canal is in line with the child's shoulders.

If the foam pad is not available, or if extra lift is needed because the child has a very prominent occiput:

- Use a folded towel, a folded sheet, or a multi-trauma dressing to achieve the desired upper-body lift.

When the child is properly positioned on the device:

- Fasten the diagonal straps, then the chest strap, and then the abdominal strap.

The chest strap can be loosened later if the local EMS protocol calls for the IV administration of a fluid or if further examination of the chest is necessary. The abdominal strap can be loosened if use of a pneumatic anti-shock garment is indicated.

If no medic is present:

- Check the child's ears for fluid and/or blood if you suspect head trauma.

Your observation at this time will be important since the child's ears will be concealed by the sections of the head immobilizer. Relate your observation to the medic when you transfer the child.

While the rescuer at the child's head continues to maintain in-line stabilization:

- Position the sections of the head immobilizer snugly against the sides of the child's head and press them against the Velcro pieces, one at a time.

When the head immobilizer is in place:

- Have the rescuer release the in-line stabilization.

Finally:

- Fasten the uppermost head strap across the child's forehead and the lower strap across the cervical collar.

The child is now secure in the Pedi-Immobilizer. Straps should be used to secure the immobilizer to the long spine board, and another set of straps should be used to secure the spine board to the ambulance stretcher.

An injured child who is strapped in a car seat can be transferred to a Pedi-Immobilizer in the following manner. You will need two assistants for the procedure.

- Direct one rescuer to hold gentle in-line manual stabilization on the child's head.

While the rescuer maintains manual stabilization:

- Apply a pediatric cervical collar.
- With the assistance of the other rescuer, carefully remove the car seat from the vehicle and carry it to an open area where the Pedi-Immobilizer and a long spine board have been placed.

While the rescuer continues to maintain stabilization on the child's head:

- Carefully remove the car seat straps from around the child.

Then:

- Slide the lower end of the Pedi-Immobilizer downward between the child and the car seat.

Obviously, the immobilizer cannot be positioned while in the stored position. The head immobilizer must be removed and the straps must be folded behind the board.

While the rescuer at the child's head continues to maintain in-line stabilization and with the assistance of the other rescuer:

- Tilt the car seat onto its back on the long spine board.
- Carefully slide the child onto the Pedi-Immobilizer until the shoulders are at the top of the diagonal straps and the head is centered between the Velcro pieces.
- Position the foam pad under the child's shoulder blades to achieve the proper spinal alignment. If necessary, use a folded towel, a folded sheet, or a multi-trauma dressing to achieve the desired upper-body lift.
- Join the diagonal straps, then the chest strap, and then the abdominal strap.

While the rescuer at the child's head continues to maintain in-line stabilization:

- Position the head immobilizer sections on the Velcro pieces to assure a snug fit.

When the head immobilizer is in place:

- Direct the rescuer to release manual stabilization on the head.

Finally:

- Fasten the uppermost head strap across the child's forehead and the lower strap across the cervical collar.

The child is now secure in the Pedi-Immobilizer. Straps should be used to secure the immobilizer to the spine board. Another set of straps should be used to secure the spine board to the ambulance stretcher.

Using a Pediatric Car Seat

All 50 states and the District of Columbia require that young children travel in car safety seats. These laws increase the probability that children, specifically those who weigh up to 40 pounds, will be properly restrained within the car seat in the event that the vehicle is involved in an accident. Being properly restrained within a federally approved car safety seat can dramatically reduce the potential for death or a life-threatening injury; however, there is no guarantee that the child will not sustain a spinal injury.

While car seats are available in many different styles, there are three basic types that rescuers and EMS personnel should be familiar with.

- The rear-facing infant seat that reclines for the young child who weighs under 20 pounds and is unable to sit up alone
- The larger forward-facing toddler seat
- The convertible seat that can be reclined and used facing rearward for infants and set upright and facing forward for an older child

The decision to immobilize a small child in a car seat should be based on an evaluation of the situation. It is recommended that the car seat be used for immobilization when:

- The child and the car seat are found properly restrained in the vehicle.
- An assessment of the child reveals no life-threatening condition.
- The restraint seat has not been damaged.
- There is a lack of specially designed pediatric equipment or a lack of adult equipment that can be modified for the child patient.

It is not recommended that a child be immobilized in a car seat when:

- The child is in severe respiratory distress or an assessment reveals other life-threatening conditions that may require better access to manage those conditions.
- If the restraint seat has lost its normal anatomical configuration or there are jagged metal edges because of damage to the tubular metal of the car seat.

The technique for car seat immobilization follows the basic principles of immobilizing an adult with a short spine board.

While another rescuer maintains the child's head in a neutral or slightly sniffing position:

- Strap or tape in place at the level of the child's hips a small folded blanket, a multi-trauma dressing, or a small pillow. Keep the padding low enough to maintain good visibility of the chest.
- Pad both sides of the child's head with a rolled towel, folded multi-trauma dressings, or a 6- to 8-inch length of stockinette that is filled with Styrofoam packing peanuts.
- Use adhesive tape applied in a criss-cross fashion from one side of the car seat to the other to secure the pads in place. Make sure that the tape contacts the padding and the child's forehead.

Sandbags of the type usually carried on an ambulance should *not* be used to stabilize the child's head. They will exert a downward force on the child's shoulders and may cause respiratory embarrassment or destabilize clavicular injuries.

When the child is properly immobilized in the seat:

- Carry the seat to the ambulance.

The safest place in the ambulance for the immobilized child is on the captain's chair or medic seat at the head end of the stretcher and facing the back door of the ambulance.

SUMMARY

The ninth phase of activity begins when mechanisms of entrapment have been removed from around patients and ends when they are packaged and ready for removal from the vehicles.

Packaging includes the reinforcement of dressings and bandages that were placed on major wounds during initial emergency care efforts, the dressing and bandaging of lesser wounds that will be hidden by immobilizing devices, at least the makeshift stabilization of skeletal injuries if the proper immobilization devices cannot be used, and immobilization of the spine.

While EMS personnel are usually responsible for packaging activities, rescuers should be able to secure patients to upper-body immobilization devices for times when medics are busy caring for individuals who have immediate life-threatening injuries. Thus squad members should know how to use the immobilization devices that are carried on local ambulances as well as those carried on the rescue unit.

While there is a different procedure for the various types of upper-body immobilization devices, the same two preparatory steps should be taken regardless of the device used:

First, items should be removed from the patient's shirt and jacket pockets. Pens, pencils, glass cases, cigarette packs, and other bulky objects can interfere with strapping operations.

Second, working space should be created between the patient and the seat by sliding the patient's hips forward just a few inches. Otherwise, the device may slip when the patient is moved, and if it does, the immobilizing effect will be lost.

A small child can be immobilized in a pediatric car seat when (1) the child and the car seat are found properly restrained in the vehicle, (2) an assessment of the child reveals no life-threatening conditions, (3) the restraint seat has not been damaged, and (4) there is no specially designed pediatric immobilization device or an adult device that can be modified for child patients.

It is not recommended that a child be immobilized in a pediatric car seat when (1) the child is in severe respiratory distress, (2) the child has a life-threatening condition that cannot be managed while the child is in the seat, (3) the car seat has lost its normal anatomical configuration, or (4) the seat has sharp metal edges because of damage.

When the decision is made to secure a child to a pediatric car seat, strapping should be done in such a way that the chest remains visible. Sandbags should not be used to stabilize the child's head; they will exert a downward force on the child's shoulders that can cause respiratory problems or destabilize clavicular injuries.

PHASE TEN

Removing Injured Patients from Vehicles

INTRODUCTION

The tenth phase of a vehicle rescue operation begins when packaging activities are completed and ends when the patients are outside the accident vehicles and ready for transfer to ambulances or helicopters.

In the Dark Ages of vehicle rescue, removing accident victims from wrecked vehicles was usually a dangerous operation—dangerous for the victims, that is! Few rescue squads had the tools or the expertise for disassembling cars; thus injured persons were often pulled through whatever openings existed in the wreckage. If a door could be opened, the resulting opening became an exitway. If doors could not be opened, people were pulled through window openings.

Today, removing windshields and rear windows, widening door openings, and folding back or removing the roof of a vehicle are common practices that create working space in which EMS and rescue personnel can carry out lifesaving and disentanglement operations. Removing mechanisms of entrapment from around occupants creates even

more working space in which rescue and EMS personnel can properly package injured patients with dressings, bandages, and immobilization devices.

Removing a patient involves much more than simply lifting and moving him from the vehicle, however. It must be accomplished in such a way that existing injuries are not aggravated nor new ones produced.

Following are suggestions that you and a team of rescuers might use in a number of situations.

REMOVING PATIENTS FROM A VEHICLE ON ITS WHEELS

An advantage of a vehicle remaining on its wheels is that patients can be removed in a number of ways.

- Ambulatory individuals can be assisted from vehicles.
- Immobilized, seated patients can be removed through door openings on long spine boards.

- Supine occupants and occupants who are lying on a side can be lifted from seats on long spine boards and scoop stretchers.
- Patients who are laying on the floor can be pulled through door openings onto long spine boards with rope slings.

On the other hand, the removal of patients from vehicles that are on a side or the roof must usually be accomplished with just one or two procedures.

Removing Patients Who Have Only Minor Injuries

When knowledge of the circumstances of an accident, observations of the vehicle and mechanisms of injury and entrapment, and a complete initial and focused exam and S.A.M.P.L.E. history assessment remove any doubt that a patient can stand and walk, there is no reason to rigidly immobilize a patient and secure him to a patient-carrying device.

A rescuer's ability to assist a minimally injured patient away from a vehicle will free EMS and rescue personnel for packaging and transfer procedures that require a number of people.

Keep in mind that a conscious individual who has complete control of his faculties has every right to refuse procedures that he may feel are unnecessary and perhaps embarrassing. This does not mean that you should simply shrug your shoulders and walk away when a patient insists that he can help himself. Stand at the door opening and offer your hand. Chances are that he will take it.

The One-Rescuer Assist

The following procedure should be used only when you are sure that a patient has no injuries that will be aggravated by twisting the body, standing, and walking.

- Help the patient to turn 90 degrees on the seat and put both feet on the ground.

- Pause for a moment until he becomes oriented.

Then:

- Assist him to the standing position.

When you are sure the individual can walk:

- Place the patient's arm around your neck.
- Grasp the hand of that arm with your nearest hand.
- Place your free arm around his waist.
- Help him walk to the ambulance. Let him set the pace.

Even the most rugged individual attempts to do more than he is able to after an accident. Be prepared to switch techniques from an assist to a drag or carry if the patient you are helping suddenly loses consciousness or if changing conditions necessitate the rapid movement of the patient.

Using a Long Spine Board

Even though there are no injuries other than superficial ones, a patient may not be able to function on his own. Much as he would like to leave the vehicle unassisted, the message from the brain does not get to the legs and feet! A minimally injured patient who does not require immobilization can be removed from a vehicle on a long spine board.

While you support the patient in the seated position with his legs in front of his body and his feet on the floorboard:

- Direct your partner to place padding between the patient's knees and loosely tie the legs together with a cravat or several turns of roller bandage.
- Then have your partner rig a long spine board with straps.

When the spine board is ready:

- Direct your partner to position one end of the board on the edge of the seat next to the patient's right hip.

- Have other rescuers outside the car support the board level with the ground.

While the other rescuers hold the spine board in position:

- Direct your partner to carefully lift the patient's legs to the seat while you turn him and lower him onto the board.

When the patient's upper body is on the spine board and while the other rescuers continue to hold the board horizontally:

- You and your partner slide the patient onto the board.

When the patient is fully on the board:

- Secure him to the board with the straps; then move him to the ambulance or helicopter.

Removing an Injured Patient Who Is Secured to an Upper-Body Immobilization Device

Unfortunately, many rescuers spend a great deal of time and effort carefully packaging a patient in a cervical collar and an upper-body immobilizing device and then try to remove him from the vehicle by simply man-handling him. They use straps, the hand-holds or handles of the immobilizing device, or no more than hands placed behind and under the patient.

Sometimes the techniques work, and the rescuers are able to deposit the patient onto an ambulance stretcher without incident. But many times the movement ends in disaster when the rescuers lose their footing because of debris or a slippery road surface or lose their grip and drop the patient. Such accidents can be avoided by using a long spine board.

Following is a procedure you might use to remove the packaged driver or left rear-seat passenger of a vehicle. Obviously, the procedure would be reversed to remove the right-side passengers.

- Have one rescuer stand behind the driver's seat and support the patient's head.
- Have another rescuer (let's call him your partner for the sake of clarity) slide onto the front seat next to the patient.

If there is a packaged person sitting on the right side of the front seat:

- Have your partner stand behind the seat next to the rescuer who is supporting the driver's head.

Next:

- Have other rescuers rest one end of a long spine board that has been rigged with straps on the seat next to the patient's left hip.
- Direct the rescuers to support the board in the horizontal position.

When the spine board is in position:

- Stand at the side of the board.
- Pass the end of a 9-foot strap (or a rolled sheet) under the patient's mid-thighs from left to right to your partner's right hand.
- Direct your partner to wrap the end of the strap around his right hand.
- Wrap the other end of the strap in your left hand.

On your command "lift":

- You and your partner lift the patient just a few inches from the seat with the strap.

While you and your partner support the patient with the strap:

- Direct the other rescuers to carefully slide the end of the long spine board fully under the person's buttocks.

On your command "lower":

- You and your partner gently lower the patient onto the board.

While the rescuers outside the vehicle continue to support the foot end of the board:

- Gently pivot the patient on the board while your partner lifts the patient's legs onto the seat.
- Then lower the driver's upper-body backward onto the board.

While your partner supports the patient's legs slightly above the board and the other rescuer holds the board level:

- You and another rescuer slide the patient onto the long board.

Then:

- Secure the patient to the board with straps.

When the patient is secure on the board:

- Carry him to the ambulance or helicopter or to a wheeled stretcher.

As you can imagine, the job of removing packaged persons from vehicles is made much easier by folding back or otherwise disposing of the roof and pushing the driver's door beyond its normal range of motion. The rescuers who are supporting the patient's head and assisting with the lift from positions behind the seat can stand up and move about as necessary, and the rescuer who helps slide the patient onto the board can do so while standing between the board and the door.

Let's change the scenario a bit and consider ways in which patients can be removed from vehicles when they are not nicely packaged and seated upright.

THE USE OF A ROPE SLING

To facilitate the removal of a patient from within or under a vehicle, we recommend using the endless rope sling as provided by Rescue Training Consultants. This sling assists in keeping the C-spine in line, while making it easier to slide the patient on a board.

Removing an Injured Patient Who Is Lying on a Vehicle's Seat

Because of the patient's position, it's highly unlikely that rescuers or EMS personnel will be able to secure him to an upper-body immobilization device without a lot of potentially harmful movement. The patient can be pulled onto a long spine board, however, with a minimum of spinal movement.

While other rescuers prepare the board with straps:

- Have another rescuer (we'll call him your partner) get into a position where he can support the patient's head.

Depending on the circumstances, your partner may have to stand at one side of the door opening or on the floor of the vehicle behind the front seat.

While your partner manually stabilizes the patient's head and neck:

- Put the patient in as anatomically straight a position as possible.
- Then lift the patient's shoulders slightly.

While you and your partner support the patient's head and shoulders in a slightly elevated position:

- Direct the other rescuers to slide one end of the spine board between the patient and the seat.

You will have to raise the patient far enough for the board to pass under his shoulder blades. If you don't, pulling the person onto the board will be difficult. The end of the board needs to be advanced only to the point where the edge is beyond the shoulder blades.

While the other rescuers hold the board level and your partner continues to support the patient's head:

- Lay the splice of the rope sling on the patient's chest at the level of his armpits.
- Carefully work the sling under the patient's arms so the rope is snug in his armpits.

If the sling is adjustable:

- Slide the adjustment rings along the rope toward the patient's head.
- Position the adjustment rings behind the cervical collar so that the parallel parts of rope will help support the patient's head as he is being pulled onto the board.

To prevent the patient's arms from moving when pull is exerted on the sling:

- Secure his hands together on his abdomen with a Velcro strap, a cravat, or several turns of soft roller bandage.

When you have the sling properly positioned and while your partner continues to support the patient's head and the other rescuers hold the board level:

- Move to the end of the board.
- Take a stance that will help you maintain your balance.
- Exert a smooth, steady pull on the sling to move the patient onto the spine board. Keep your hands as close to the board as possible to prevent the sling from lifting the patient's shoulders off the board.

When the patient is secure on the board:

- Carry him to the ambulance or a wheeled stretcher.

Removing an Injured Patient from the Floor Ahead of the Front Seat

Imagine that the driver of a four-door passenger car, the only occupant of the vehicle, is lying on his right side on the front-seat floor. His head is next to the right-side door opening and his feet are at the driver's door opening. The man either dove to the floor when he saw that the crash was inevitable, or he was propelled there when the crash occurred.

The front doors of the vehicle have been moved beyond their normal range of motion, the roof has been folded back, and the right side of the front seat has been pulled off the track and moved backward with a hand winch.

A rigid cervical collar has been applied by ambulance personnel, and a medic is kneeling at the right door opening supporting the man's head. Because of the close quarters, it is not possible to package him in an upper-body immobilizing device. Manhandling him from the vehicle is likely to aggravate injuries.

In this case, you can use a rope sling to pull him onto a long spine board with minimal movement of body parts.

- With the windshield removed, direct a rescuer to lay prone on the hood of the car and use his hands to support the patient on his side.

While he continues to support the patient's head:

- Have other rescuers insert a long spine board through the right side door just to the point where the end is resting on the transmission hump next to the patient (or the midpoint of the floor if there is no transmission hump).
- Direct them to hold the board level with the ground.

When the board is in place and while one rescuer continues to support the patient's head:

• You and the rescuer on the hood work together to ease the patient to a supine position on the board.

While the rescuer continues to support the patient's head and the rescuers support the foot end of the board:

• Lay the splice of the rope sling over the patient's arms and then work the sling under the patient's arms so that the rope is snug in his armpits.

If the sling is adjustable:

• Slide the adjustment rings along the rope toward the patient's head.
• Position the rings behind the cervical collar, if possible, so that the parallel parts of rope will help support the patient's head as he is being pulled onto the board.

To prevent the patient's arms from moving when pull is exerted on the sling:

• Secure his hands together on his abdomen with a Velcro strap, a cravat, or several turns of roller bandage.

When you have the sling properly positioned and while one rescuer continues to support the patient's head and the other rescuers hold the board level:

• Move to the other end of the board.
• Take a stance so you can maintain balance.
• Exert a smooth, steady pull onto the sling to move the patient onto the board. Remember to keep your hands as close to the board as possible to prevent the sling from lifting the patient's shoulders from the board.

When the patient is fully on the board:

• Place the board on the wheeled stretcher or the ground.

• Secure the patient to the board with straps.
• Further immobilize his head with cravats, tape, or an immobilization device appropriate for the board.
• Then transfer the patient to the ambulance.

Removing an Injured Patient from the Floor Behind the Front Seat

Suppose that in the scenario just completed, the driver is not the only patient. Suppose that a rear seat passenger is lying on the floor of the vehicle behind the front seat, thrown there upon impact.

Having seen the patient on the floor, you and the other rescuers would have created working space at the sides of the vehicle by either removing the rear doors or pulling down the B-pillars and doors together. Take one more step to create additional working space within the vehicle.

First:

• Have a rescuer apply a rigid cervical collar; next
• With the help of another rescuer, remove the rear seat of the vehicle.

Then:

• Have the rescuer take a position in the vehicle next to the patient's head.

While the rescuer supports the patient's head:

• Have rescuers place one end of the long spine board in the door opening near the patient's head.
• Have other rescuers support the foot end of the board and hold it level.

When the board is in position and while the rescuer continues to support the patient's head:

• Have the rescuers at the door opening gently lift and support the patient's head and shoulders.

Then:

- Direct the person who is supporting the foot of the board to slide the board under the patient's shoulders.

How far the rescuer inserts the board doesn't really matter as long as its end is beyond the patient's shoulder blades. Insertion may be easier if the board-handler raises the foot end of the board slightly.

While the rescuer at the foot end continues to hold the board in place:

- Have the rescuers who are kneeling at the door opening lay the splice of the rope sling over the patient's chest at the level of the armpits.

The rescuer holding the head may have to transfer the support of the patient's head to another rescuer at this point, in order to allow the positioning of the sling. The patient's head should be supported until he is secured to the backboard.

- Direct the rescuers to work the sling under the patient's arms so that the rope is snug in the armpits.

If the sling is adjustable:

- Have the rescuers slide the adjustment rings along the rope toward the patient's head and position them behind the patient's neck.

To prevent the patient's arms from moving when pull is exerted on the sling:

- Have a rescuer secure the patient's hands together with a Velcro strap, a cravat, or several turns of roller bandage.

When the patient is ready for moving:

- Have the rescuers at the door opening kneel by the side of the board and support it.

- Direct another rescuer to kneel at one side of the foot end of the board and have the rescuer who was supporting the foot end take a position at the opposite side.
- You stand at the foot end of the board with the free end of the sling.

When everyone is in position:

- Direct one rescuer to raise the patient's legs slightly.

Then:

- Pull the patient onto the board with the rope sling. Keep your hands as close to the board as possible to prevent the sling from lifting the patient's head as it pulls him onto the board.

While the two rescuers at the door opening support the board on the rocker panel:

- Secure the patient to the board with straps.

Then:

- Transfer the patient to the ambulance.

It will be necessary to make a third door when an injured person is lying on the floor behind the front seat of a two-door sedan. Making the opening and removing the rear seat will create as much working space as in a four-door sedan.

Removing an Injured Patient from Underneath a Vehicle That Is on Its Wheels

Let's return to the business of caring for the weekend mechanic who was trapped under his car when the makeshift supports collapsed.

The side of the car has been lifted and is supported by jacks or cribbing. The man has a rigid cervical collar in place. He has no penetrating wound of the chest or abdomen. If the man has a lower back injury or rib or extremity fractures, pulling him from under the car by his arms, shoulders, or clothing is likely to aggravate those injuries. In this case, use a rope sling to pull the man onto a long spine board with minimal movement of body parts.

- Instruct two rescuers to kneel, one on each side of the patient's head but with enough room between them for the spine board.

While they are getting into position:

- Have two other rescuers position the spine board on the ground with one end close to the patient's head and the board aligned with the patient's body.

When the rescuers at the patient's head are in position:

- Direct them to lift the patient's head, neck, and shoulders just a few inches from the ground.

While those rescuers support the patient:

- Have the other rescuers slide the board under the patient until the end is just past the shoulder blades.

When the board is in place:

- Instruct the rescuers at the side of the patient to gently lower the person onto the spine board.

Next:

- Have those rescuers lay the splice of the rope sling on the patient's chest at the level of his armpits.
- Tell them to work the sling under the person's arms so that the rope is snug in his armpits.

  If the sling is adjustable:

- Have the rescuers slide the adjustment rings along the rope parts toward the

patient's head and position the rings behind the cervical collar so the parallel parts of the rope will help support the head and prevent it from sliding on the board as he is pulled onto the board.

To prevent the patient's arms from moving when pull is exerted on the sling:

- Have the rescuers secure his hands in place over his abdomen with a Velcro strap, a cravat, or several turns of roller bandage, if possible.

When the sling is in place:

- Kneel at the foot end of the board in a position that will allow you to pull on the rope.

Kneeling is important; it will allow you to keep the sling flat against the board. If you pull on the rope while you are standing, the sling will form an angle with the board. Since the patient's head is supported by the sling, the angled rope will cause his head to tilt severely.

When you are in position and everyone is ready:

- Exert a smooth, steady pull on the sling to move the patient onto the board.

When the patient is on the board:

- Initiate lifesaving measures as necessary.

Before you have the rescuers move the board to the ambulance:

- Secure the patient with straps.

REMOVING INJURED PATIENTS FROM A VEHICLE THAT IS ON ITS SIDE

Let's say that a patient must be removed from a car that has rolled onto its side after the driver swerved sharply to avoid a collision. The car is stable in the vertical position, and the roof has been folded down to expose the entire interior of the vehicle. Sharp-edged roof stubs and sheet-metal edges have been shielded. Two medics are supporting the victim.

While it was possible for the medics to fit the victim with a rigid cervical collar, there was no way that they could package him with an upper-body immobilization device because of a position against the car door that could best be described as "crumpled." As is usually the case when a person cannot be rigidly immobilized, manhandling the victim from the vehicle will certainly aggravate injuries. In this case removal onto a long spine board with the help of a rope sling is indicated.

- Have four rescuers, two to a side, support a long spine board between them so it is at a right angle to the car and resting on the "hinge" that exists between the folded down roof section and the body of the vehicle.

When the rescuers with the board are in position:

- Have the medics lift and support the patient's head and shoulders in a slightly elevated position.

Then:

- Direct the rescuers to insert the end of the spine board carefully into the space between the patient and the car door.

Ideally, the end of the board should be inserted to a point just above the level of the patient's waist. If this is not possible, be sure that the end of the board is at least a few inches beyond the patient's shoulder blades.

When the board is in position:

- Instruct the medics to lower the patient's upper body gently onto the spine board.

Then:

- Have them make adjustments as necessary to center the person on the board.

Next:

- Instruct one of the medics or another rescuer to lay the splice of the rope sling over the patient's chest at the level of his armpits.

Then:

- Have the EMT or rescuer work the sling under the patient's arms so the rope is snug in his armpits.

If the sling is adjustable:

- Direct the medic or rescuer to slide the adjustment rings along the rope toward the patient's head and position the rings behind the cervical collar.

When the sling is in place on the patient:

- Lay the remainder of the sling along the length of the board.

To prevent the patient's hands from moving when pull is exerted on the rope sling:

- Have the rescuers secure them together with a Velcro strap, a cravat, or several turns of roller bandage.

When the sling is in position and the patient's hands are secured:

- Take a position at the end of the board. Be sure of a firm footing and take a stance that will allow you to remain balanced while you are pulling on the sling.

When everyone is ready:

- Exert a smooth, steady pull on the sling to move the patient onto the board.

Work in close concert with the medics; listen for their signals. Keep in mind that they will have to straighten the patient's legs gently while you are pulling the person onto the board.

When the patient is fully on the board and while the rescuers continue to hold the board steady:

- Secure the patient to the board with straps.

When the patient is secure:

- Have the rescuers carry him to the ambulance.

Let's say that instead of just one patient in the vehicle that is on its side, there are four, two in the front of the passenger compartment and two in the rear. The removal procedure is essentially the same as the one just described. Simply remove them one at a time, starting at the top of each stack and working down.

REMOVING INJURED PATIENTS FROM AN OVERTURNED VEHICLE

Many parts of a vehicle rescue operation are a bit more difficult when a vehicle is upside down: Fuel leaks are hard to stop; stabilization requires just about every piece of cribbing that the squad vehicle has, and then some; doors are hard to open because of the positions in which rescuers have to work; and disentanglement is usually troublesome because of the lack of working space. It stands to reason, then, that removal operations should be difficult as well, and they usually are!

The ideal way to remove injured patients from an overturned vehicle is to bring them out together on the roof after the vehicle has been lifted with medium- or low-pressure air bags and stabilized with pneumatic jacks. Not every squad has this capability, however.

Our best advice for removing people from an overturned vehicle is to pull them out one by one onto a long spine board with a rope

sling. A rescuer inside the vehicle will have to untangle arms and legs carefully as the operation progresses.

SECURING INJURED PATIENTS TO LONG SPINE BOARDS AND OTHER IMMOBILIZATION AND PATIENT-CARRYING DEVICES

An injured patient should be secured to a long spine board with at least three straps as soon as the individual is moved onto the board. Only in extreme cases when lives are at risk should an injured person be carried on a spine board (or other patient-carrying device, for that matter) without first being secured to the device.

Using a Conventional Long Spine Board

An injured patient can be secured to a conventional long spine board with 9-foot web straps in a number of ways. The straps could simply be passed around the stretcher and buckled over the patient, but this is not a good procedure. Since the straps are under the board's runners, they could become snagged and displaced and even damaged when the board is slid over a rough surface.

When dangling straps are not likely to be in the way of rescuers or to become snagged during a removal operation, they can be threaded through handholds in the board. One end is passed through a handhold from underneath, carried across the board to the opposite handhold, and passed through the handhold from the top down. When the patient is on the board, the ends of the straps are buckled and tightened.

A third strapping technique can be utilized when dangling straps will be a problem for rescuers working in close quarters. In this technique, the patient is moved onto the board and the buckle is laid on the patient with the quick-release device facing up. While one rescuer holds the buckle in place, another rescuer passes the end around and through a handhold from the bottom up, carries the strap over the patient (under the buckle), passes the end through the opposite handhold from the top down, carries the end of the strap around the handhold, joins the end with the buckle, and tightens the strap to secure the patient. A good rule to remember is to strap across the upper chest, the pelvis, and the thighs.

Several commercially available long spine boards can be used to remove injured patients from vehicles in the ways just described. In each case, assume that:

- The patient is supine and centered on the board.
- A rigid cervical collar is in place.
- The board is resting on level ground.
- A rescuer is supporting the patient's head throughout the strapping operation.

Using a Scoop Stretcher

A scoop stretcher can be used to remove and carry an injured patient from the front or rear seat of a vehicle, from under a vehicle (if there is sufficient working space), and from the ground (as when a patient has been thrown from a vehicle or when a pedestrian has been struck). Following is the procedure that you might use with another rescuer.

Before doing anything else:

- Be sure that the stretcher halves are locked together and that the system is complete. In addition to the scoop stretcher, there should be three one-piece, 7-foot patient-restraint straps and three strap retention clips.

With your partner at the head of the stretcher and you at the foot:

- Place the stretcher next to the patient and align the head panels with the person's head.

To adjust the stretcher to fit the patient:

- Loosen the length-adjustment collets by rotating them clockwise (as you view them from the foot of the stretcher).

The next step is to extend the length of the stretcher, if necessary.

While your partner holds the head end of the stretcher so that the panels remain aligned with the patient's head:

- Pull on the foot end of the stretcher until the center of the foot panels are aligned with the patient's feet.

Then:

- Tighten the adjustment collets by turning them clockwise.

To prepare the stretcher:

- Release the patient-restraint strap buckles and lay the straps on the ground away from the stretcher. Be sure that the straps are out from underneath the stretcher.

Scissors-type Application. Because of the space needed, use of this procedure may be limited to situations where an accident victim is on the ground or roadway.

- Open the foot end of the stretcher by depressing both sides of the latch release.

The scoop latches are designed for safety and will release only when both scoop latch fingers are depressed together. The other end latch will act as a hinge as the parts of the stretcher are moved away from each other.

- Lift the stretcher and separate the ends far enough to allow you and your partner to lower it around the patient without making contact.
- Lower the stretcher to the ground with the halves on each side of the patient. Be sure that the head panels are aligned with the patient's head.

- Carefully begin to close the scoop by bringing the open latch sections together.
- Continue to close the scoop until the sides of the stretcher contact the patient. Do not attempt to close the scoop at this time.

While your partner lifts and rolls the patient slightly onto one side:

- Move the half of the stretcher that is under the lifted portion of the patient until that half is in proper alignment.

Then:

- Direct your partner to lower the patient gently onto the properly positioned stretcher half.
- Repeat the procedure to get the other half of the stretcher in proper alignment under the patient.

The slight lifting and rolling of the patient will allow you to position the halves of the stretcher under the patient without any binding or pinching.
    When the stretcher halves are properly aligned under the patient:
- Join the latch parts. Be sure that the latch fingers snap into the locked position.

Two-Piece Application. This procedure might be used when space limitations prevent you from opening the stretcher like a pair of scissors. Both halves of the stretcher must be completely separated before starting the procedure.
    With your partner at the head end and you at the foot end:

- Place the two halves of the stretcher on the ground while maintaining the alignment of the head panels with the patient's head.

With a gentle rocking action:

- Ease the stretcher parts under the patient. Keep the latches in alignment to facilitate their connection.
- Snap the foot end latches together and then the head end latches.

After snapping both latches closed and verifying that both have closed completely:

- Have your partner lift the head end of the stretcher just far enough for you to reach under the stretcher for the lower halves of the straps.

The stretcher should not be lifted any more than is absolutely necessary; otherwise, the patient will slide toward the foot.
    When the lower portions of the straps are in place under the stretcher:

- Instruct your partner to lower the head end of the stretcher.

Then:

- Buckle the upper and lower portions of the straps.

Be sure that the straps connect only to the corresponding buckles; do not cross them. When properly applied, the straps should be straight across the patient and wrapped completely around the patient and the stretcher.
    When the straps are in place:

- Tighten each strap by applying tension to the loose end while holding the buckle.

Proper tensioning is important. Pulling on the loose end of the straps without holding the buckle will apply undue pressure to the patient.
    If you elect to lift and carry a scoop stretcher by the ends:

- Do not lift while grasping the latch; instead

- Use the handhold spaces provided on each side of the latch.

If you elect to lift and carry the stretcher by the sides:

- Position yourself and your partner more toward the upper body of the patient than the middle of the stretcher. Thus it is more likely that the person will be balanced when you lift the stretcher.
- Do not lift with one hand on the adjustment collets. To do so may loosen them and allow the stretcher to lengthen; instead
- Get a firm grip on the side rails of the stretcher.

On your signal:

- Lift with your legs to avoid back strain.

Scoop stretchers are manufactured with various adjustment mechanisms; some have spring pin connectors and others have threaded collets. This is another reason that you should be familiar with the equipment you have available.

SUMMARY

The tenth phase of activity begins when patient packaging operations are complete and ends when all patients have been removed from the accident vehicles.

Patients must be removed from vehicles in such a way that existing injuries will not be aggravated and new ones will not be produced. This is why the steps of creating working space and exitways in a vehicle are so important.

Patients can be removed from an upright vehicle in a number of ways. An ambulatory individual who has only minor injuries can be assisted from the vehicle. An immobilized seated patient can be removed through the adjacent door opening on a long spine board. A patient who is lying on a seat can be removed on a long spine board or scoop stretcher. A patient who is on the floor of the vehicle can be pulled onto a long spine board with a rope sling.

Patients can be removed from a vehicle that is on its side with a long spine board and a rope sling. Patients who are piled on top of each other can be removed one at a time from the top down.

The ideal way to remove patients from an overturned vehicle is to separate the roof from the body of the vehicle and pull the occupants free on the cut roof section. If tools are not available for the job, the patients can be pulled through door and window openings onto a long spine board with a rope sling.

Regardless of the manner in which they were removed from a vehicle, patients should be firmly secured to a rigid patient-carrying device as soon as possible. If this cannot be accomplished in the vehicle, it should be done as soon as they are clear of the wreckage.

PHASE ELEVEN

Transferring Injured Patients to Ambulances

INTRODUCTION

The eleventh phase of a vehicle rescue operation begins when injured patients have been properly packaged and removed from the vehicles.

When an accident has occurred on smooth, level ground and it has been possible to park the ambulance at the edge of the minimal danger zone, the transfer of an injured person from a wrecked vehicle to the ambulance may involve nothing more than carrying a full-body immobilization device or rolling a wheeled stretcher.

When a vehicle is surrounded by debris, however, or when it is situated on rough terrain or at the bottom of a steep hill, transfer may be a difficult task that requires rescuers to perform specific procedures with specific equipment.

Before we discuss any special procedures, let's have a few words about what has become a usual, albeit dangerous, technique: moving a loaded multi-level wheeled ambulance stretcher in the fully raised position.

Moving a multi-level stretcher in the fully raised position may be acceptable when the surface under the wheels is a smooth, absolutely level hospital corridor. But when the surface is cracked concrete, uneven asphalt, or soft or uneven ground, or when a road surface is littered with debris, to wheel a patient on an ambulance stretcher in the fully raised position is to invite disaster. One wheel passing over a crack in the pavement or a stone can wrench the stretcher from rescuers' hands, and, because of the high center of gravity, tipping over is likely. The impact of a 3-foot fall will certainly aggravate injuries even when a person is rigidly immobilized and, in fact, may even be fatal.

So, be extremely careful when you are moving a patient on an ambulance stretcher in the "up" position. You should have at least four hands holding the stretcher, and more if the patient is obese or the route is extremely rough. Be extremely careful when moving a stretcher in the "down" position as well. Even without a patient on the stretcher, it is easy to injure your back when working in this "hunched over" position. The use of handles and straps found on most stretchers will allow you to move the stretcher while in an upright position.

TRANSFERRING AN INJURED PERSON OVER DEBRIS OR ROUGH TERRAIN

The following hypothetical accident situation demonstrates the need for rescue personnel to know special transfer procedures.

In an effort to beat the traffic light change, the driver of an 18-wheel dump truck entered the intersection and attempted to make a left turn at too great a speed. The rig rolled onto its right side and crushed the front end of a car that was stopped in the opposing lane for the red light. When the rig turned onto its side, 44,000 pounds of baseball-sized stones spilled from the trailer and flowed around the cars like a viscous fluid. The car has been opened up, mechanisms of entrapment have been displaced, and the driver is packaged on a long spine board and ready for transfer to an ambulance.

The layer of stones, as much as 12 inches deep in some places, makes walking near the vehicles both difficult and dangerous. Several rescuers fell and suffered bruises during the gaining access and disentanglement operations. The risk of squad members dropping the stretchers while carrying them to the ambulances is high.

You are responsible for transferring the patient to the ambulance. You must utilize a patient movement procedure whereby emergency service personnel can pass the stretcher from hand to hand while they maintain a safe and firm footing.

The Eight-Person Shift

At least eight individuals are needed for the procedure. If there are not enough rescuers and firefighters immediately available for the job, you will need to either call in additional emergency service units or recruit able-bodied, apparently responsible persons from the ranks of the spectators.

While the stretcher handlers are moving into position:

• Direct EMS personnel to move their wheeled ambulance stretcher to the edge of the area made dangerous by the debris.

When you have at least eight stretcher handlers:

• Form the individuals into two lines that lead away from the vehicle to the ambulances or where the wheeled stretcher is located. The lines must be parallel, but they need not be straight.
• Direct the handlers in each line to stand shoulder-to-shoulder and face the handlers in the other line.
• Instruct the stretcher handlers to shuffle their feet or do whatever else is necessary to obtain and maintain a firm and safe footing.
• Tell the handlers that they will be moving the stretcher from hand to hand while they maintain a firm footing.
• Emphasize the importance of not shifting their feet while supporting the stretcher.
• Explain that as soon as the stretcher passes a pair of handlers, those individuals should leave the line and quickly take a new position at the head of the line.

When everyone is in position and understands your instructions:

• Have the first pair of handlers pull the end of the stretcher from the vehicle. It doesn't really matter whether the patient is removed head first or feet first.
• Direct the handlers to continue to ease the stretcher from the vehicle until it is supported by six people.

When all six people have a firm grip on the stretcher:

• Direct them to stand and lift the stretcher to the level of their shoulders.

Keeping the stretcher at this height is important. It will allow the handlers to support and move the injured person with minimal back strain.

When the six handlers are supporting the stretcher stationary at the level of their shoulders:

- Take a position behind one line of handlers from which you can direct the stretcher movement operation.

When you are in position:

- Instruct the handlers to pass the stretcher from hand to hand.
- Reemphasize that they should not move their feet; to do so may cause them to lose their footing.

As soon as the trailing end of the stretcher clears the pair of handlers closest to the car:

- Tell those two individuals to leave their position and move to the head of the line.
- Continue to leap frog the handlers in this manner until the stretcher is away from the debris area.

When the stretcher is out of the debris area:

- Direct the handlers to lower the stretcher onto the wheeled ambulance cot.
- Repeat the procedure until all injured persons have been removed.

This maneuver can be accomplished with more than eight bearers, but it should not be attempted with fewer than six since only four people will be supporting the stretcher at any given time. If one person loses his footing and thus loses his grip on the stretcher, it's likely that the sudden imbalance will cause the other three bearers to lose their footing and grip as well.

The eight-person shift can also be used to move stretchers over ice-covered or muddy ground, over obstacles, or in any other level-ground situation where rescuers cannot safely carry a stretcher because of treacherous footing.

TRANSFERRING AN INJURED PERSON UP A MODERATELY STEEP HILL

Here's a problem that requires a different situation. A car has veered off the road, rolled down a hill on its wheels, and struck a tree with sufficient force for the occupants to be injured. The occupants have been removed from the vehicle and are immobilized on a variety of patient-carrying devices. They are ready to be moved to the ambulances that are parked on the road at the top of the hill.

Just because a vehicle is at the bottom of a hill does not mean that the transfer of an injured person will be overly difficult. Six stretcher bearers should be able to climb a gently sloping hill with ease. It is when the angle of the slope is so great that a hill cannot be safely climbed by a stretcher team that special procedures are required.

Using People to Move the Stretcher

Passing a stretcher from hand to hand in the manner of the eight-person shift just described is a quick and easy technique to use when a number of people are available to help and when footing and balance can be maintained on the hill while standing at a right angle to the slope.

If you have enough people to move the stretcher(s) with just one or two leap frog maneuvers, take advantage of your good fortune. Have the two lines of people remain in place after the last stretcher has been moved to the top of the hill. Then have the people move the rescue equipment up the hill hand to hand. A lot of tired rescuers will be forever grateful!

Using Ropes for Guidelines

Let's say that when you arrived on the scene you decided that the hill was a bit too steep to descend without assistance, so you had squad members rig two descent lines. If they rigged the ropes correctly—about 6 feet apart and high enough on the anchor points at the top of the hill to assure that they will be about 4 feet from the ground when under tension—the descent lines can be used as ascent lines as well.

You will need eight people for this procedure. Two will anchor the descent lines and six will carry the stretcher.

- Position the two anchor persons at the bottom of the hill.
- Instruct them to form a loop in each end of the ascent lines with a figure-eight knot or bowline.
- Have each anchor person step into the loop, face uphill, position the loop against his buttocks, and lean back to put tension on the rope.

When the anchor persons are in position:

- Direct the stretcher bearers to carry the stretcher to the bottom of the hill.
- Have them pass between the ascent lines.

When the stretcher bearers are in position:

- Instruct them to face uphill and grip the rope with their free hand.

When everyone is in position and the lines are taut:

- Take a position alongside one of the ropes, and
- Tell the stretcher bearers to start their ascent.

Movement is accomplished when each stretcher bearer grips the rope, pulls himself forward, acquires balance, loosens his grip, slides his hand forward, grips the rope again, and pulls himself forward and thus up the hill. Your close coordination of these actions assures smooth movement.

If anyone loses his grip on the rope and slips during the movement:

- Have everyone stop and grip the rope until the person regains his footing and grips the rope again.

When the team is at the top of the hill:

- Have the bearers carry the stretcher to the ambulance.

Using a Tow/Haul Line

When a hill is too slippery to climb even with guidelines, a third rope can be used to pull the stretcher up the hill while six bearers support the stretcher and pull themselves up with the two guided ropes.

The rescue and EMS personnel who have been freeing the patients from the vehicle will serve as stretcher bearers.

- Instruct two rescuers to take positions as anchor persons at the bottom of the hill.
- Tell them to keep the lines taut by leaning against a loop formed in the end of each rope.

It should be noted here that if trees or other suitable anchor points are available at the bottom of the hill, rescuers will not be required to anchor the lines with their bodies for this or the preceding procedure. The ropes can be tied to the anchor points.

While the anchor persons are getting into position:

- Have the stretcher team move the stretcher to the bottom of the hill near the anchor persons.

As soon as one of the descent/ascent lines is taut:

- Pull yourself up the hill by means of the rope.

When you are at the top of the hill:

- Acquire a rope, a length of webbing, a carabiner, and a single-sheave pulley from the rescue unit.

- Recruit five or six rescuers and firefighters (and spectators, if necessary) to man the tow line.
- Have the tow line team members uncoil the rope and lay it on the ground so it will lay out freely as the end is carried down the hill.

With webbing and a carabiner:

- Secure the pulley to an anchor point between and level with the two anchor points for the descent/ascent lines.

When the pulley is in place:

- Pass one end of the tow line through the pulley.
- Form a loop in the end of the tow line with a figure-eight knot or a bowline.

Next:

- Position one rescuer at the top of the hill where he will be able to see the stretcher and the tow line handlers. This rescuer will be the tow line team leader.
- Have the tow line crew members pick up the rope.

When the tow line crew is ready:

- Step into the loop that you have formed in the end of the tow/haul line.
- Have the line handlers lower you down the hill.

When you are at the bottom of the hill:

- Direct the stretcher team to take a position between the taut ascent lines.

When the stretcher is in position:

- Secure the end of the tow/haul line to the head of the stretcher.
- Have the stretcher bearers grip the ascent line with their free hand.

When the stretcher bearers are ready:

- Signal the tow/haul line team leader to direct the team members to haul on the line slowly and thus pull the stretcher up the hill.

The tow/haul line team leader will have to watch the ascent closely to assure that the line handlers do not move the rope so quickly that the stretcher bearers will not be able to keep up.

If a stretcher bearer loses footing during the ascent:

- Stop the operation until the person can regain footing and get a new grip on the rope.

When the stretcher is at the top of the hill:

- Untie the tow/haul line; and
- Have the bearers carry the stretcher to an ambulance.

This is the simplest of towing/hauling techniques. If there are not enough people for the task or if the hill is quite steep or very slippery, mechanical advantage can be gained by threading the end of the line through the pulley at the upper anchor point, then through another pulley that has been secured to the head of the stretcher, and then securing the end of the tow/haul line to the anchor point.

MOVING A STRETCHER UP A STEEP HILL BY MEANS OF ROPES AND LADDERS

Let's consider a situation where an injured person must be transferred from the bottom of a hill to the top of the hill where an ambulance is located. In this case the hill is too steep for any of the hand carries or rope-assisted carries, so firefighters have placed ladders against the side of the hill as the means for rescue personnel to descend to the wreckage. You are in charge of the operation.

Any number of rigid patient-carrying devices can be used for this operation; however, the plastic basket stretcher is best suited to the task. Depending on whether it will be moved horizontally or vertically, this stretcher will slide either on the beams of the ladder or on the rungs between them.

A rope pad can be wrapped around the rung over which the hoisting line is passed. The pad will prevent the rope from being damaged by metal spurs and sharp metal edges.

EVACUATING INJURED PERSONS BY MEDIVAC

Helicopter medical evacuation was first widely used during the Korean conflict. There, and later in Vietnam, helicopters carried seriously wounded military personnel from front-line aid stations to Mobile Army Surgical Hospitals (M.A.S.H.) where "save" rates often exceeded 90%.

The first civilian hospital-based air medical team was established in Denver, Colorado, in 1972. Today, more than 160 helicopter programs serve many urban and rural areas of the United States. Modern air ambulances are safe and efficient, and their crews provide a high level of pre-hospital emergency care.

As helicopter ambulance programs continue to grow, so does the number of emergency medical service personnel who use them. More EMS providers than ever before can request helicopter transportation of seriously sick and injured persons. For a helicopter program to be absolutely safe and effective, however, it must be integrated into the local and regional EMS system.

This section has been prepared to acquaint you with helicopter ambulance operations in general. If your EMS system has a helicopter service or if it utilizes a helicopter service from another EMS system, attend an orientation program as part of your training course. Then become completely familiar with the standard operating procedures developed for the system, and follow those pro-

cedures when you need a helicopter at the scene of a vehicle accident.

Medivac-Helicopter Ambulances

The single-engine Bell Long Ranger is the rotary-wing aircraft most often used for helicopter evacuations. Long Rangers are usually configured and equipped for one patient. As helicopter programs have grown and expanded, twin-engine helicopters have become the standard. Among the larger aircraft that are popular now are the Aerospatiale Dauphin, the MBB BK117, the B0105, the Sikorsky S76, the Bell 222, and the Ball 412.

Size, rotor lengths, loading systems, medical interiors, and other features vary among helicopters. Thus you should become familiar not only with the make and model that usually flies within your EMS response area but also with helicopters that might be called into your area in the event of a multiple-casualty incident.

Helicopter Medical Personnel— Flight Medics

Hospital-based helicopters generally carry two advanced life-support personnel. One is usually a registered nurse; the other may be a flight-medic, another nurse, or a physician. Specialty teams for neonates, organ donors, and complicated cardiac patients are also available in some areas. Approximately 60% of helicopter operations involve transferring patients from one hospital to another. The remaining 40% are responses to the locations of sick or injured persons. These are called scene pickups. It is during these responses that rescuers assist helicopter personnel with landing zone coordination, radio communications, patient packaging, and transfer to the aircraft.

Indications for Helicopter Transport

Obviously, not every sick or injured person needs to be transported to a medical facility by helicopter. While local protocols vary, it is usually the patients that fit within the following categories who are considered for helicopter transportation when an advanced life support (ALS) unit is unavailable or unable to reach the location of the patient within a reasonable time, and when travel time to a medical facility where the patient can be cared for properly will exceed 20 minutes.

Consider helicopter transportation when any patient exhibits:

- Severe respiratory distress
- Blood pressure of 90 systolic or less
- Heart rate of less than 60 in an adult
- Injuries requiring special care facilities (major burns, smoke inhalation, amputations, etc.)

Your ability to recognize potentially lethal mechanisms of injury is important. Consider an injured person to be a prime candidate for helicopter transportation when the individual has been:

- In a motor vehicle that collided with another vehicle or object at a speed greater than 30 miles an hour
- In a motor vehicle where another person was killed
- In a motor vehicle that rolled over
- In a motor vehicle that exhibits passenger compartment intrusion of greater than one foot
- Ejected from a vehicle
- Thrown from a motorcycle
- Trapped in a vehicle during a lengthy extrication procedure

The nature of the injury should also be considered when evaluating a patient for helicopter transportation. A patient should be transported to a medical facility quickly when he or she has:

- A penetrating injury to the head, neck, or torso
- Severe blunt trauma to the head, neck, or torso

- Uncorrected complete or partial airway obstruction
- An amputation above the wrist or ankle
- Evidence of intrathoracic injury such as chest wall bruising or tenderness, absence of breath sounds, or asymmetrical expansion of the chest
- A head injury with an altered or decreasing level of consciousness
- Suspected fractures with absent distal pulses and/or a cold or cyanotic extremity
- Major burns, and major burns associated with injuries

Seriously injured young children are often transported by helicopter, as are persons over the age of 65 years who have multiple injuries.

A number of medical problems warrant helicopter transportation when an ALS unit is not available or when ground travel time is likely to be long, including:

- Chest pain with hypotension, respiratory distress, or cardiac dysrhythmias with or without cardiac history
- Suspected intracerebral emergency with altered level of consciousness or localizing neurologic findings
- Overdose with respiratory depression or seizures
- Obstetrical emergency or complicated delivery
- Suspected or diagnosed aortic aneurysm with severe pain, hypotension, pallor, or shock
- Uncontrolled seizure activity
- Severe respiratory emergency [asthma, chronic obstructive pulmonary disease (COPD), airway obstruction] with respiratory distress

Other times when rapid helicopter transportation may be instrumental in saving a life are when a sick or injured person is in a remote or inaccessible location, in hazardous material emergencies, and in multiple-casualty incidents.

The above guidelines are offered as an example of the types of patients that may require medivac transportation. Become familiar with the medivac guidelines in your area, so you will be able to use them in determining if a helicopter should be utilized.

Your Role as a Rescuer in Helicopter Ambulance Operations

While you may not participate in the actual transportation of an injured person to a medical facility, there is much you can do to prepare the person for transfer. You must initiate basic emergency care measures, and you may have to supervise the preparation or assist with the preparation of a landing zone suitable for the helicopter.

Preparing a Patient for Transport by Air

Following are some of the steps that you or a medic might take to prepare the patient for transportation:

- Extricate the person in the safest and most expeditious way.
- Apply a rigid cervical and upper-body immobilization device.
- Assure an open airway by inserting an endotracheal tube (ETT), or other airway device.
- Ventilate and suction the patient as necessary, and administer oxygen.
- Dress and bandage wounds and immobilize skeletal injuries.
- Put the patient in a pneumatic anti-shock garment.
- Completely immobilize the patient on a rigid, full-body patient-carrying device.

If the weather is cold:

- Protect the patient from hypothermia.
- Place the patient in a warm ambulance until the helicopter arrives.

If you are trained and authorized to do so:

- Start one or two 14- or 16-gauge IV infusions and draw blood samples. Be sure that the IV lines are well secured.

If your patient has a medical problem and is not injured, in addition to packaging the person for transportation:

- Obtain a history and the name of the patient's physician, and gather any medications.

An easy way to obtain a history is to use the letters S.A.M.P.L.E. as a guide:

S= Signs and symptoms
A= Allergies
M= Medications
P= Pertinent past history
L= Last oral intake (solid or liquid)
E= Events leading up to chief complaint

Preparing the Landing Zone

Contrary to popular opinion, helicopters do not swoop down from the sky onto any piece of ground, scoop up a sick or injured person, and zoom off to a medical facility. They sit down on specially selected and prepared areas designated as landing zones.

Following are suggestions that you might follow if you are in charge of preparing a landing zone for a helicopter ambulance.

- First, select a landing zone appropriate to the size of the helicopter.

During daylight hours, the landing zone for a small helicopter landing should be a square with 60-foot sides. At night the square should have 100-foot sides. The landing zone for a medium-size helicopter landing in daylight should be a square with 75-foot sides. The square should have 125-foot sides at night. A large helicopter needs even more room. The landing zone should be 120 feet square, and at night the sides should be increased to 200 feet.

The landing surface should be flat and firm and clear of people, vehicles, stumps, brush, posts, large rocks, and obstructions such as trees, poles, and wires. Rescuers and firefighters should pick up loose debris that might be blown up into the rotor system.

The landing zone should be at least 50 yards from the accident vehicles, if possible, so that noise and rotor wash will not be a problem for rescuers.

If the helicopter will land on a divided highway, traffic must be stopped in both directions even though the aircraft will land on only one side of the highway.

Next:

- Consider the wind direction when selecting a landing site.

Helicopters usually land and take off into the wind; they make vertical descents and ascents only when it is absolutely necessary. If the approach and departure paths have obstructions such as wires, poles, antennae, and trees, notify the crew about wind direction and obstructions by radio.

- Mark the touchdown area.

Each corner of the square touchdown area should be marked with a highly visible device (such as a flag, flares, or surveyor's tapes) during daylight hours and a flashing or rotating light at night. Flares can be used day or night, but only in areas where sparks from the flares will not ignite dry vegetation.

- Designate the wind direction.

Place a fifth warning device on the upwind side of the square to designate the wind direction.

- Create a safe environment.

Spectators should be kept at least 200 feet from the touchdown area and emergency service personnel who are not directly involved with the landing should remain at least 100 feet from the touchdown zone. A fire apparatus should be standing by in a safe place, and if the ground is extremely dusty, firefighters should wet down the touchdown area.

Personnel who will be near the helicopter when it touches down should be wearing protective clothing and safety goggles; debris dislodged by the rotor wash can blow under pull-down helmet shields. Helmet chin straps should be securely fastened. Baseball caps should not be worn; they can be blown from the wearer's head and drawn into the rotor system.

- Light the touchdown area at night.

Low-beam headlights, vehicle-mounted spotlights and floodlights, portable floodlights, and hand lights can be used to define the touchdown area at night. All other non-essential lights should be turned off, and no lights should be directed toward the helicopter. White lights can ruin a pilot's night vision and temporarily blind him. Prohibit photographers from using flashbulbs and video lights during landings and takeoffs.

- Assign personnel to keep spectators and non-essential emergency service personnel from wandering into the landing zone at any time until the helicopter departs.

Even when they have been asked to remain in a safe place, spectators and non-essential emergency service personnel have a tendency to approach the landing zone as a helicopter approaches, if for no other reason than to get a better view. Properly dressed (and thus easily identifiable) rescuers or firefighters should be assigned to locations around the landing zone to keep people from wandering into the danger area. These people should keep their eyes on the periphery of the landing zone, not on the helicopter.

When you see the helicopter:

- Assign one person to guide the pilot to a safe landing.

The guide should wear eye protection, and he should stand at the location of the wind direction marker with his back to the wind and facing the touchdown area. He should stand with his arms raised over his head to indicate the landing direction. As the helicopter turns into the wind, the ground guide should begin to direct the approach with appropriate hand signals while maintaining eye contact with the pilot.

Ground Operations

Safety remains the prime consideration even when the helicopter has landed.

- Do not approach the helicopter, and do not allow anyone else to approach it. The crew will leave the aircraft and approach you when it is safe to do so.
- Have the landing zone crew members prohibit smoking anywhere within 50 feet of the aircraft.

If the helicopter is to remain running while at the scene:

- Station a landing zone crew member in a position to protect the rear of the helicopter to prevent anyone from approaching the tail rotor.

The tail rotor of a helicopter is generally 3 to 6 feet from the ground (if the ground is level) and spins so fast that it cannot be seen. Someone who inadvertently walks into a spinning rotor can be killed.

When the helicopter is ready for loading:

- Give the helicopter crew only the people they need to move the patient to the aircraft and assist with the loading.
- Instruct those people to follow the directions of the crew members without question.

If you are part of the transfer and loading team or if you will accompany the team to the helicopter:

- Approach the helicopter only from the front or side, never from the rear. No one should ever be aft of the rear landing skid support tubes.
- Approach and depart from the helicopter on the downhill side if the helicopter is on uneven ground.
- Keep low when you are approaching the helicopter; a sudden gust of wind can cause the main rotor to suddenly dip to the point where the tip is only 4 feet off the ground.
- Do not carry anything to the helicopter that is over head high, including IV poles and bags.
- Have all equipment secured. Caps, loose blankets and sheets, or other objects can be blown off by the wind or propwash of the helicopter's blades.
- Do not duck under the body, boom, or tail section of the helicopter if you must move from one side of the aircraft to the other. Go around the front.

When the patient is loaded:

- Allow only the flight crew to close and lock the doors. A broken door will prevent a takeoff.

When the helicopter is ready for departure:

- Be sure that the departure path is free from vehicles and spectators; if an emergency occurs during takeoff, the aircraft will land in that area.

Hazardous Material Situations

Accidents involving hazardous materials require the special attention of fire and rescue units on the ground. The hazardous materials of concern are those that are toxic, poisonous, flammable, explosive, irritating, or radioactive in nature. Helicopter ambulance crews normally do not carry special suits or breathing apparatus to protect them from hazardous materials.

A helicopter ambulance crew must be warned that hazardous materials are present at the location so that they can take special steps to prevent contamination of crew members and the aircraft. Sick or injured persons who are contaminated by hazardous materials may require special protection before loading on the aircraft.

Please note: Much of the information contained in this section has been compiled from the pamphlet *Preparing a Landing Zone,* edited by Jim Whitman and published by the National EMS Pilots Association.

SUMMARY

The eleventh phase of a vehicle rescue operation begins when injured patients have been removed from the vehicles and ends when those persons have been transferred to ambulances.

When vehicles are on level ground, transferring injured persons to ambulances may involve nothing more than rolling or carrying stretchers 25 feet to the edge of the danger zone. But when a vehicle is at the bottom of a hill, rescuers may have to use specific equipment and special techniques to accomplish the transfer.

When a hill is just steep enough that a stretcher cannot be safely carried by a team of six rescuers but is not so steep that people cannot stand upright, a stretcher can be moved up the hill by the eight-rescuer shift (or a modification of that technique). Eight rescuers pass the stretcher from hand to hand while they maintain a safe footing. When the stretcher passes one pair of rescuers, they leave the end and go to the head of the line. This leap-frogging continues until the stretcher is on level ground.

When there are sufficient personnel, a stretcher can be passed hand-to-hand between two lines of people standing side-by-side on the hill.

The chance that a severely injured patient will survive is dramatically increased when the person can be transported to a trauma center by helicopter. While rescue personnel may not participate in the actual transfer of an injured person to a medical facility, they can assist with the transfer by initiating emergency care prior to the arrival of the helicopter and preparing the landing zone.

PHASE TWELVE

Terminating the Rescue Operation

INTRODUCTION

The final phase of a vehicle rescue operation begins when the last patient is in transit to a medical facility. The final phase ends when the rescue squad is fully prepared to respond to the next call for help.

Contrary to popular opinion, the termination phase of a vehicle rescue operation is much more than a short period of time during which rescuers pick up equipment, pack it on the rescue truck, return to quarters, have a cup of coffee, and go home. In fact, concluding on-scene activities may take several hours, and carrying out a plan of in-quarters activities may take several hours more.

CONTINUING ON-SCENE ACTIVITIES

Depending on the circumstances of a motor vehicle accident, rescuers, firefighters, and support personnel may also have to:

- Move and anchor downed wires.
- Extinguish fire in or under a vehicle.
- Pool spilled fuel and arrange for removal.
- Initiate fire prevention efforts.
- Stabilize vehicles.
- Illuminate the scene.
- Control the movements of spectators.
- Control traffic at the scene.

These activities have one thing in common: Once started, they may have to be continued until the scene is secure and the rescue squad is ready to return to quarters.

If it was necessary to remove downed wires from the wreckage, to anchor them by some means, and then to keep rescuers and spectators away from the wires, those particular hazard management activities must be continued until a power company crew can make the scene safe. The equipment that is anchoring the wire cannot be recovered, and the personnel who are guarding the wire cannot be withdrawn.

Fire-prevention efforts must be continued until there is no longer a danger of fire. Rescue personnel should resist the temptation to downgrade fire-prevention efforts just because victims have been removed from the wreckage and the operation is drawing to a close. It is usually when defenses are down that disasters occur.

It may be necessary to leave a vehicle that is on its side stabilized until a tow vehicle is ready to remove it from the scene.

During a nighttime operation, power distribution and lighting equipment cannot be dismantled until all rescue operations are concluded. Emergency service personnel who are working around the wreckage depend on lights. Police officers need lights for their investigation. The wrecker operator may need lights to prepare the accident vehicles for removal. Floodlights may be helping squad members in their effort to locate tools and equipment. Floodlights, in addition to providing light to work by, also warn oncoming drivers of the accident scene.

Crowd control and traffic control measures may have to be continued until the wreckage has been removed and all emergency service personnel are ready to leave the scene.

DEALING WITH DEBRIS

The problem of scene debris is often considered lightly by rescue personnel, if it is considered at all. Many rescue officers shrug off questions about their responsibility for debris clean-up with comments such as "Let someone else take care of debris. We're rescuers, not street cleaners."

It's true that rescue personnel are not street cleaners; nor are they movers and haulers. Squad members should not be expected to move large amounts of debris from a roadway. Nor should they be expected to move large quantities of loose or packaged cargo from one vehicle to another, or perform any other task that will delay preparations for a prompt return to service.

Nonetheless, there are some debris removal tasks that rescuers can and should do

with equipment that is usually carried on a rescue truck—the removal of broken glass and metal parts from the roadway, for example. If rescuers are willing to pitch in and help clear away minor debris, roadways can be opened quicker, and everyone can go home. This does not mean that rescue personnel should perform minor clean-up procedures as a matter of course, however.

Police officers are trained to consider many things during an accident investigation, including the location, nature, and amount of collision-related debris. While clumps of dirt, trails and pools of fluids, and vehicle parts may appear to be trash in the eyes of rescue personnel, these bits of debris may provide an accident reconstruction specialist with clues as to the cause and effect of a collision.

Categories of Debris

Listed below are several kinds of debris that can be found in many places at an accident location.

Underbody Debris. When a vehicle is involved in an accident, collision forces can cause accumulations of dirt, mud, and road tar to dislodge from under the floor pan and fenders and fall onto the roadway. An investigator can often determine the point of impact, the approximate speeds of the involved vehicles, and the direction that the vehicles took after the collision from the patterns and distribution of underbody debris on a roadway.

Vehicle Parts. Metal, plastic, and glass components often break away from a vehicle at the time of impact. Some metal and plastic parts will slide or roll a considerable distance; in fact, investigators have found vehicle parts hundreds of feet from points of impact. The distribution of broken parts often tells an investigating officer the direction in which accident vehicles rolled or slid after collision.

Vehicle Fluids. Coolant from the radiator, oil from the crankcase, gasoline or diesel fuel, automatic transmission fluid, brake fluid, battery acid, and fluid from power steering and power brake reservoirs can be spilled onto the highway as the result of an accident. The form of a spill is important to investigators. Splatters of liquid may identify the point of impact if collision forces were sufficient to break fluid containers and lines. Dribbles of liquid between the point of impact and the point where a vehicle has come to rest show the pathway that the vehicle took after collision—not always a straight line. Runoff is fluid that has collected in a puddle and is generally found adjacent to the point where the vehicle has stopped.

Liquid Cargo. Gasoline, fuel oil, milk, acid, chocolate, and water are just a few of the liquid cargoes carried by trucks. In addition to flammability and explosion hazards, a problem that this type of cargo creates for investigators is that a large amount of the liquid may flood the area around a vehicle and obliterate other clues.

Granular Cargo. Loose stone, gravel, grain, fertilizer, coal, cement, and other dry materials can be released from a damaged dry cargo carrier. A trail of granular material may show investigators the path that the vehicle took from the point of impact to its final resting place.

Miscellaneous Cargo. Luggage, packaged goods, crates, and rolls may litter the highway after an accident, but these items are seldom considered significant in investigations.

Road Materials. Gravel, cinders, and pebbles are often dislodged and scattered by the tires of vehicles. The pattern of dislodged road materials may show the direction of vehicle travel following a collision, and that a vehicle ran onto the shoulder before or after the accident.

Clothing. An investigating officer can learn much about an accident by observing clothing. An article of clothing may mark the spot where a pedestrian was struck. It is not uncommon for a pedestrian's shoes to remain where he was standing when struck by a vehicle. Bits of clothing may mark the place where a person struck the roadway after being thrown from a vehicle. Shreds of cloth-

ing may mark the path that a body took while sliding along a roadway.

Blood. A pool of blood on the roadway generally indicates the place where a patient came to rest after exiting or being thrown from a vehicle. Tissue and bone fragments in a pool of blood may suggest that the patient sustained injury at that point after being struck by or thrown from a vehicle. A trail of blood may indicate that a body was removed from a vehicle or that the patient crawled away from the wreckage.

Because a conscientious job of debris removal may ruin an investigator's chances of ever knowing exactly how an accident happened, rescuers should always wait for police approval before moving debris.

Debris Removal Procedures

Following are some suggestions as to how the various types of debris can be removed from the scene.

Underbody debris does not usually present a problem. It can be swept up with a stiff broom, shoveled into a container, and disposed of away from the scene.

Glass fragments should not be swept against the curb or onto the shoulder of the road where particles can be picked up by tires and scattered back onto the roadway. Instead, glass fragments should be swept into a pile and shoveled into a container for disposal elsewhere. This requires a little extra effort, but remember: Extra effort distinguishes a good rescue squad from a mediocre one.

Unbroken windshields and rear windows and large pieces of broken windshields should be removed from accident locations, especially if the accident has occurred in an area where children play. Large pieces of glass are attractive nuisances that can cause severe injuries. Large pieces of automotive glass can usually be placed in a vehicle before it is towed away. Metal parts and metal and plastic trim can also be placed in a wrecked vehicle.

Pooled fluids should be absorbed with an absorbent granular material or special absorbent pads, bagged, and safely deposited away from the scene. Flushing liquids into sewers and open areas alongside of roads is a dangerous practice that should be discontinued.

The transfer of a large quantity of liquid cargo from one vehicle to another is not something that should be undertaken by emergency service personnel even when the cargo is not hazardous; transferring cargo is a job for material handling specialists.

The responsibility for pooling large amounts of a spilled liquid cargo may fall to a fire department or rescue squad simply because the job must be done quickly. However, transferring the liquid from the pool to containers or a transfer truck should be done by other individuals. When confronted with a large spill, whether dangerous or not, a rescue officer should contact a representative of the local environmental protection agency for advice and assistance. Calling for technical help does not indicate a weakness in a rescue officer; it signifies good judgment.

Small amounts of gravel, grain, coal, stone, and other granular debris can be shoveled into containers or moved to the side of the road for pickup later. When a large amount of granular cargo has spilled, a front-end loader should be used to load it into a dump truck.

Luggage, boxes, crates, and other miscellaneous cargo should be moved by rescuers to the side of the road where the items can be guarded until they can be removed from the scene.

Gravel, cinders, dirt, and other road construction materials can be swept together and shoveled into a container or, when there are large amounts of debris, swept to the side of the road for later collection.

Personal effects and articles of clothing should be collected and turned over to the police. A receipt should be obtained for valuables.

While the technique is just about obsolete, washing the highway with a hose stream may still be necessary in certain situations. Such might be the case when a truck loaded with dirt has turned over during a rainstorm, and a film of slippery mud has remained on the road after most of the dirt has been transferred to another truck with a front-end loader. When it is necessary to flush a road surface during cold weather, provisions must be made to have the road sanded. A coating of ice may be far more dangerous than a coating of mud.

When debris removal operations are completed and there is no longer a need for scene support, the officer-in-charge can wind down the rescue operation.

RECALLING PERSONNEL AND RECOVERING EQUIPMENT

It's not unlikely for squad members to be spread over a wide area when on-scene activities are terminated, especially when several emergency services have been involved in a large-scale operation. Some rescuers may be directing traffic a considerable distance from the actual scene. Others may be guarding downed wires, and still others may be disposing of debris. The rescue officer must know where all his people are and he must have some means to recall them. If every squad member has a portable radio, recall is no problem. Voice commands from the rescue unit's public address system usually carry for a considerable distance, and some squads use horn signals to summon rescuers. In some cases, it may be necessary to send a police car or another vehicle to round up squad personnel. Lacking any other means, a rescue officer may have to send runners to recall distant squad members.

A thorough recall procedure is important. More than one rescue officer has been embarrassed by a phone call to the station from a squad member who had been left at an accident location. And more than one rescuer has been embarrassed by the necessity of hitchhiking back to the station after discovering that the rescue unit left the scene without him.

If equipment was staged near the rescue vehicle at the start of a rescue operation, it should be returned to the staging area. Thus the driver (or other squad member responsible for the staging area) will be able to return the equipment to its proper place on the unit. A quick check of the compartments after all of the tools have been put away and a comparison of the contents to the inventory lists posted on the compartment doors will reveal any shortages.

RETURNING TO QUARTERS

When all rescuers are present or accounted for and tools and equipment are in place, the rescue unit is ready to return to quarters. The emotional moment has passed. Rescuers are tired, perhaps to the point of exhaustion. But however tired they may be, the driver of the rescue truck, the officer, and the squad members can be no less alert when returning to quarters then they were while responding to the emergency.

The driver must practice the rules of defensive driving on the way back to the station, and he must drive with complete regard for the safety of the squad personnel on the rig and other motorists. The officer must be alert for dangerous traffic conditions. And just as they did while responding to the alarm, squad members must wear protective clothing and be protected by safety belts. Nothing should change on the return to quarters except the speed at which the rescue truck travels.

CLEANING AND SERVICING EQUIPMENT

As a trained rescuer, you should be aware of the importance of having a variety of supplies and equipment for the tasks associated with vehicle rescue. However, the tools and appliances that were often acquired at considerable expense to your fire department or squad will be of little value if they are not cleaned, serviced, and properly stored.

Cleaning and servicing equipment after use, inspecting tools and appliances on a regular basis, and carrying out periodic testing and preventive maintenance procedures are quickly done tasks that produce long-term benefits. The efforts significantly reduce the incidence of costly professional repairs. Moreover, they assure that every piece of equipment is in a safe operating condition and ready for immediate use when it is needed most: at locations of accidents where the saving of lives may depend on the rescuers' ability to operate quickly and efficiently with available equipment.

Rescue tools and equipment are made of many different materials. Wood is the most commonly used material. Fiberglass is being used more and more in the construction of hand tools since it is not as susceptible to damage from moisture and chemicals as is wood. There are a number of bare-metal and chrome-plated tools, and many tools have painted metal parts. Rubber and plastics are used in the construction of tools, and it is likely that graphite, ceramics, and other by-products of space technology will be used in the foreseeable future. It should stand to reason, then, that if so many materials are used for the construction of tools used for rescue operations, there should be a number of ways to care for them.

Following are suggestions for the cleaning and servicing of many of the tools used for vehicle rescue operations. Also included are suggestions for periodic inspection and testing, and preventive maintenance programs.

Tools with Bare Wood Handles

Drilling hammers, engineer hammers, sledgehammers, axes, and pike poles are among the wood-handled tools most often used during vehicle rescue operations. Because of the many ways that these tools are used both properly and improperly, the wood handles should be carefully inspected after each use.

Since dirt can hide cracks in wood handles:

- Brush any loose dirt from the tool with a dry, stiff-bristled brush such as a scrub brush.

If a film of dirt remains on the tool after brushing deposits away:

- Do not immerse the tool in a container of water and let it soak with the expectation of floating the dirt away; moisture cracks can form if wood fibers remain saturated with water for a long period.

Instead:

- Wipe the dirt film from the tool with a cloth dampened with clear water.

If the handle is coated with oil or transmission fluid:

- Wipe the coating from the tool with a rag wet with soapy water.
- Wipe the wood handle with a cloth damp with clean water.
- Then dry the handle with a clean cloth.

If the handle is partly coated with heavy grease or tar:

- Wipe it down with a rag wet with a solvent such as bug and tar remover or a degreaser, but not gasoline!

The use of solvents on bare-wood-handled tools should be limited to removing the most stubborn coatings. The wood will absorb the solvent, and the chemical may damage wood fibers.

When the handle is clean:

- Inspect it for cracks, fracture lines, indentations, and chips.

If you find any signs of damage that may make the tool unsafe for future operations:

- Either replace the handle immediately, or remove the tool from service until the handle can be replaced.

Don't put a tool with a cracked handle back in service just because the handle cannot be replaced immediately. You or another rescuer may have to use the tool during a rescue operation, perhaps with disastrous results. Think of the potential for injury if the handle of a 3-pound drilling hammer breaks and the head flies while the tool is being used to forcefully drive a panel cutter while making an opening in the roof of a vehicle. Worse yet, think what might happen when the 8-, 10-, or 12-pound head of a sledgehammer flies after the handle breaks!

Tools with Coated Wood Handles

Tool manufacturers often coat the wood handles of tools with varnish or another clear coating to protect the tool from water and chemicals.

To clean the coated handles of tools:

- Remove any buildup of dirt with a stiff brush.
- Wipe away any remaining film of dirt with a cloth moistened with clear water.

If a foreign substance on the handle (such as road tar) resists this effort:

- Remove the substance with a cloth wet with an appropriate mild solvent.

Normal use of a wood-handled tool, accidental impact with an object being struck, and cleaning with an inappropriate solvent will eventually remove some of the protective covering. This does not mean that the tool should be discarded, however.

If the tool is otherwise serviceable:

- Thoroughly clean the handle, rough the surface with steel wool or a fine sandpaper, and re-coat the handle with a preparation recommended by the tool manufacturer.

As is the case for wood cribbing, do not paint the wood handles of hand tools in an effort to improve appearance, identify ownership, or hide unpleasant-appearing damage.

Paint hides damage that signals an unsafe tool.

Tools and Equipment Made of Fiberglass, Plastic, or Rubber

Tools and equipment made of fiberglass, plastic, and rubber or tools with parts made of those materials are easily maintained.

To clean a fiberglass, plastic, or rubber tool or part:

- Remove any buildup of dirt with a stiff brush.
- Clean the tool or part with soap and water applied with a sponge or rag. Use a scrub brush to remove a stubborn substance.

You should be able to remove dirt and even grease and oil in this manner; the soap should be a suitable solvent.

If you encounter a substance that is not easily removable with soap and water:

- Use a solvent that is designed for the particular material.

Be careful! Make sure you use a solvent that is compatible with the material being cleaned. Some plastic and rubber materials are susceptible to damage from petroleum products, and fiberglass, plastics, and rubber can be damaged by some commercial solvents. Most manufacturers include on the label a statement as to what materials the solvent can be used with. Follow the recommendations. Failure to do so may result in damage sufficient to make the tool or piece of equipment unsafe for further use.

Bare Metal Surfaces

Many different kinds of metal are used in the manufacturing of hand tools, power tools, and other equipment used for rescue operations, including cold-rolled steel, hardened steel, steel alloys, aluminum and aluminum alloys, brass, nickel, and even some exotic alloys that include magnesium and tita-

nium. This does not mean that different metals need different care, however. A number of cleaning and servicing procedures can be used for all metal tools.

Your first concern should be for cleanliness. Grease, oil, dirt, and other foreign matter can hide damage and can even interfere with the operation of some tools. The first step, then, is to:

- Remove deposits of dirt with a stiff brush; then
- Wash the tool with soap and water applied from a rag or sponge. Use a scrub brush on hard-to-remove deposits.

If the tool has a wood handle:

- Wash only the metal parts.

When the tool is clean:

- Rub the tool dry with a clean rag.

After thoroughly drying the tool:

- Lubricate it to prevent the bare metal from rusting.

Any of a number of lubricants can be used to protect steel tools. Machine oil, petroleum products such as Three-in-One Oil and Mystery Oil, silicon-based lubricants, and synthetic lubricants such as WD-40 and CRC-56 work very well, but they tend to be expensive. An inexpensive lubricant that is almost always found in a fire station or squad garage is ordinary 30-weight motor oil. It does the job well at a significantly lower cost than other lubricants.

The secret of properly protecting a steel metal tool is to clean the tool thoroughly, apply a lubricant sparingly, and wipe off any excess. Too much lubricant creates two problems. First, it makes the tool slippery and hard to handle. Second, the excess lubricant attracts dirt.

When you are lubricating a metal tool that has a wood handle:

- Take care not to get any lubricant on the handle, and if you do, wipe it off immediately.

The problem is not severe when a lubricant is applied with a rag. But when a spray can is used, lubricant is likely to cover much of the handle. Quick removal is important. Remember that petroleum products can damage wood.

Cutting Tools

Special attention should be paid to cutting tools during cleaning and inspection activities. Replaceable-blade cutting tools such as hacksaws, reciprocating saws, chain saws, abrasive disc saws, circular saws, and panel cutters should be closely examined.

If you see uneven teeth, nicks, cuts, gouges, and/or missing pieces in the cutting edges:

- Replace the blade prior to putting the tool back into service.

Saw blades that appear to have been rubbed smooth, blades that have teeth missing, and blades with teeth that appear "welded" together should be replaced. Moreover, rescuers should be reminded of proper cutting procedures when this sort of damage appears frequently. Ground-down saw teeth or teeth that have a welded appearance almost always indicate that a variable-speed tool has been operated too fast, or that too much force was used rather than letting the tool do the work.

Cutting tools that have permanent or semipermanent cutting edges (knives and axes, for example) require cleaning, inspection, and maintenance. Cutting edges should be cleaned and inspected for cracks, nicks, and dullness. Dull cutting edges should be sharpened and dressed with a honing stone. Exceptionally dull edges may require filing and then sharpening and honing.

Using a file to dress a cutting edge is usually undertaken only by a person who is experienced in sharpening cutting tools.

Likewise, the repair of severe damage (such as a nick) is best left to a professional tool sharpener. Indiscriminate use of a grinder can cause additional damage that may go unnoticed until the tool is used again.

Impact Tools

Tools that are used to strike other tools, and tools that are routinely struck may require maintenance other than cleaning.

If you see that a hardened-steel striking tool such as a hammer has cracks or that pieces of the tool are missing:

- Replace the tool with a new one.

It is far better to replace a damaged hardened tool than to attempt to repair it or, worse yet, to ignore the damage and return the tool to service.

Chisels, flat-head axes, and panel cutters are often damaged during use when they are struck a glancing blow rather than a straight-on blow to the impact surface. The resulting damage is called "mushrooming" (Figure 12.01). Mushrooming presents a hazard to future rescue operations if the damage is not repaired. Pieces of the mush-

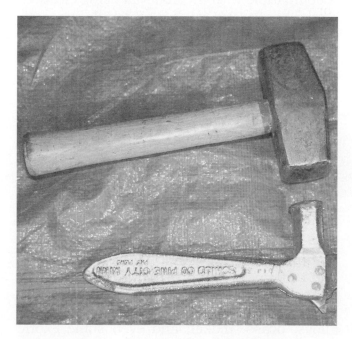

FIGURE 12.01   Peening Over on Schild Tool

roomed head can break off and become projectiles with sufficient force to injure unprotected body parts.

If you see that a tool has a mushroomed impact surface:

- Use a file to dress the irregular edges.

If the impact surface is severely mushroomed:

- Dress the tool with a grinder.

Keep in mind that a grinding wheel can cause additional damage to an impact tool just as it can cause additional damage to an edged tool. If you have any doubt as to your ability to dress a tool with a grinder, let a professional do the job.

As with the other tools and equipment discussed thus far, suppress any urge you may have to paint the cutting edge and striking surface of metal tools. Paint can hide damage that, if unnoticed, may pose a serious threat to the user of that tool during future rescue operations.

Painted and Chrome-Plated Tools

Tools are usually painted or chrome-plated to make them more resistant to wear and corrosion, although one can't help but wonder whether some tools are painted or chrome-plated just to make them more attractive. Whatever the reason for application, a good coat of paint and a proper plating job will last a long time with minimal maintenance.

To clean painted and chrome-plated tools:

- Remove deposits of dirt with a stiff brush.
- Wash the tools with soap and water.
- Rinse the tools with clear water and dry them thoroughly with a towel.

If significant deposits of grease, grime, or dirt cannot be removed with soap and water:

- Remove the deposits with a solvent suitable for the particular tool. Follow

the solvent or tool manufacturer's recommendations.

When the tool is clean and dry:

- Lubricate any parts of the tool that are not protected by paint or chrome; for example, the cutting edge.

A word of caution about using water to clean tools: Water may be harmful to some parts of complex tools and equipment. Water in the fuel system, a wet carburetor, or wet ignition points can render a power tool inoperative. Use only as much water as you need to clean the tool and to rinse it after the cleaning.

Some tools and equipment require more than a simple cleaning and lubrication. Following are some suggestions that you should find helpful not only for post-incident care and maintenance but also for storing, periodic inspection, and testing.

Cribbing

Wood cribbing and wedges are among the most important pieces of equipment for vehicle rescue operations. Cribbing and wedges are used to stabilize and support vehicles and other mechanisms of entrapment. Cribbing is used as a rigid base for power tools such as hydraulic spreaders and rams. Yet while rescuers depend on wood cribbing for so many things, there is no more misused and abused tool. Lengths of cribbing are often used as striking tools, and more often than not, cribbing is piled into a carrying case or into the compartment of a rescue truck even though it is wet with water or chemicals, coated with oil, caked with dirt, chipped, or cracked. The tool that is often used to make operations safer for victims and rescuers alike deserves better.

To clean and service cribbing after use:

- Dump the cribbing onto a salvage cover to make cleanup easier.
- Inspect all sides of each piece of cribbing. Look for cracks and deep

indentations caused by impact, excessive compression, and stress.

If any of the cribbing is obviously cracked or if pieces are missing:

- Do not attempt to join cracked pieces with nails or corrugated fasteners or, worse yet, by wrapping them with duct tape!

Instead:

- Discard the damaged pieces and replace them with new serviceable lumber.

If the cribbing has been contaminated with a hazardous material other than oil, gasoline, or transmission fluid:

- Dispose of the contaminated cribbing in a safe manner and replace it with new stock.

If any of the cribbing is caked with dirt but is dry:

- Remove deposits of dirt with a stiff brush.

If cribbing is coated with oil or transmission fluid, and for economic reasons it cannot be replaced:

- Do not use gasoline or another solvent; instead
- Wash the cribbing with soapy water.

You will not be able to clean away any fluid that has seeped into the wood, but you will be able to remove any coating that will make the cribbing slippery for subsequent operations.

After brushing or washing the cribbing:

- Inspect each length closely for less-than-obvious cracks that might have been missed on the initial inspection. Dispose of any pieces that are damaged.

- Repair rope handles or straps if damaged (if the cribbing is so-equipped).

If the cribbing is wet with water (from rain or snow or from washing it):

- Stack the wet cribbing so that air can circulate around the pieces.
- Let the pieces dry thoroughly; then replace them in the carrying box or apparatus compartment.

Suppress any urge that you might have to create "parade-grade" cribbing by painting it. While paint will make the cribbing prettier, it will also hide cracks that will make the cribbing dangerous for subsequent operations.

If you feel it necessary to mark cribbing so that it can be identified as belonging to your unit, simply paint one end, preferably the end that has the rope or strap handle.

Sectioned Clampsticks and Telescoping Hotsticks

A lineman's clampstick and a telescoping hotstick enable trained rescuers to safely relocate downed wires at accident locations. While these tools are rated for high voltages, they can be rendered unsafe by a coating of dirt or grease, both of which can conduct current down the outer surface of the tool to the user's hands. Following are cleaning and servicing operations that should be scrupulously undertaken after each use.

If you have a sectional clampstick:

- Bump gently, use a small brush, or use an air hose to dislodge dirt from the quick-disconnect fittings and the open ends of the clampstick sections. If you are using an air hose, be sure to wear safety goggles.

It's important that this step is undertaken before the tool is washed. If water contacts dirt in the fittings, the resulting "mud" will harden. If it is not removed, the caked mud will prevent assembly of the clampstick sections.

- Thoroughly clean the clampstick and hotstick with warm soapy water.
- Dry the tools thoroughly with a towel or clean dry rag.

When the sections of the clampstick are completely dry:

- Assemble the sections and check the moving parts for proper operations. Make adjustments as necessary.

When the telescoping hotstick is completely dry:

- Extend the sections fully, making sure that the spring-loaded latches operate correctly to make the tool a rigid device.

Do not under any circumstances apply a lubricant to any part of a sectioned clampstick or telescoping hotstick. Lubricants attract dirt that can conduct current.

Chain Hand Winches

Chain hand winches rated for 2 tons and less are often mildly stressed during normal operations. They can be stressed to the point of failure when a rescuer attempts to get more pull from the winch by using a cheater bar. Unfortunately, you can't tell whether the mechanism of a hand-held chain winch has been damaged by stress without disassembling the gear housing. However, you can tell when the chain itself is damaged and thus unsafe by examining the chain and hook.

Before you do anything else:

- Thoroughly clean the chain with soap and water or a suitable degreaser and dry it.
- Lay the chain out straight in a well-lighted place.

If you have a record of the length of the chain when the winch was new, or if you have a new winch of the same make and model as a spare:

- Compare the length of the chain of the winch that is being serviced with the record or the chain of the new winch.
- Closely examine the chain link by link. Look for excessive wear, gouges, nicks, bending, and elongation of the links.
- Inspect the hook. Look for twisting or expansion of the metal at the opening. Examine the throat, saddle, and neck of the hook for excessive wear and cracks.

If you find that the chain is stretched and/or that the links and hook are damaged:

- Remove the hand winch from service until it can be inspected and damaged parts replaced.

If there does not appear to be any damage that will make the winch unsafe during future rescue operations:

- Have someone hold on to the hook or capture an anchor point with the hook; then operate the winch in the usual manner.

Check for proper freewheeling and operate the handle to check the raising and lowering movements.

If the winch does not operate properly:

- Remove it from service and take it to an authorized repair facility.

If the winch operates properly:

- Apply a light film of lubricant to the housing, chain, and hook to protect them from rust and corrosion.
- Store the winch in a dry compartment on the rescue unit.

Cable Hand Winches

A cable hand winch is easier to inspect because of its open construction.

- Pull out all the cable and clean the entire assembly with soap and water.
- Dry the assembly with a towel or a clean dry cloth.
- Lay the cable out straight in a brightly lighted area.
- Inspect every inch of the cable. Look for excessive wear; broken, cut, sheared, or crushed wires; a marked reduction in the diameter of parts of the cable; kinks; and rust.
- Inspect the hook. Look for twisting or expansion of the metal at the opening. Examine the throat, saddle, and neck of the hook for excessive wear and cracks.
- Inspect the ratchet for broken teeth.

If there does not appear to be any damage that will make the winch unsafe for future rescue operations:

- Have someone hold on to the hook or capture a rigid anchor point with the hook and operate the winch.

If the winch does not operate properly:

- Remove it from service and take it to an authorized repair facility.

If the winch operates properly:

- Apply a light film of lubricant to protect the metal parts from rust and corrosion.
- Store the winch in a dry compartment on the rescue unit.

Rescue Chain Set

There is little probability that a 1/4-inch chain set will be damaged during rescue operations if the chains are used with a 2-ton or smaller hand winch. One-quarter-inch chains have a working strength of 4100 pounds. Nonetheless, they should be inspected after each use.

The manufacturers of top-quality chains place on each chain before delivery a permanent metal tag that shows the length of the chain when new. Having such a tag will enable you to tell by just a single measurement whether a chain has been stretched.

Before you inspect the chain:

- Clean it thoroughly with soap and water or a degreaser. Remember that an accumulation of dirt hides damage.

When the chain is clean and dry:

- Lay it out straight in a brightly lighted place.
- Measure the chain and compare the measurement with the metal information tag if one is affixed to the chain (Figure 12.02).

If the chain has been stretched:

- Remove it from service. You have no way of telling what load the chain can be expected to bear during future rescue operations.

If the chain does not have an information tag:

- Closely examine the chain link by link. Look for excessive wear, gouges, nicks, bending, and elongation of the links.

Then:

- Inspect the hook. Look for twisting or expansion of the metal at the opening. Examine the throat, saddle, and neck of the hook for excessive wear and cracks.

If you see damage and suspect that the chain may not be safe for future rescue operations:

- Remove the chain from service.

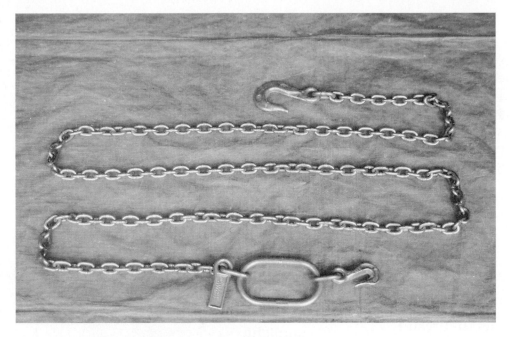

FIGURE 12.02   Metal Tag on Chain Set

If there are no signs of damage:

• Coat the chain with a thin film of lubricant and return it to its storage place on the rescue unit.

Rescue Strap Set

Two-inch web straps that have a steel triangle at one end and a steel choker triangle at the other are stronger and more versatile than 1/4-inch rescue chains. The manufacturers of certified straps use webbing that has red threads woven into the interior of the strap. Red threads that can be seen through a cut or abrasion signal that the strap should no longer be used. It may not be able to support the rated load.

Wire Rope Slings

Wire rope slings are sometimes used during vehicle rescue operations to stabilize unsteady vehicles or to move one vehicle away from another vehicle or an impacted object. Because of the nature of its use, there should be no question as to the integrity of a wire rope sling.

Standard B30.9 of the American National Standards Institute (ANSI) states that a wire rope sling should be removed from service anytime any of the following conditions are present:

• Ten randomly distributed broken wires in one rope lay or five broken wires in one strand in one rope lay.
• Kinking, crushing, bird caging, or any other damage resulting in distortion of the wire rope structure.
• Evidence of heat damage.
• End attachments that are cracked, deformed, or worn.
• Hooks that have been opened more than 15% of the normal throat opening measured at the narrowest point or twisted more than 10 degrees from the plane of the unbent hook.
• Corrosion of the wire rope or end attachments.

If you see any of these conditions during your inspection of a wire rope sling, remove the sling from service. You cannot be sure of the load that it will bear during future rescue operations.

Rope

Synthetic fiber ropes that are used in rescue operations are strong, to be sure, but like any other rope they can be damaged. A number of chemicals can damage synthetic fiber ropes, as can dirt and grit. Passing a nylon rope at high speed over an object made of nylon can cause rope fibers to melt. A rope passing over a rough object can be abraded. And rope can be severely stressed by heavy loads and shock loading. Thus it is vitally important that you carefully inspect rescue ropes.

After every use:

- Inspect every foot of a rope as you pass it through your hands.
- Look for heavy abrasions that result when a loaded rope is passed over a rough object.

Don't be concerned about a small amount of surface fuzz. It appears naturally after a rope has been used, and a small amount of surface fuzz may actually help guard the rope against further abrasion.

- Look for indications that the rope has been damaged by contact with a chemical or heat, indications like discolored sections and melted portions.
- Feel for hard lumps and soft mushy places in the core, indications of core damage.
- Feel for changes in flexibility as the rope passes through your hands.
- Simultaneously look and feel for changes in diameter, another indication of core damage.

If you see things that cause you to suspect that the rope may not be safe for future rescue operations:

- Remove the rope from service.

If the rope does not appear to be damaged:

- Wash it with cool clear water.

A synthetic fiber rope can be washed in two ways: in a washing machine, although it is likely to come out badly tangled, or with an inexpensive rope washer that attaches to the end of a garden hose. Commercial cleaners are available that will remove dirt, grit, and minor stains. Bleach should never be used on a synthetic fiber rope as it will weaken the rope fibers.

After a synthetic fiber rope has been washed:

- Allow it to dry in air away from direct sunlight.

When the rope is completely dry:

- Store it in a dry place away from sunlight.

Hydraulic Rescue Tool Systems

Hydraulic rescue tools add power, speed, and efficiency to vehicle rescue operations. Today's rescuers are able to perform tasks with hydraulic rescue tools that could be performed only with great difficulty not too many years ago, if they could be performed at all. Even so, hydraulic rescue tool systems are often so poorly maintained that they are unusable at the time of an emergency. This is unfortunate, for just a few simple procedures undertaken after each use, and a few more procedures undertaken periodically between uses will assure that hydraulic tools are always ready for service.

Post-Use Maintenance

Every component of the tool system that was used during the rescue operation should be cleaned, inspected, and serviced as necessary, starting with the spreading and pulling tool itself.

- Brush deposits of dry dirt from the tool.

If a dirt film remains or if parts of the tool are coated with oil or grease:

- Clean the tool with soap and water; use a scrub brush, if necessary.

Then:

- Dry the tool with a towel or dry rags.

When the tool is clean and dry:

- Closely inspect the tool for excessive wear and damage.
- Check to see that all nuts, bolts, retainer rings, screws, and pins are in place and securely fastened.
- Make sure that hose fittings are clean and operable.

If any part of the tool is unquestionably damaged, appears damaged, or appears to be unsafe:

- Remove the tool from service and notify the proper authority who can arrange for service by an authorized tool distributor or service agency.

If the tool is ready for service:

- Protect the tool surface with a thin coat of lubricant. Be sure to coat all surfaces.
- Join the hoses and move the control in both directions to equalize pressure in the tool.

A cutting tool should be cleaned, inspected, and serviced in the manner just described. In addition to those steps:

- Closely inspect the cutting edges. Look for cracks and large nicks that may have been produced when the tool was used in an improper manner or when the tool was used to cut an especially hard object.

If you see damage that may make future operations unsafe:

- Remove the tool from service and notify the proper authority, who can arrange for service by an authorized tool distributor or service agency.

Special attention should be given to the hoses that carry hydraulic fluid under pressure between the power unit and the tool(s). Generally, the more powerful the hydraulic tool, the greater the pressure within the hoses.

- Clean the hydraulic hoses thoroughly with soap and water. Dirt and deposits of oil and grease will hide damage.
- Dry the hoses with a towel or dry cloth.
- Closely inspect the hoses and couplings. Look for abrasions, lacerations, sharp kinks, bulging that indicates a weak spot in the wall of the hose, and "alligatoring," a change in the appearance of the hose that occurs when the hose is contacted by a corrosive material.

If there is any indication of damage:

- Replace the hoses with new ones. Do not leave a damaged hose in service with the thought that it will probably last for a few more operations.

If the hoses are ready for service:

- Roll them into a coil large enough that the hoses will not kink while in a storage compartment.

Don't forget to remove the chains and accessories from the storage compartment and inspect and service them if they were used.

- Clean the chains and accessories as necessary, and check them for damage.
- Inspect the accessories for cracks and missing pieces.
- Inspect the chains for stretched and damaged links and the hooks for stretching and twisting.

If any of the accessories or chains appear damaged to the point where you suspect they may be unsafe during future rescue operations:

- Remove the accessories or chains from service.

Don't neglect the power unit. If it will not operate properly during a rescue operation, all your efforts to assure that the rest of the system is operable will have been in vain.

- Fill the fuel tank to the proper level.
- Check the level of the hydraulic fluid reservoir.
- Check the starter rope or cable for defects. Replace the rope or cable if necessary.
- Do not wash the power unit with a hose.

Instead:

- Clean dirty components with a cloth dampened with water, soap, and water or a suitable degreaser, depending on the nature and extent of soiling.
- Replace the components of the hydraulic rescue system in their proper storage places.

Even though the metal parts are coated with a light film of lubricant, hydraulic rescue equipment should be kept in compartments that are usually dry. Moreover, the compartments should be large enough that the hoses will not be kinked and that the tools and accessories will not be damaged by continual contact with each other.

Daily Maintenance and Inspection

The following steps should be taken when the rescue vehicle, tools, and equipment are inspected daily or at the beginning of each shift:

- Carefully inspect the tool(s) for hydraulic leaks.

- Check inside the frame of each tool for dirt and debris.
- Inspect the hoses and couplings for wear and damage.
- Check the control valve operation for easy movement and free return.
- Be sure all parts are clean.
- Check the blades of cutting tools for damage.
- Check to see that all nuts, bolts, retainer rings, and screws are in place and securely fastened.

All components of a hydraulic rescue tool system should be inspected annually and serviced by an authorized tool distributor or service agency.

Air-Operated Cutting Tools

The manufacturers of air-operated cutting tools usually do not recommend that any major repairs be attempted by a user unless the individual is specially trained. The following steps will assure that a properly operating tool is always ready for service.

- Clean the components of the cutting system with a rag dampened with water or soap and water, depending on the nature and degree of soil.
- Inspect the tool, the regulator, the hose line(s), and accessories for obvious damage.

If parts are damaged and it appears that the system cannot be operated safely during future rescue operations:

- Replace parts, as necessary, or remove the tool from service.

When the components appear intact and serviceable:

- Check the level of the in-line oiler (if provided), and refill it as necessary.
- Lubricate the air-operated tool according to the manufacturer's instructions.

- Lubricate the tool bit retainer, if necessary.

When an in-line oiler is not used, lubrication usually involves squirting a small amount of lubricant into the air supply nipple of the tool. Follow the tool manufacturer's suggestions.

Don't neglect the tool bits. The finest air-operated cutting tool is of no value when tool bits cannot be inserted into the retainer or when tool bits are so dull that efficient cutting is virtually impossible.

- Examine the cutting edge(s) of each tool bit.

If the edge(s) are dull or broken:

- Resharpen and dress the edges with a grinder. Take care not to overheat the bits.
- Examine the shanks of every tool bit.

If any of the shanks have burrs that may prevent the bit from being seated in the tool retainer:

- Remove the burrs with a file or a power grinder. Again, take care not to overheat the bit with the grinder.

When all the components have been inspected and serviced:

- Coat the air-operated tool and the tool bits with a thin film of lubricant to prevent rust and corrosion.
- Store the equipment in its carrying case in a dry compartment of the rescue unit.

Air Bags

All components of an air bag system should be thoroughly cleaned after each use, especially when the parts were exposed to sand, dirt, sludge, oil, and gasoline. Then the units should be properly stored.

Post-Use Cleaning Procedures

Soap, water, and "elbow grease" are used to clean air bags. Never use a solvent, even when bags are heavily coated with grease, oil, and dirt.

- Prepare a solution of warm water and a mild detergent in a bucket.
- Brush sand and dirt from the controller and hoses.
- Wipe off any buildup of grease or oil; then use a rag wet with the detergent solution to wipe the controller and hoses clean.
- Set the controller and hoses aside to dry.
- Lay the air bags on a flat surface and use a brush or broom to scrub the surface of each bag with the detergent solution.
- Rinse the bags with clear water and set them aside on an edge with the air supply nipple facing up.

Never use a rubber preservative or black tire paint to improve the appearance of scuffed air bags. The coating will make the bags slippery when wet.

Storing Air Bags

Correct storage procedures are important to the maintenance of an air bag system.

- Adjust the regulator handle to the neutral (zero-pressure) position.
- Store the regulator where it will be secure. Be sure that the regulator hose is not kinked.

While they are sturdy, regulators are not designed to take much abuse. Sliding around with other tools in the bottom of a compartment can damage the gauges.

If you have a fitting controller:

- Loosen the caps at the top of the relief valves prior to storage.

- Turn the controller valves to the open position to prevent the washers from becoming bonded to their seats during lengthy storage periods.

Since the valves of the dead-man controller remain in the neutral position when not being operated, the preceding valve adjustment steps are unnecessary.

- Store either type of controller where it will not be contacted by cribbing or tools. If you have a fitting controller, store it in such a way that the plastic ball valve handles are protected.
- Store air supply hoses in a coil secured with a belt or length of cord. Be sure that heavy objects are not stored on top of the coils; they may crush or cut the hose side walls.

If you can store the air bags flat:

- Do so, with the nipple facing the compartment door. Thus when the bags are unloaded the nipples will always be in the uppermost position where they are least subject to damage.

If you must store the bags standing on an edge:

- Be sure that the nipples are pointing up, not down in a position where they will bear the weight of the bag.

Periodic Maintenance and Testing

To assure that an air bag system is kept in peak operating condition, maintenance and safety checks should be performed at least every six months, and every three months when the bags are used often.

Following is a maintenance-testing procedure designed to assure that an air bag system is always ready for immediate use. The procedure involves assembling the components of the system in order.

- Connect the regulator to the compressed air supply cylinder and tighten the nut.

If the regulator has a hand wheel:

- Tighten the nut by hand.

If the regulator does not have a hand wheel:

- Use the correct-sized open-end wrench or an adjustable wrench to assure a tight seal. Do not use a pipe wrench or the wrong sized open-end wrench.

Next:

- Inspect the end of the hose that extends from the regulator. Look for dirt or corrosion on this fitting.

If necessary:

- Clean the fitting with a rag or soft wire brush.

Next:

- Check the air inlet coupling on the controller for corrosion and for a buildup of sand or dirt between the collet and the barrel.

If necessary:

- Use a stream of compressed air to clean the fitting.

Next:

- Connect the hose from the regulator to the controller. Assure that the hose is securely plugged into the controller.
- Close the control valve on the regulator (the small valve that controls air flow from the regulator to the controller).
- Open the cylinder valve and adjust the regulator pressure to the setting specified by the manufacturer.
- Check for leakage from the nut that connects the regulator to the supply cylinder.

If air is leaking:

• Tighten the nut with the hand wheel.

If turning the hand wheel does not stop the leak:

• Close the cylinder valve, bleed air from the regulator by opening the control valve, disconnect the nut from the cylinder fitting, and replace the nylon seat washer on the gland.

If a wrench-tightened regulator nut is leaking and gentle turning with a wrench does not stop the leak:

• Close the cylinder valve, bleed air from the regulator by opening the control valve, disconnect the regulator from the cylinder, and check the gland for burrs or nicks.

If there are burrs or nicks and there is not a replaceable seat, the gland will have to be carefully smoothed with a file.

When you have reconnected the regulator to the supply cylinder and repressed it:

• Check the regulator gauges for operation.

If they are not indicating pressure:

• Lightly tap the side of the gauge; the needle may have become stuck in place as the result of a lengthy storage period, or the gauge may be defective.

If the gauges do not operate smoothly or function correctly or if the liquid is gone from a liquid-filled gauge:

• Stop the test, dissemble the components, and contact the manufacturer for repair or replacement.

If the gauges are operating properly:

• Check for air leakage from the gauges, the seat valve, and the shut-off valve.
• Close the cylinder valve. A decrease in pressure in the low-pressure gauge

indicates a leak somewhere in the regulator.

If there does not appear to be a leak:

• Open the cylinder valve.

If you have a fitting controller:

• Close the ball valves. If you have a dead-man controller, the valves will be in the closed position.
• Slowly open the air flow valve to charge the hose that extends from the regulator to the controller.
• Turn the regulator hand wheel until the low-pressure valve indicates the manufacturer's recommended setting.
• Check the regulator hose for nicks, cuts, creases, and folds that may have resulted from storage.
• Check around the pressed couplings for hose cuts. Run your fingers over the entire length of hose and feel for bubbles and bulges that warn of internal defects.

If the check is positive:

• Shut off the air supply, disassemble the system, and contact the manufacturer for a new hose.

If the test is negative:

• Go on to the next step.

If you have a fitting controller:

• Check the pipe joints for air leaks.

If you find any air leaks:

• Mark the leading fitting so that it can be repaired after the test.

To assure that the controller will not lose its shape or develop leaks, the components of most fitting controllers are joined with either a hard-drying epoxy cement or a Teflon compound when they are assembled. Nonetheless, fittings can loosen, especially during periods of hard use. Repairs can be made with a liquid epoxy cement or a product such as Loctite. If you have any questions regarding the repair of a fitting controller, contact the manufacturer.

Before opening the valves and allowing air to flow from the controller, be sure the relief valves are closed.

- Turn the notched knobs clockwise as you look at the end of the knobs. On dead-man units, the reliefs are always closed.

If you have a fitting controller:

- Be sure that the lead seal is attached to the top of each relief valve.

If a seal is missing:

- Stop the test.
- Shut off the air supply and disassemble the components.
- Send the controller to the manufacturer for testing and recertification.

Remember: The relief valve is the heart of the safety system. If it does not operate properly, an air bag can be seriously overinflated, perhaps with terrible consequences.

After closing the controller relief valves:

- Check the hoses that join the controller to the air bags.
- Look for cuts, creases and folds, and dirt in the couplings.
- Clean the couplings with a stream of compressed air, if necessary.

If they appear satisfactory:

- Connect the hoses to the controller and the air bags.
- Slowly inflate the bags, one at a time, to 50% of their rated pressure.

- Close the valves and check each hose for cuts and nicks and for bubbles and bulges indicative of internal defects.

The hoses that join the air bags to the controller are manufactured to be a specific size with a specific elasticity. Thus, if an air bag is overinflated or if a load shifts and/or shock occurs, air will be relieved from the controller.

If the hoses appear to be defective:

- Shut off the air supply, disassemble the components, and contact the manufacturer.

If the hoses appear to be intact:

- Continue with the test.
- Examine the air bags.
- Check for air leaks at the nipples, and check the surfaces of the bags for bulges and bubbles.
- Brush the surfaces of the bags with soapy water to check for air leaks.

Nicks, cuts, and abrasions are of no major concern unless the steel or fabric cords of an air bag are exposed. When cords are evident, the bag should be returned to the manufacturer for testing and evaluation.

If the bags appear to be in good shape:

- Adjust the position of each so that the bags, hoses, and controller are in straight lines.
- One at a time, operate the controller valves until the bags are inflated to the maximum recommended pressure as indicated by the red line on the controller gauges.
- Check to see that the relief valves open when the gauge needle passes over the red line.

If the relief valves don't open:

- Determine whether they are merely stuck.

If you have a fitting controller:

- Turn the notched knob of the nonfunctioning relief valve counterclockwise.

If you have a dead-man controller:

- Push the joystick to the deflate position and then allow it to return to the neutral position. It may be possible to free a seat washer by opening and closing these valves several times.

Relief valve sticking in a fitting-type controller usually results from storing the controller with a relief valve in a tightly closed position. Dead-man controllers have a spring override that will not allow the relief valve to become bonded to the brass seat.

If these efforts do not result in the relief valves operating satisfactorily:

- Shut off the air supply, disassemble the equipment, and contact the manufacturer.

If the relief operates properly:

- Continue with the test.

After closing the relief valves again (if you have a fitting-type controller):

- Fill the bag to the maximum operating pressure again and recheck the bags and hoses.
- Test the remaining bags and spare hoses in the same manner.

It takes time to test an air bag system, to be sure. But when the test is done, you can be sure that your air bags are not likely to fail when they are needed most during a critical rescue operation!

The Jimmi-Jak System

Very little effort is required to keep the components of the Jimmi-Jak System in good working order. After each use:

- Brush dirt and any other dry materials from the Jacs and the accessories.

If any of the Jacs or accessories are soiled with oil or grease:

- Wash the dirty parts thoroughly with soap and water.
- Dry the parts with a towel or dry cloth; then
- Protect the steel parts with a thin coating of lubricant.

The only steel parts of the Jimmi-Jak System that are susceptible to rusting are the points of the attachments, the serrated jaws of the V-blocks, the chains, and the J-hooks. All other parts are aluminum or stainless steel.

To service the rest of the components:

- Wipe the hoses, the regulator, and the controller with a damp cloth.
- Check to see that the fittings are free from dirt.

Storage

The regulator and controller should be stored in a place where they are not likely to be contacted and damaged by other tools. Attachments should be stored in a box rather than loose in a compartment; thus there is less of a chance that the shafts of the attachments will become burred. Air supply hoses should be coiled, and the coils should be secured with a belt or length of cord. Be sure that heavy objects are not stored on top of the coils; they may crush or cut the hose side walls.

If the Jacs are stored horizontally and are not used often, they should be rotated a half-turn so the piston cups will not flatten on one side.

Periodic Inspection and Maintenance

There is no requirement to assemble the components and make a complete system check; little can happen to the various parts if they are properly stored. However, to do so gives squad members a chance to set up and break down the system and thus gain proficiency. The following procedures should be undertaken regardless of whether the components are assembled periodically.

Every six months:

- Check to see that the self-locking nut on the piston retaining rod is tight. The nut is located inside the piston as viewed from the top.

If the nut is loose:

- Turn it clockwise with a 3/4-inch socket on the end of an extension.

Next:

- Manually operate the piston of each Jac to assure that it moves easily within the body of the cylinder.

If the piston does not easily slide in and out:

- Remove the three 1/4-inch Allen set screws that secure the shell of the cylinder to the base.
- Invert the Jac and rap it hard against a block of wood to drive the base away from the shell and allow access to the interior of the shell.
- Spray the inside wall of the shell with a dry molybdenum lubricant.
- Coat the piston retaining rod with a wet molybdenum lubricant to assure that the piston cup will move easily up and down on the rod. Do not use an oil-based lubricant; it will damage the piston cup.

To reassemble the unit:

- Press the base onto the shell so the screw holes of the base are lined up with the screw holes of the shell.
- Insert the set screws and tighten them.

Finally:

- Re-coat the steel parts with a thin film of lubricant.

The attachments of the Jimmi-Jak System should also be checked during a periodic inspection and maintenance program.

- Join each attachment to the piston of one of the Jaks.

If the attachment will not easily seat and lock in place, or if you have difficulty in inserting the shaft of the attachment into the receptacle in the end of the piston:

- Check the shaft of the attachment for burrs.
- Remove any burrs with a fine file.

Personal Protective Gear

As with all rescue tools and equipment, your personal protective envelope—the gear that you wear—should be cleaned and inspected after each use. You need to pay close attention to the gear because it is your body that the equipment is designed to protect. Faulty equipment creates gaps and weaknesses in the personal protective envelope, and gaps in protection can contribute to injury and even death. Clean gear is safer, and therefore affords the wearer more and better protection.

All the components of the personal protective system require inspection and care: helmet, coat, pants, boots and shoes, gloves, eye protection, and respiratory protection.

The Helmet

A protective helmet is really a system of protection that has several components that must be intact and properly functioning to afford protection to the wearer. The three components are the shell, the suspension, and the liner. All three should be inspected after every use and serviced and repaired as necessary.

- Clean the shell thoroughly with soap and water.
- Rinse the shell with clear water and dry it with a clean towel or rag.

After cleaning:

- Closely examine the shell for significant damage. Look for cracks, deep nicks, missing pieces, and deformation.

If yours is a multiple-layered (laminated) composition shell:

- Look for bubbles in the shell, indicators that the laminates have separated.

If you find any significant damage:

- Replace the shell with a new one and discard the old shell.

A damaged shell is unsafe and will afford the wearer only reduced, if any, protection.

The helmet suspension is designed to support the entire helmet system on your head.

- Closely examine the suspension. Look for frayed or torn tapes.
- Make sure that the adjustment straps and tabs are in proper working order.
- Adjust the suspension, if necessary, to assure the proper headroom between the shell and your skull.

The suspension should maintain the shell in a position 1/4 inch to 1/2 inch above the top of the head. This space is important; it keeps the shell from contacting your skull when the helmet impacts with something. For this reason, do not use the space between the top of the suspension and the shell for storing spare gloves, extra socks, cravats, candy bars, and the like.

Next:

- Adjust the suspension to assure the proper fit. The helmet should fit snugly and should not slip or twist during normal activities.

Proper fit is important to the safe operation of the helmet system. The suspension may stretch a little over a period of wear. This is a normal occurrence, however, and is not cause for concern as long as you periodically check the suspension for a proper fit and make adjustments as necessary. A damaged suspension should be replaced immediately to assure that the helmet system affords maximum protection.

The helmet liner may be an integral part of the suspension or it may be a separate item. Like the other parts of a helmet, the liner should be cleaned regularly and inspected for wear and damage.

To clean your helmet liner:

- Simply give it a normal laundering with mild soap and gentle agitation, or follow the recommendations of the manufacturer.
- Inspect the liner for damage.

If you discover damage that will make the liner unsafe:

- Replace the damaged liner with a new one.

Remember: A helmet is a system of three components that must be present and in good working order if the wearer is to be properly protected. You should not wear a helmet that is damaged, a helmet that does not fit your head properly, or a helmet that is not complete.

CLEANING CONTAMINATED TOOLS AND EQUIPMENT*

Vehicle rescue activities often raise the concern for the possible exposure of personnel involved in the extraction of injured persons or

*Written by Katherine West, BSN, MSED, CIC, Infection Control Consultant.

contamination of equipment used during the extraction. First, it is important to note that turnout gear offers protection to the wearer that is greater than that required under the Occupational Safety and Health Administration (OSHA) regulation for protection of workers from bloodborne pathogens. Second, should blood get onto your turnout gear, that is *not* considered to be an exposure. Only blood on non-intact skin would be considered a reportable incident or exposure. Should blood come into contact with non-intact skin during extrication activities, the area should be washed with waterless handwash solution at the scene and the department's designated officer should be notified ASAP. Any event in which blood is splashed into your eyes, nose, or mouth should also be reported to the designated officer as an exposure incident. These areas should be flushed with water as soon as possible. The designated officer for infection control will advise you of any additional follow-up as per your department's Exposure Control Plan. Third, it should be noted that the risk for exposure does and will always exist in the emergency response work environment.

However, the risk for acquiring a bloodborne disease remains low based on current data obtained from the Centers for Disease Control and Prevention (CDC). (1) See Figure 12.03 of this section for a listing of what constitutes an exposure and the associated risk factors. The bloodborne disease that poses the greatest risk is hepatitis B, and this disease is preventable by participation in your department's hepatitis B vaccine program. Diseases such as hepatitis C and HIV also pose a risk, but risk can be reduced by washing or flushing the area and seeking post-exposure medical follow-up as defined by the OSHA regulations and the CDC guidelines. (2) It is important to remember that risk for infection is low and that the risk for exposure cannot be completely eliminated. It is also important to remember that exposure *does not* mean infection.

Turnout gear that has become contaminated with blood can be easily cleaned following the manufacturer's recommendations for care and cleaning. Contaminated gear does *not* need to be destroyed or sent out for special cleaning because of blood contamination. Blood is very different from chemical agents and blood does not pose the same type of risk as chemical agents. If small amounts of blood are present on gear, it can be spot cleaned using soap and water followed by washing with your available disinfectant. Figure 12.04 of this section reflects the general recommendations for cleaning grossly blood-contaminated turnout gear. (3) Blood on boots, helmets, and visors may be washed off with soap and water followed by a disinfection agent such as bleach and water at a 1:100 dilution (1/4-cup bleach in one gallon of water). (2) No stronger solution is necessary! (4) At the 1:100 dilution, metals will not corrode, there is no strong odor, and it is very effective and nontoxic. Remember, hepatitis B is the only bloodborne virus that is known to be able to survive for any length of time once exposed to the environment. (2,4) And this risk is removed by receiving the vaccine. Contaminated station uniforms may be washed in the station washer and dryer, if available. No special additives need to be added to the wash water. Just run a routine cycle and place in the dryer. There is no need to run an empty load

FIGURE 12.03

Defining Exposure	Risk Assessment
1. Contaminated needlestick injury	0.32%
2. Blood/OPIM* into the eye, inner surface of the nose, or mouth	0.09%
3. Blood/OPIM in contact with an open area of the skin	0.00–0.09%
4. Cuts with sharp objects covered with blood/OPIM	0.00–0.09%

*OPIM (Other potentially infectious materials)—csf, synovial fluid, amniotic fluid, plural fluid, pericardial fluid, abdominal fluid.
Adopted from: *HIV Transmission in the Health-Care Setting*, Infectious Disease Clinics of North America, June 1994: 319-329.

FIGURE 12.04   Cleaning Procedures for Firefighter Protective Clothing; Section 1—Washing Instructions

---

Protective clothing should be washed separately from other garments. All hooks and eyes should be fastened and the garment turned inside out or placed in a large laundry bag that can be tied shut to avoid damage to the wash tub. A stainless steel tub should be utilized if available.

These instructions can be used for cleaning any of the following washloads in a large capacity (16 gallon) top-loading or front-loading washing machine.

(a) One protective coat + one protective trouser

(b) Two protective coats

(c) Two protective trousers

Prior to washing, heavily soiled garments should be pretreated

1. While the washing machine is filling with hot water [temperature between 120° F and 130° F (49° C and 55° C)], add 1/2 cup (4 oz.) of liquid oxygenated bleach (do not use chlorine bleach) and 1 cup (8 oz.) of liquid detergent. These products are readily available in supermarkets around the country.

2. Fill washing machine to highest water level.

3. Add garments to be washed.

4. Set washing machine for normal cycle, cotton/white, or similar setting.

5. Machine should be programmed for double rinse. If the machine will not automatically double rinse, a complete second cycle can be run without adding detergent or oxygenated bleach. Double rinsing helps remove any residual dirt and ensures detergent removal.

6. Remove garments from washing machine and dry by hanging in a shaded area that receives good cross ventilation or hang on a line and use a fan to circulate the air. A water extractor may be used.

---

after washing a contaminated load. There is no need for any special washer or dryer for washing contaminated station uniforms. It is important to note that there are no scientific studies noting that contaminated clothing poses a risk for the transmission of bloodborne diseases. (5) The reason that contaminated clothing cannot be taken home is because OSHA requires that the employer control personal protective equipment and it cannot be controlled if taken home. (6)

If tools or equipment becomes contaminated with blood during rescue activities, the item should be rinsed with water at the scene if possible. If not possible, then the item(s) should be placed or wrapped with plastic for transport to the station for proper cleaning and disinfection. Disposable gloves should be used for rinsing. Upon arrival at the station, the item(s) should be taken to the designated decontamination area as identified in your department's exposure control plan. In most cases, this will be the Bay Area. Rubber utility

(dishwashing) gloves should be worn for all cleaning activities because they offer a thicker material which is more resistant to puncture and tearing. (2,4) Reference your department's exposure control plan for specific cleaning recommendations for cleaning various types of equipment and what personal protective equipment is indicated because of the chemical cleaning agents that might be used. (2,7) All cleaning activities need to be documented.

Any injury that might occur during the cleaning and decontamination process should be reported to the designated officer ASAP to ascertain whether or not an exposure occurred. Research has shown that most bacteria and viruses are removed after the simple use of soap and water cleaning. (5) Therefore, risk in the cleaning process is significantly reduced after initial cleaning with soap and water.

Your department's exposure control plan is an important document which will outline clearly how to reduce the risk for exposure in the emergency care environment. The contents of this document should be presented in education and training programs upon hire and updated on at least a yearly basis. A copy of this plan should be available to all members. Become familiar with your depart-

ment's plan with special attention to the sections on cleaning contaminated equipment, clothing, and post-exposure procedures for medical follow-up should an exposure occur. Remember risk is present but risk is low.

References to "Cleaning Contaminated Tools and Equipment"

1. HIV/Aids Quarterly Surveillance Report, Centers for Disease Control, December 1994.

2. Guidelines for Prevention of Transmission of Human Immunodeficiency Virus and Hepatitis B Virus to Health-Care and Public Safety Workers, Centers for Disease Control, February 1989.

3. National Fire Protection Association Standard 1581-Infection Control, NFPA, Quincy, MA, 1992.

4. Bond, W.W., Activity of Chemical Germicides against Certain Pathogens: Human Immunodeficiency Virus (HIV), Hepatitis B Virus (HBV), and Mycobacterium Tuberculosis (MTB), *Chemical Germicides in Health Care*, Polyscience Publications, Canada, 1995:139.

5. Occupational Exposure to Bloodborne Pathogens; Final Rule, Department of Labor, *Federal Register*, December 6, 1991.

6. Occupational Safety and Health Administration, Interpretive Quips, January 1994:63.

7. West, K.H., *Infectious Disease Handbook for Emergency Care Personnel*, ACGIH, Cincinnati, OH, 1994.

8. Favero, M.S., Chemical Germicides in the Health Care Field: The Perspective from the Centers for Disease Control and Prevention, *Chemical Germicides in Health Care*, Polyscience Publications, Canada, 1995:35–36.

PREPARING THE RUN REPORT

There are probably as many varieties of run reports as there are rescue squads to prepare them. Some reports show little more than the date, times out and in, and location of the accident. Others have the means to collect a wealth of information about an accident response.

The improvement of any system of people and machines often depends on data-collection practices. A well-written rescue report can provide a database from which the officers of a rescue squad can determine needs and plan squad upgrading activities.

In 1969, the Autonetics Division of North American Rockwell prepared a model information-collection system to be used in the report *Extrication Methods and Ambulance Operational Guidelines*, published by the U.S. Department of Transportation. The report forms illustrated in this chapter have been adapted from that model and are as valid

today as they were at the time of preparation. The forms provide the means for collecting data on the different aspects of a vehicle rescue operation. The information may be used for a variety of purposes, including the development of statistics, critiquing of operations, improvement of training programs, and planning of equipment purchases.

The Motor Vehicle Accident Report

The form shown in Figure 12.05 provides general information about an accident, including the location, time, and circumstances relating to the accident. Information on the environment, which is shown in the middle of the form, is important to statisticians. The street diagram is important to the critique that should follow every significant vehicle rescue operation. It can be used to recall the positions of vehicles and the locations of emergency vehicles. Problems of traffic flow, hazards, and difficulties in

MOTOR VEHICLE ACCIDENT REPORT

GENERAL INFORMATION

Report number_____   Date of accident _____

Location of accident (street address, road, and nearest intersection)

_____

City_____County_____State_____

Time alarm received _____A.M. _____P.M.   Time in service _____A.M. _____P.M.

Time in quarters _____A.M. _____P.M.   Total time in service _____ hrs. _____ mins.

Motor vehicles involved (indicate by number)

☐ Passenger car(s)   ☐ Trucks   ☐ Motorcycle(s)   ☐ Bus(es)

Other conveyances involved (indicate by number)

☐ Bicycle   ☐ Train   ☐ Other (specify) _____

Other objects involved (check)

☐ Animal   ☐ Fixed object   ☐ Other _____

People involved (indicate by number)

☐ Driver(s)   ☐ Passenger(s)   ☐ Pedestrian(s)

ENVIRONMENT

Check appropriate boxes

Location
☐ Urban
☐ Suburban
☐ Rural

Type of road
☐ Unimproved
☐ Paved
☐ Single lane
☐ 2-Lane
☐ 3-Lane
☐ 4-Lane
☐ 4-Lane divided
☐ Freeway/turnpike

Road Condition
☐ Dry
☐ Wet
☐ Snow-covered
☐ Icy

Weather
☐ Clear
☐ Cloudy
☐ Fog
☐ Mist
☐ Rain
☐ Sleet
☐ Hail
☐ Snow
☐ Windy

Lighting
☐ Dawn
☐ Daylight
☐ Dusk
☐ Night

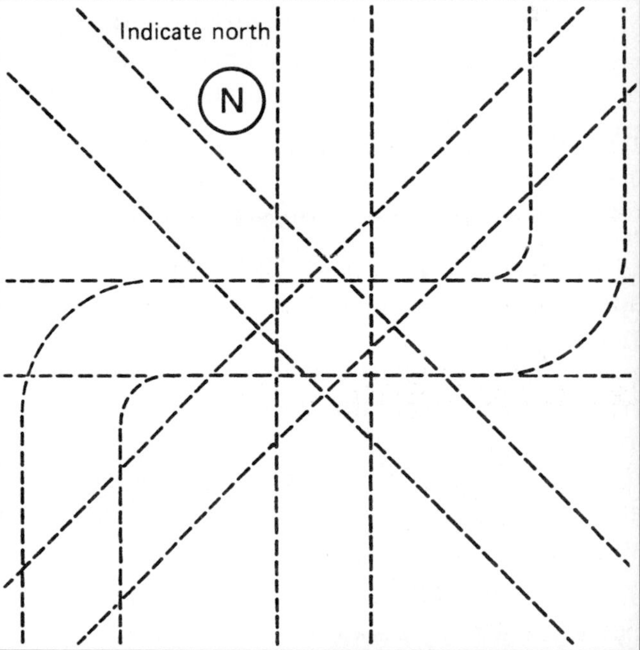

Indicate north

N

Show street names. Show position of vehicles and patients. Number vehicles as (1) etc., patients as ① etc. Show placement of emergency vehicles.

EMERGENCY SERVICE UNITS ON SCENE

List by organization

Fire _____
Rescue _____
Ambulance _____
Police _____
Civil defense _____
Other_____

Community resources used

_____
_____
_____
_____
_____
_____

Report prepared on _____ By _____ Title_____

FIGURE 12.05   Motor Vehicle Accident Report

reaching access roads should all be indicated in the diagram; it should be made as complete as possible. The list of responding emergency service organizations and community resources will give an accurate picture of the forces needed to handle the emergency.

The Accident Vehicle Report

The form shown in Figure 12.06 should be completed for each vehicle listed on the diagram on the motor vehicle accident report. The first section of the report provides data for statistics. The middle section of the form describes the vehicle's location, orientation, and condition. This information is important during a critique of stabilization and gaining access procedures. The bottom section of the form provides data on the hazards present in or around the vehicle.

The Patient Extrication Report

The form shown in Figure 12.07 provides a complete picture of the access and disentanglement activities. The orientation and location of the victim are described in detail, as are the degree of entrapment and the extrication procedures that were used. The information generated is useful in critiquing, training, and planning equipment purchases.

The Patient Injury Report

The form shown in Figure 12.08 is an example of a form used to collect information on the emergency care procedures used. The data can be used to pinpoint any deficiencies in patient care procedures.

While they appear complex, the report forms usually require little more than checking appropriate blocks. A two-car accident that results in two people being injured will require the completion of several forms. The work will take a little time, but it will provide all of the information that one needs to know about the incident and the rescue operation. Most areas of the country have standardized

forms that are used for the purpose of providing a "pre-hospital care report form." In most instances these forms are completed by the medics giving care to the patient. No matter what forms you use, fill them out carefully as they may be subpoenaed and used as legal documents.

CRITIQUING THE OPERATION

A critique is a review of an operation. It is a meeting designed to promote efficiency in future operations. Physicians hold critiques so they can discuss causes of death and disability. By means of presentations and discussions, the doctors attempt to determine whether a patient may have survived if treatment had been undertaken in a different way. Most pre-hospital medical providers have their pre-hospital care report forms (runsheets) routinely reviewed by a "quality assurance" review process to assure that the patient care provided was appropriate. Fire chiefs hold critiques to assess firefighting operations. They discuss techniques that worked and those that failed in an effort to improve their operations.

Nowhere is a critique more important than in the rescue service. Rescue personnel should hold critiques of accident scene operations so they can establish what was and was not done properly.

A critique should be held as a fact-finding conference, not a faultfinding one. Its purpose is to examine the various points that constitute a rescue operation, with an eye toward improving future rescue activities.

Not all critiques will involve negative criticism. There will be conferences in which participants will find nothing wrong with the operation being examined. These critiques are as important as those that find faults. They will reinforce the confidence of the squad members in themselves, their officers, their equipment, and the techniques they employ during rescue operations. Moreover, these critiques will point up the value of training, discipline, and cooperation.

ACCIDENT VEHICLE REPORT

VEHICLE NUMBER (from diagram)

Report number _____   Date of accident _____

Make _____ Model _____ Year _____

License number _____ State _____

Type of vehicle
- ☐ 2-Door sedan
- ☐ Limousine
- ☐ Tractor-trailer
- ☐ Other (specify) _____

- ☐ 4-Door sedan
- ☐ Recreation vehicle
- ☐ Bus

- ☐ Convertible
- ☐ Pick-up truck
- ☐ Motorcycle

- ☐ Station wagon
- ☐ Straight truck
- ☐ House trailer

Equipment
- ☐ Bench seats
- ☐ Bucket seats

- ☐ Lap belts
- ☐ Shoulder belts
- ☐ Air bags

- ☐ Rigid steering column
- ☐ Collapsible steering column

VEHICLE LOCATION, ORIENTATION, AND DAMAGE

Vehicle location
- ☐ On roadway
- ☐ On shoulder
- ☐ In ditch/gulley
- ☐ Downhill
- ☐ Uphill
- ☐ Over bridge
- ☐ Over cliff
- ☐ In water

Vehicle orientation
- ☐ Upright
- ☐ On right side
- ☐ On left side
- ☐ Front end up
- ☐ Rear end up
- ☐ Overturned

Damage to vehicle

P — Penetrated   C — Crushed   O — Off, out

	P	C	O
Right front			
Left front			
Right side			
Left side			
Right rear			
Left rear			
Right top			
Left top			
Windshield			
Rt. front window			
Lt. front window			
Rt. rear window			
Lt. rear window			
Rear window			

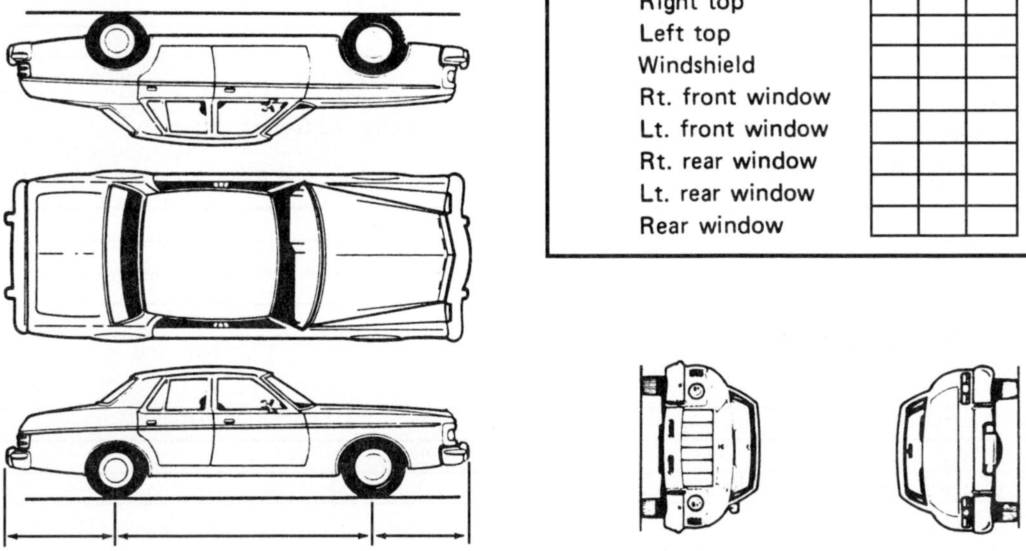

Indicate crushed area of vehicle by shading

HAZARDS

Hazards involving vehicle
- ☐ Electric wires
- ☐ Fire
- ☐ Hazardous commodity (specify) _____
- ☐ Other (specify) _____

- ☐ Smoke
- ☐ Submerged

- ☐ Buried under debris

FIGURE 12.06   Accident Vehicle Report

PATIENT IDENTIFICATION

ACCIDENT PATIENT EXTRICATION REPORT

Report number _____   Date of accident _____

Patient number (from accident diagram) _____

Name (or other identification) _____

Patient was found in, on, under or near vehicle number _____ (from diagram)

Patient was ☐ Driver ☐ Passenger ☐ Pedestrian ☐ Bicyclist ☐ Motorcyclist

ORIENTATION/LOCATION OF PATIENT

Situation
Insert appropriate code in boxes

S – Seated on
L – Lying on
P – Protruding from

	Seat	Floor	Windshield	Rear window	Side window	Door	Roof
Front right							
Front center							
Front left							
Rear right							
Rear center							
Rear left							

CAUSE OF RESTRAINT

Patient was ☐ Not trapped
        ☐ Trapped by

☐ Windshield   ☐ Door
☐ Dashboard   ☐ Roof
☐ Engine   ☐ Steering wheel
☐ Lap belt   ☐ Shoulder belt
☐ Pedal   ☐ Other

Patient was pinned
☐ Under vehicle
☐ Between vehicle and object

ACCESS TO PATIENT

Access was gained through ☐ Door ☐ Window ☐ Body of the vehicle

Tools and techniques used to gain access

_____
_____
_____
_____

Ease of gaining access ☐ No difficulty ☐ Moderate difficulty ☐ Severe difficulty

Describe any problem in gaining access

_____
_____
_____
_____

DISENTANGLEMENT

Tools and techniques used to disentangle patient

_____
_____
_____
_____

Ease of disentanglement ☐ No difficulty ☐ Moderate diffculty ☐ Severe difficulty

Describe any problem in disentanglement

_____
_____
_____
_____

FIGURE 12.07   Patient Extrication Report

PATIENT INJURY REPORT

INITIAL CONTACT

Report number _____   Date of accident _____

Patient number (from diagram) _____   Name (or other identification) _____

When first reached, patient was apparently
☐ Uninjured   ☐ Slightly injured   ☐ Severely injured   ☐ Dead

Primary survey
☐ Patient breathing   ☐ Patient not breathing   ☐ No apparent heart action
☐ Patient conscious   ☐ Patient unconscious
☐ Patient bleeding slightly   ☐ Patient bleeding moderately   ☐ Patient bleeding severely
☐ Apparent spinal injury from: _____ Survey   _____ Mechanisms of injury

Livesaving measures
☐ Opened airway   ☐ Initiated pulmonary resuscitation   ☐ Initiated CPR
☐ Controlled major hemorrhage
☐ Inmobilized cervical spine
☐ Other (specify) _____

EMERGENCY CARE MEASURES

Using the codes shown below, indicate on the figures the location and nature of injuries and the emergency care measures provided.

Injuries

A — Abrasion   L — Laceration
B — Burn   P — Puncture
F — Fracture   S — Swelling
H — Hemorrhage   X — Amputation
I — Internal injury   Z — Pain

Emergency care measures

1 — Airway
2 — Tourniquet
3 — Dressing and bandage
4 — Splint

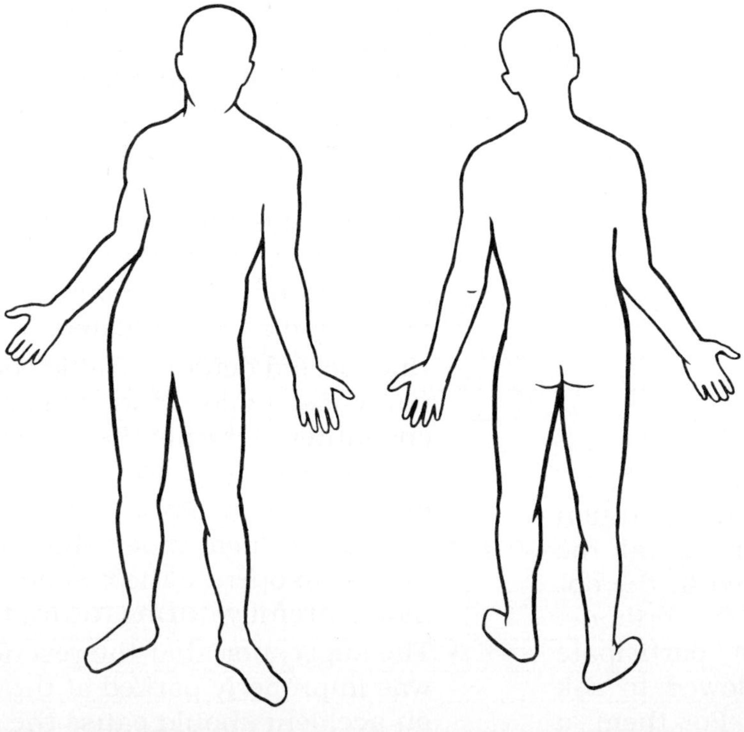

Immobilization
☐ Patient immobilized on spine board
☐ Patient immobilized on full backboard

Problems encountered during immobilization

_____
_____
_____
_____
_____
_____
_____

Emergency care equipment used

_____
_____
_____
_____
_____
_____
_____
_____
_____

FIGURE 12.08   Patient Injury Report

When a Critique Should Be Held

Ideally, the critique of a rescue operation is held as soon after conclusion of the operation as possible while events are still fresh in the minds of the participants. Unfortunately, this will not always be possible. Certainly, it will be difficult to hold a meaningful critique at 4 A.M. when squad members are both physically and mentally tired.

In the career service, a critique might be held during the next daily training session or just before the end of the shift. In volunteer organizations, a critique might be held at a regularly scheduled training session or at a specially convened evening meeting. Training sessions are especially well suited for critiques. If new or different techniques are proposed and if the facilities are available, the techniques can be tried out immediately.

Where a Critique Should Be Held

A critique can be held anywhere that a number of people can gather, but a critique is much more effective when held in a room that has a chart stand or a blackboard on which the reviewer can draw diagrams and list ideas. An overhead projector is an ideal accessory for a critique. With a projector, a screen, a few sheets of clear acetate, and a wax pencil, a reviewer can diagram the accident scene and show the positions of accident vehicles, emergency units, hazards, and so on. With overlays, the reviewer can also show how the rescue operation might have been done differently.

Who Should Participate in a Critique

The officer-in-charge of the rescue operation should be the discussion leader, and all the squad members who participated in the operation should participate in the critique. Squad members who did not participate should also be invited and allowed to ask questions about the operation. For them, a critique will not be a review, but a training experience, and they may be able to pick up ideas that can be put into practice during the next rescue operation.

The unit's training officer should also attend a critique if he was not a part of the actual rescue team. He will gain valuable insight into skill areas in which squad personnel may be weak, and from his observations he will be able to plan future training activities.

How a Critique Should Be Conducted

A critique should be based on facts, not hearsay or secondhand information. The accident report should always be the basis for a critique (which points up the need for a complete and comprehensive report). A critique can be an informal, feet-on-the-table discussion, or it can be a structured meeting built around a prepared incident critique sheet. Whatever method is selected, the critique leader should attempt to develop information in the same sequence that the rescue operation was conducted. Although objections may be raised that this approach is unnecessarily lengthy, rescuers should consider its overwhelming value in planning for future rescue operations. The following list provides examples to illustrate how such information gathering might benefit a rescue squad.

- If it was apparent that the rescue vehicle was not ready for service, an improved preventive maintenance program may be indicated.
- Unexpected detours, traffic congestion, new construction, and similar problems encountered during the response point out the need for drivers to be continually alert for changing conditions.
- A reported "near miss" should inspire drivers to operate the rescue vehicle more carefully during future runs.
- The suggestion that the rescue vehicle was improperly parked at the scene of an accident should cause the officer-in-

charge and the driver to think more seriously about traffic and other hazards when approaching the next accident scene.

- If the conference establishes the fact that traffic was a hindrance to effective rescue operations, there appears to be a need to retrain squad members in effective control measures, or to gain better police participation.
- If the critique shows that some of the accident victims were not found immediately, there is a need to reacquaint squad members with search procedures.
- If difficulties in hazard management or support are brought to light, there may be a problem caused by a lack of either training or proper equipment.
- If squad members report problems in gaining access or disentanglement, they may need training in additional techniques.
- When conferees feel that removal and transfer operations might have been better, it may be time to review and upgrade patient-handling techniques.
- A discussion of cleanup operations and vehicle maintenance activities can lead to procedures for getting the rescue vehicle ready for service sooner.

Everyone who attends a critique should be given opportunities to contribute to the discussion. Drivers should tell of problems experienced in getting the rescue vehicle to the scene. The officer in charge should discuss his decisions; he should tell the squad members why he made these decisions and what he might do differently during future operations. Squad members should comment on their activities. If they feel that they were not adequately prepared to perform a particular operation from the standpoint of training or equipment availability, they should bring this out during the discussion. Admitted shortcomings are always the basis for improvement.

Everyone should remember that a critique should not be a session devoted to faultfinding, blame placing, and name-calling. When this happens, the effectiveness of the critique is compromised, dissension is created, and confidence in the squad's leadership is damaged if not destroyed. The discussion should be objective. Participants should have only one thing in mind as they critique a rescue operation: the improvement of squad activities during future rescue operations.

COPING WITH POST-INCIDENT STRESS

If a rescue operation did not last long but was particularly stressful, a Critical Incident Stress Debriefing team member can come to the station to conduct "defusings." A debriefing gives the rescuers a chance to relax for a few minutes and catch their breath and allows CISD team members to assess how the rescue personnel are doing emotionally and work with those who need immediate help.

Critical Incident Stress Debriefing

A Critical Incident Stress Debriefing is a psychological and educational process designed to lessen the impact of major events on emergency service personnel and to accelerate *normal* recovery in *normal* people who are experiencing *normal* stress after participating in a highly *abnormal* event. A CISD can be held for a group, the rescue team that just returned from an accident, for example, or a single individual who is in need of help.

A CISD affords emergency service personnel an opportunity to talk about what happened, what they saw, and how they felt about the incident, and to learn how to cope with the stress that they may be experiencing. A debriefing without the educational component is not very useful and may even be detrimental to the mental health of some individuals. A CISD is not a time to talk about who did what during the rescue operation, either well or poorly; that should have been done during the critique. A CISD should be conducted by qualified mental health professionals—people trained in crisis intervention and posttraumatic stress disorders.

The CISD Team Network

Critical Incident Stress Debriefing teams are in place in many parts of the United States, and new teams are being formed and trained every day. If you are unaware of a CISD team in your area, call the International Critical Incident Stress Debriefing Team Coordination Center, at (410) 313-2473, which provides a 24-hour referral service. You will be given the number of a team in your general area.

Why Rescuers Should Participate in a CISD

To put it simply, it will make them feel better! The opportunity to talk about what happened and how they felt during the rescue operation and afterward has helped a large number of emergency service personnel cope with stress. Those who did not feel better by the time the debriefing was over reported that they felt better within a short period of time.

A debriefing also gives the CISD team the opportunity to identify persons who may be in need of individual mental health counseling; the referral process is an important part of a debriefing. You may fit within that category and never know it until the problem is identified by a mental health professional.

What to Do If There Is No CISD Team in Your Area

The fact that there is no CISD team in your immediate area or within a reasonable travel distance does not mean that rescuers must go on without counseling. Squad chaplains, local ministers, and professionals from community mental health agencies can help rescuers get through stressful incidents. An individual squad member can sit down and vent his or her feelings with a trusted friend.

Respected older members are often used as sounding boards after bad incidents.

Remember. Stress is a normal part of everyday life and is common to every rescue event. The information included in this book should help you to understand what is happening when you experience the symptoms of stress. It may also help you to understand your co-workers both at the scene of a rescue operation and afterward as they deal with the stresses imposed by their work.

The old notion that "real rescuers" do not suffer from stress or have emotional reactions to death and destruction is one that has no place in modern emergency services.

SUMMARY

The final phase of a vehicle rescue operation begins when the last injured person is transferred to an ambulance and ends when the rescue squad is once more ready for service.

Rescue personnel are not usually responsible for removing accident debris from a roadway. Nonetheless, most squad members will pitch in so that the road can be opened and the squad released from the scene.

Debris should not be moved until clearance is given by the police officer in charge. What appears to be a piece of junk to a rescuer may be an important piece of evidence in the eyes of a trained accident investigator.

Debris removal is not necessarily the last step in on-scene activities, however. Hazard management operations initiated by rescuers may have to be continued until the hazards are eliminated or management responsibilities are assumed by other agencies. Support operations (lighting the scene, for example) may have to be continued until everyone is ready to leave the scene.

When there is no longer a need for the squad, rescuers can recover equipment and return to quarters. The driver and the squad members should be no less alert and careful during the return than they were during the response.

Tools and equipment are cleaned, serviced, and returned to their place on the rescue vehicle, broken equipment is repaired or replaced, expendable items are replaced, and the vehicle is cleaned and serviced as soon as possible.

The rescue officer or a designated squad member prepares a complete report of the incident. As soon as it is practical after the operation, participating squad members and the unit training officer should assemble and critique the operation. The critique should be a fact-finding exercise, not a fault-

finding one. Facts, comments, and recommendations should be recorded and filed.

If the operation was particularly stressful, a critical incident stress debriefing should be conducted. If a CISD team is not available, squad members should be given the opportunity to talk with the squad chaplain, local ministers, or community mental health professionals, people trained to counsel individuals who are experiencing stress.

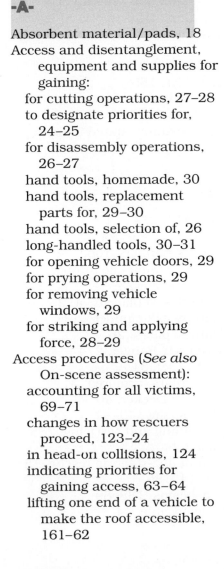

INDEX

-T-

Tags, colored string and triage:
  description of, 25
  for priority marking, 64
Talcum powder used with
    gloves, 20
Tape:
  barricade, 24
  fabric-backed, 19
  fluorescent surveyor's, 24–25
Tape measure, retractable, 11
Tarpaulin, lightweight, 14
Termination phase:
  cleaning and servicing
    equipment, 285–306
  continuing on-scene
    activities, 281–82
  coping with post-incident
    stress, 313–14
  critiquing the operation, 308,
    312
  dealing with debris, 282–84
  preparing run reports, 306–8
  recalling personnel and
    recovering equipment,
    284–85
  returning to quarters, 285
Thermal mask:
  for rescuers, 11
  for victims, 15, 191
TK Simplex jacks, 33
Tools (See Equipment, cleaning
    and servicing; Equipment
    and supplies)
Topography, selection of rescue
    vehicles and, 4
Topper Rescue Axe^R, 31
Tow/haul line, 272–73
Traco Distributors, 31
Traffic cones, 24
Traffic control equipment and
    supplies:
  audible warning and
    signaling, 24
  for controlling the movement
    of spectators, 24
  Cyalume^R Lightsticks, 11, 23,
    25, 26
  to designate priorities for
    gaining access, 24–25
  flags, 23
  flares, 23

flashlights, 23
  for power generation,
    distribution, and
    illumination, 25–26
  traffic cones, 24
Traffic vests, 10
Transferring victims:
  eight-person shift, 270–71
  helicopters for, 274–79
  ladders and ropes for, 273–74
  over debris or rough terrain,
    270–71
  problem with moving in fully
    raised ambulance
    stretcher, 269
  ropes as guidelines, 271–72
  up steep hills, 271–74
  tow/haul line for, 272–73
Trouble light, 25, 91
Trousers, Nomex^R, 10
True Craft, 27
Trunks, car, 125
  access procedures through,
    163–64
Tunnel vision, 60
Turnout coat,
    firefighter's/rescuer's, 8–9
Turnout pants, firefighter's, 10

-U-

Umbrellas, golf or doorman's,
    13
Underbody debris, 282, 283
U.S. Department of
    Transportation (DOT), 21,
    306
Universal Clip-On Light
    Bracket, 11
Upper-body protection, 8–9
Utility companies, obtaining
    help from, 67

-V-

Vehicle(s): (See also Rescue
    vehicles):
  air bags, conflict over,
    116–21
  anatomy of, 124–26
  catalytic converters, dangers
    of, 113–14

components hazardous to
    rescuers, 112–16
  controlling traffic at
    accidents, 86
  disabling electrical system,
    112–13
  drive shafts, dangers of, 114
  energy-absorbing bumpers,
    dangers of, 115–16
  fires, 90
  fluids, use of in termination
    phase, 282–83
  parts, use of in termination
    phase, 282
  searching for unaccounted
    victims in nearby, 71
  struts, dangers of, 114–15
Vehicle accident reports,
    preparing, 308
Vehicle recovery companies,
    66–67
Vehicles, equipment and
    supplies used on (See also
    Access and disentangle-
    ment, equipment and
    supplies for gaining):
  for disassembly operations,
    26–27
  for identifying hazardous
    material transport, 21–22
  for off-road rescue, 37–38
  for opening doors, 29
  for stabilizing, 16–17
  for stopping the flow of
    flammable fuel, 17–18
Vehicles, gaining access to (See
    under Access procedures)
Vehicle stabilization (See
    Stabilizing vehicles)
Vepro, 45
Vertabrace Extrication Collar,
    175, 177–78
Vetter Systems, 43, 44, 45
Victim extrication reports,
    preparing, 308
Victims (See also Protecting
    victims during
    disentanglement
    procedures; Protection
    equipment and supplies for
    victims; Removal of
    victims):
  accounting for all, 69–71